Cystic Fibrosis
Medical Care

D1561541

Cystic Fibrosis
Medical Care

David M. Orenstein, M.D.
Professor of Pediatrics
School of Medicine;
Professor of Health, Physical,
and Recreational Education
School of Education
University of Pittsburgh;
Director, Cystic Fibrosis Center
Children's Hospital of Pittsburgh
Pittsburgh, Pennsylvania

Beryl J. Rosenstein, M.D.
Professor of Pediatrics
School of Medicine
Johns Hopkins University;
Director, Cystic Fibrosis Center
Johns Hopkins Hospital
Baltimore, Maryland

Robert C. Stern, M.D.
Professor of Pediatrics
Case Western Reserve University;
Associate Pediatrician
Rainbow Babies and Children's Hospital
Cleveland, Ohio

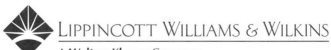

LIPPINCOTT WILLIAMS & WILKINS
A **Wolters Kluwer** Company
Philadelphia · Baltimore · New York · London
Buenos Aires · Hong Kong · Sydney · Tokyo

Acquisitions Editor: Joyce-Rachel John
Developmental Editor: Kristen Kirchner
Production Editor: Frank Aversa
Manufacturing Manager: Kevin Watt
Cover Designer: Catherine Lau Hunt
Compositor: Lippincott Williams & Wilkins, Desktop Division
Printer: Edwards Brothers

© **2000 by LIPPINCOTT WILLIAMS & WILKINS**
530 Walnut Street
Philadelphia, PA 19106 USA
LWW.com

Printed in the USA

Library of Congress Cataloging-in-Publication Data
Orenstein, David M., 1945–
    Cystic fibrosis : medical care / David M. Orenstein, Beryl J. Rosenstein,
      Robert C. Stern. p. ; cm.
    Includes bibliographical references and index.
    ISBN 0-7817-1798-1
    1. Cystic fibrosis.   I. Stern, Robert C., 1938–   II. Rosenstein, Beryl J.   III. Title.
    [DNLM: 1. Cystic Fibrosis—diagnosis.   2. Cystic Fibrosis—complications.
3. Cystic Fibrosis—therapy. WI 820 O66c 2000]
    RC858.C95 IO743 2000
    616.3'7–dc21   99-055489

Care has been taken to confirm the accuracy of the information presented and to describe generally accepted practices. However, the authors and publisher are not responsible for errors or omissions or for any consequences from application of the information in this book and make no warranty, expressed or implied, with respect to the currency, completeness, or accuracy of the contents of the publication. Application of this information in a particular situation remains the professional responsibility of the practitioner.

The authors and publisher have exerted every effort to ensure that drug selection and dosage set forth in this text are in accordance with current recommendations and practice at the time of publication. However, in view of ongoing research, changes in government regulations, and the constant flow of information relating to drug therapy and drug reactions, the reader is urged to check the package insert for each drug for any change in indications and dosage and for added warnings and precautions. This is particularly important when the recommended agent is a new or infrequently employed drug.

Some drugs and medical devices presented in this publication have Food and Drug Administration (FDA) clearance for limited use in restricted research settings. It is the responsibility of the health care provider to ascertain the FDA status of each drug or device planned for use in their clinical practice.

10 9 8 7 6 5 4 3 2 1

Contents

Preface

Cystic fibrosis (CF) has been recognized for over 60 years, and what a remarkable transformation it has undergone in these years, especially the past three decades. While these decades have seen the elucidation of the molecular and cellular underpinnings of CF, the most dramatic changes have been in the improved length and quality of life of CF patients. These improvements have resulted not from the dramatic cellular and molecular biologic discoveries, but from the widespread application of therapeutic principles laid out in the 1950s and 1960s. The dawning of the new century brings the promise of a new therapeutic era. Unfortunately, even if there were a cellular or molecular cure tomorrow, all but newly born (or perhaps newly conceived) patients would require continued application of the standard therapies, to keep their lungs healthy enough to benefit from these new treatments.

What we hope to accomplish in *Cystic Fibrosis* is to introduce the physician and medical community to the principles and practices of CF medical care. We have tried to keep the book practical and easy to use. We chose not to give exhaustive, in-depth references, but rather to supply suggested reading at the end of each chapter. This is not meant to be a "recipe" book, and it will not make a novice into a CF specialist, but it will help familiarize those new to the field with the important aspects of CF care.

We feel strongly that CF care is best carried out in CF centers, in conjunction with primary care physicians working in the community. Neither can work successfully alone to deliver excellent care to the CF patient and family. We hope that this book may improve the cooperation between the center physicians and care team and the primary care physicians. Although there are those with more expertise in many specific topics covered in this book, as CF generalists, we have some 80 years of combined experience, a love for our work, an abiding gratitude for the opportunity to work with the patients, their families, and the CF community at large, and a commitment to improve our patients' care as much as possible.

After chapters on the molecular and cellular bases of CF and its diagnosis we cover the major organ systems affected by CF, and deal with surgery for CF patients, transplantation (lung and liver), hospitalization, and terminal care. We have included chapters on special populations (adolescents and adults), exercise, and laboratory testing.

We hope to make the work of our professional colleagues easier, and thereby make the lives of the many CF patients and their families easier, and longer, as well.

David M. Orenstein
Beryl J. Rosenstein
Robert C. Stern

Acknowledgments

I am delighted to take the opportunity to acknowledge my sister Miriam Sumner, for contributions without number. She has logged more hours on the telephone with me during the writing of this book than I can ever adequately thank her for. I also acknowledge my brother Herbert who was my coach when we were growing up, and though we live half a planet apart, we've grown ever closer—for this I am extremely grateful. No one has ever been given better siblings than I have. And thanks to Shosh, Joel, Anna, and Black Orenstein, Willy and Dory Sumner, and Jim Maloni.

David M. Orenstein

My participation in writing this book was made possible only because of the lessons learned from so many wonderful patients, families, and colleagues. I also recognize the support, encouragement, and patience of my wife Carolyn, who graciously endured the many hours I spent on this project, and the outstanding secretarial support of Linda Packham, who had the uncanny ability to transform random thoughts into meaningful text. Lastly, I have been blessed by Amanda, Annie, Ariel, Benjamin, Matthew, and Zachary (and their parents) who make it all worthwhile.

Beryl J. Rosenstein

1
Introduction

Cystic fibrosis (CF) is the most common profoundly life-shortening inherited disease among white populations, and is found in every ethnic and racial group. The clinical syndrome was first described in the medical literature in 1938 by Dr. Dorothy Andersen, but an ancient folk saying suggests that it has been in existence at least since the Middle Ages ("Wehe dem Kind, das beim Kuss auf die Stirn salzig schmeckt, es ist 'verhext' und muss bald sterben": "woe the child who tastes salty from a kiss on the brow, for he is hexed, and soon must die"). Although the sweat gland defect referred to in this saying seldom causes life-threatening morbidity, it remains the diagnostic hallmark of the disease and was at least partly responsible for unlocking the cellular underpinnings of this multisystem disorder, beginning in the early to mid-1980's.

In the 1950's and 1960's, when clinical treatment programs began to change CF from a devastating condition (life expectancy less than 1 year) to a chronic disorder affecting children and adults (median survival currently exceeds 30 years), it had been assumed that CF was primarily a disorder of mucus production, perhaps caused by a circulating "CF factor." It seemed obvious that the scourge of CF resulted from thick mucus: after all, thick mucus seemed to clog bronchioles and bronchi, causing the progressive airway obstruction, infection, and inflammation that led to the eventually fatal fibrosis and cyst formation of the lungs; thick mucus led to newborn (and later) intestinal blockage; mucus clogged the hepatobiliary tree, causing fatal cirrhosis in those few patients who did not die of their lung disease; and mucus blocked the vas deferens, rendering 98% of men with CF sterile, while thick cervical mucus contributed to the decreased fertility in women with CF. It was of course disconcerting that there was no mucus in sweat, and careful studies showed that CF bronchial mucus was not particularly thick at birth.

Then, beginning in the early 1980s, cell physiologists began to discover that CF epithelial cells—from all the affected organ systems, including the sweat glands—were characterized by abnormal ion transport. Studies in cell culture and in the upper and lower respiratory tract of patients showed an abnormally high (higher negative charge) basal bioelectric potential difference across these epithelia. It appeared that a chloride channel was particularly affected, with chloride exit from the cells blocked, and also that sodium reabsorption was accelerated. In one of many dramatic discoveries, investigators then demonstrated that the CF-associated abnormal bioelectric potential difference across tracheal and bronchial epithelia did not appear in lungs transplanted into the first CF patient to receive a lung transplant. His nose and upper trachea remained physiologically abnormal, but the new bronchi did not show the characteristic CF ion transport abnormalities, finally laying to rest the already discredited theory of a circulating factor and demonstrating that the CF abnormalities were resident in the affected tissues themselves.

In 1989, as physiologists continued to hone in on the exact epithelial cell ion transport abnormalities, molecular geneticists used a combination of positional cloning techniques (in an almost unprecedented cooperation among several potentially competing laboratories) to locate (long arm of chromosome 7) and clone the CF gene. From this ground-breaking work, the structure of the protein that the CF gene was predicted to encode appeared very similar to a class of proteins known to be important in regulating membrane transport, fitting in perfectly with the burgeoning understanding of the cellular defect. The protein, and its guiding gene, were dubbed the cystic fibrosis transmembrane conductance regulator (CFTR). CFTR has subsequently been shown to be the main epithelial cell chloride channel, and to have other important regulatory functions, including a role in sodium transport.

At the same time, the comprehensive clinical treatment programs introduced by pioneers like LeRoy Matthews and Carl Doershuk in the late 1950's and 1960's were bearing fruit: patients were living longer and more productive lives. The various components of these treatment programs, based in multidisciplinary centralized treatment centers, were—and still are—directed at secondary and tertiary effects of the molecular and cellular defects but have been surprisingly successful. Survival has improved dramatically since the introduction of these programs and the spread of centers accredited by the National Cystic Fibrosis Foundation in the United States and similar programs throughout the developed world. Center care has been shown clearly to be associated with better survival than care outside centers. In addition to providing comprehensive multisystem care, the centers are now the setting for clinical trials of new therapies based on the emerging understanding of the basic CF defect or defects. As these new therapies are introduced, it is likely that the outlook for patients with CF will improve even more dramatically than it has until now. In the meantime, we hope that this book will help medical professionals understand a comprehensive approach to treating patients with CF, an approach that we anticipate will remain the foundation of CF care well into this new century, even as new therapies emerge to supplement those presented in this book.

2

The Cystic Fibrosis Gene and the Molecular and Cellular Bases of Cystic Fibrosis

Cystic fibrosis (CF) has been thought to be inherited as an autosomal recessive disorder virtually since its original description decades ago, and it is almost always referred to as the most common inherited life-shortening disease among white populations. This description is not strictly accurate, because the incidence of CF (roughly 1 in 3,200 live births among those of northern European extraction) is low compared with that of the familial hyperlipidemias, which cause early death from coronary atherosclerosis. However, CF is the most common profoundly life-shortening inherited disorder (median survival of 31 years in the United States in 1998).

The gene for CF was localized to the long arm of chromosome 7 in 1985 and was cloned in 1989. It encodes a protein of 1480 amino acid residues. This protein, the CF transmembrane conductance regulator (CFTR), is a chloride channel, resident in the apical membrane of epithelial cells. In addition to its function as the epithelial cells' primary chloride channel, CFTR helps regulate transepithelial transport of other ions and water (Fig. 2–1). Specifically, CFTR downregulates an amiloride-sensitive epithelial sodium channel and also upregulates an alternate (outwardly rectifying) chloride channel. Thus, it helps regulate the water and ion content of luminal secretions.

In culture, CF cells show decreased chloride secretion and increased sodium absorption, compared with non-CF cells. The

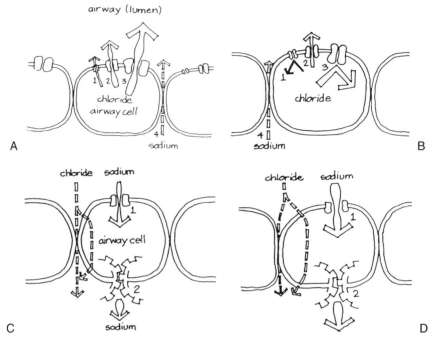

FIG. 2–1. Chloride and sodium transport in non-CF and CF airway epithelial cells. **A:** Airway epithelial cell (non-CF), showing three types of chloride channels: 1, calcium-dependent channel; 2, outwardly rectifying channel (ORCC), and 3, (most important) CF transmembrane regulator (CFTR) protein. Sodium is shown passing between cells. **B:** CF airway epithelial cell, with nonfunctional CFTR, preventing chloride exit, and calcium-dependent channel also not open, while the ORCC works minimally. **C:** Sodium absorption into non-CF epithelial cells. **D:** Sodium absorption into CF epithelial cells greater than normal.

sodium channel overactivity can be (partly) blocked with addition of amiloride (a diuretic). These effects can be demonstrated indirectly both *in vitro* and *in vivo* through the measurement of transepithelial bioelectric potential differences (PD). Three electrophysiologic features distinguish CF (Fig. 2–2): (a) higher-than-normal (negative) basal PD, which reflects enhanced Na^+ transport across a relatively Cl^--impermeable barrier; (b) greater inhibition of PD after perfusion with the Na^+ channel inhibitor amiloride, which reflects inhibition of accelerated Na^+ transport; and (c) little or no change in PD in response to perfusion of the epithelial surface with a Cl^--free solu-

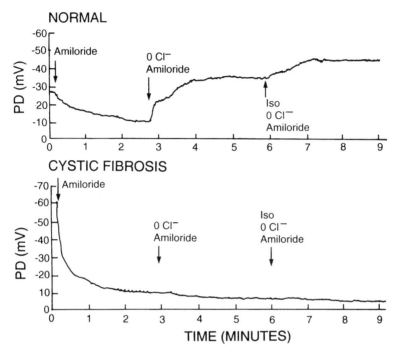

FIG. 2–2. Nasal bioelectric potential difference (PD). The tracings illustrate the response of the PD to perfusion with amiloride (10^{-4} M), the addition of a Cl^--free solution to amiloride, and the addition of isoproterenol (10^{-5} M) to the Cl^--free solution containing amiloride. **Top:** In a healthy (non-CF) subject. **Bottom:** In a patient with CF (see text for explanation). (Adapted from Knowles MR, Paradiso AM, Boucher RC. In vivo nasal potential difference: techniques and protocols for assessing efficacy of gene transfer in cystic fibrosis. *Hum Gene Ther* 1995;6:445, with permission.)

tion in conjunction with isoproterenol, which reflects an absence of CFTR-mediated Cl^- secretion.

With such a large gene and protein product, it is not surprising that things can go awry in many different ways, and in fact, over 800 different mutations have been identified in CFTR, each leading to CF. The types of defects fall into four or five pathophysiologic groupings, depending on where and how they interfere with CFTR production and function (Table 2–1). CFTR is produced in the cell nucleus and is folded, or packaged, in the endoplasmic reticulum to prepare it for transport to the cell membrane. Once at the cell mem-

TABLE 2–1. *CFTR Mutations and Their Role in CFTR Production and Function**

Class 1 production	Class 2 folding; trafficking	Class 3 regulation	Class 4 conduction	Class 5 reduced production
G542X	ΔF508	G551D	R117H	3849+10 kB C→T
W1282X	ΔI507	(ΔF508)	R347P	A455E???
3905insT	N1303K		R334W	
R553X	S549R			
	G480C			
	A455E???			

*Classifications are not exclusive; that is, ΔF508 has abnormal processing, so that little of it reaches the cell membrane, *and* the protein that does reach the cell membrane shows limited response to signals.

brane, it responds to signals by opening long enough to conduct chloride through its channel. Mutations that interfere with production of CFTR protein are considered to be in Class 1. Class 2 mutations are those like ΔF508, the most common mutation, wherein the CFTR protein is degraded in the endoplasmic reticulum instead of being folded into the proper configuration to be able to traffic to the apical cell membrane. Class 3 mutations create protein that reaches the cell membrane but then cannot respond appropriately to activation signals. In Class 4 mutations, the protein reaches its appropriate position in the cell membrane and responds to signals, but the chloride channel does not seem to remain open long enough to accomplish adequate chloride conduction. In some classification systems, there is also a Class 5 defect, which—like Class 1—interferes with protein production, but results in reduced synthesis of protein, whereas Class 1 results in no synthesis of protein.

HOW DOES THE CELLULAR DEFECT CAUSE THE CYSTIC FIBROSIS SYNDROME?

The absence or underfunctioning of CFTR in CF patients is the basis for the cellular defects and ultimately explains (or will explain) the various organ dysfunctions of CF. Not all of the mechanisms are fully understood, but many are. For example, the diagnostic and physiologic hallmark of CF, namely, the high salt content of sweat, is explainable on the basis of absent or faulty CFTR in the largely absorptive sweat duct epithelium. Sweat glands produce precursor fluid that is isotonic to serum, and as this fluid passes along the sweat duct toward the skin surface, salt is absorbed, resulting in hypotonic sweat. With absent or faulty chloride channels, chloride ions cannot be absorbed through the sweat duct epithelial cells, and remain intraluminal, retaining sodium ions as well (to maintain electrical neutrality). Thus, the fluid that emerges at the skin as sweat is relatively high in sodium and chloride.

Despite our relatively sophisticated understanding of the epithelial ion transport properties of CF and healthy cells, and of the process by which CF sweat becomes abnormal, the exact ionic composition of airway fluid is still unknown, as is the reason for the airways' being such a hospitable environment for microorganisms, such as *Hemophilus influenzae, Staphylococcus aureus,* and particularly *Pseudomonas aeruginosa.* This lack of understanding comes in part from our not knowing the balance of secretory and absorptive epithelia within the airways (in secretory cells, the chloride block would keep chloride within cells more than normal, whereas in absorptive cells, chloride entry would be lower than normal). It is clear that in order for there to be any airway fluid, this fluid must be secreted in the most peripheral airways. And because the volume of the thousands of peripheral airways is much greater than that of the few proximal airways, there must also be absorption. Where the absence of a functional chloride channel and the presence of an overactive sodium channel influence the composition of airway fluid remains undefined. Some investigators have claimed that airway fluid salt concentrations are raised, thus inactivating host salt-sensitive antibacterial polypeptides (defensins). Other investigators have postulated that the ionic composition of airway fluid is normal and that the problem that leads to airway infection is overabsorption of airway fluid, leading to relative depletion of the periciliary liquid layer, rendering the cilia incapable of accomplishing their normal airway mucus clearance (Fig. 2–3). The propensity for *P. aeruginosa* to colonize CF airways could result from an effect of CFTR on pseudomonas adherence to airway cell receptors, separate from its ionic regulatory functions. Further, it is possible that CFTR has an independent effect on the airways' immune response to various

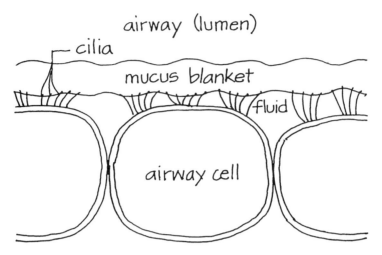

FIG. 2–3. Normal cilia and fluid. With depletion of the periciliary fluid, the cilia cannot beat effectively.

insults, real or imagined, explaining the exuberant and potentially injurious inflammatory component of CF airway disease.

GENOTYPE-PHENOTYPE RELATIONSHIP

The clinical syndrome we recognize as CF has considerable variability, and at least some of this variability seems to be associated with specific gene mutations. It has long been recognized that only 85% to 90% of CF patients have pancreatic insufficiency, whereas 10% to 15% of CF patients are pancreatic sufficient and do not require supplemental enzymes for adequate fat digestion and absorption. With the discovery of the multiple CFTR mutations, it became clear that some of these mutations (unfortunately referred to as "mild") are usually associated with pancreatic sufficiency. It also became clear that the "mild" mutations are dominant over the more common "severe" mutations. Thus, ΔF508, the most common CF mutation, is considered a severe mutation, because it is associated with pancreatic insufficiency, but patients heterozygous for ΔF508 and R117H (a mild mutation) are usually pancreatic sufficient.

Some patients with two severe mutations are pancreatic sufficient early in life, but most of them can be expected to become pancreatic insufficient. Table 2–2 lists the most common severe and mild CFTR mutations, as well as some epidemiologic features of the mutations. It is worth repeating that these labels apply only to pancreatic func-

TABLE 2–2. *Characteristics of the Most Common Cystic Fibrosis Mutations*

Mutation	Geographic/ ethnic incidence	Other characteristic
ΔF508	70–75% in North America	Pancreatic insufficiency
W1282X[1]	50–60% in Ashkenazi Jews; 2.1% worldwide	Pancreatic insufficiency
G542X[1]	3.4% worldwide	Pancreatic insufficiency; ?more meconium ileus
G551D[1]	2.4% worldwide	Pancreatic insufficiency
3905insT[1]	2.1% worldwide	Pancreatic insufficiency
N13031K[1]	1.8% worldwide	Pancreatic insufficiency
R553X[1]	1.3% worldwide	Pancreatic insufficiency
621+1G→T[1]	1.3% worldwide	Pancreatic insufficiency
1717-1G→A[1]	1.3% worldwide	Pancreatic insufficiency
A455E[1]	3–7% in Netherlands; 0–0.2% in North America	Pancreatic sufficiency;† mild lung disease
3849+10 kb C→T[1]	1.4% worldwide; 4% in Israel	Pancreatic sufficiency;† normal sweat chloride; most males not sterile; lung disease varies from mild to severe
R117H[1]	0.8% worldwide	Pancreatic sufficiency;† slightly lower sweat chloride; older age at diagnosis
R334W[1]		Pancreatic sufficiency;† older age at diagnosis
R347P[1]		Pancreatic sufficiency†
P574H[1]		Pancreatic sufficiency†
Y563N[1]		Pancreatic sufficiency†

[1]Compound heterozygotes, in most cases, meaning these patients had one copy of the mutation noted and one other CF mutation (usually ΔF508).
†Pancreatic sufficiency in most, but not all, cases. (Modified from Orenstein DM. *Cystic fibrosis: A guide for patient and family,* 2nd ed., Philadelphia: Lippincott-Raven, 1997;210.)

tion. With few exceptions, there is not a good correlation between genotype and degree of pulmonary disease.

The most common and typical cases of CF have early-onset chronic and progressive respiratory disease, pancreatic insufficiency, salty sweat, and male infertility (resulting from obstructive azoospermia). There are other affected patients with two CF mutations, typical lung disease, abnormal sweat electrolytes, and male infertility but with normal fat absorption (pancreatic sufficiency). Additional patients have been recognized with two CF mutations, typical lung disease, pancreatic sufficiency, and normal sweat chloride concentrations (e.g., some patients with ΔF508/R117H); and others with two CF mutations, delayed-onset lung disease, pancreatic sufficiency, and abnormal sweat chloride concentrations (e.g., ΔF508/A455E). Still others, for example, some patients with ΔF508/3849 +10 kb C→T, have delayed-onset lung disease, pancreatic sufficiency, and normal sweat chloride concentrations. In recent years, it has been recognized that some patients who carry two CFTR mutations have apparently normal pancreatic, sweat gland, and lung function but have obstructive azoospermia from congenital bilateral absence of the vas deferens (CBAVD; e.g., some patients with R117H). From these observations and from analysis of the specific mutations associated with these different expressions of the CF phenotype (and the amount of functional CFTR expected to reach cell membranes for each mutation), researchers have speculated that there exists a hierarchy of organ sensitivity to deficits in functional CFTR. Genotypes that result in a reduction of functional CFTR to 1% of normal values cause classic CF, consisting of pancreatic insufficiency, lung disease, abnormal sweat electrolyte concentrations, and CBAVD. Genotypes that result in a reduction of functional CFTR to 5% of normal values lead to CF with typical lung disease, sweat electrolyte abnormalities, and CBAVD but without pancreatic insufficiency. Genotypes that result in a reduction of functional CFTR to 10% of normal values cause CBAVD alone. This factor suggests that each manifestation of CF is caused by a reduction of functional CFTR levels below a tissue-specific threshold. It is also possible that tissue sensitivity varies with the qualitative alterations in CFTR and not just with the absolute quantity of CFTR that reaches the cell membrane.

POSSIBLE ROLE OF OTHER GENES IN CF DISEASE

Despite the importance of CF genotype in determining pancreatic functional status, the severity of CF lung disease has shown very little relationship to CF genotype. This variability is clearly related in part to environmental factors, including smoke exposure, viral respiratory infections, and probably intensity of treatment. There are probably also non-CFTR genes that influence CF disease severity. Airway inflammation and damage in CF have been attributed in part to high levels of neutrophil-derived proteinases (Berger, 1991). These proteinases are thought to be held in check by antiproteinases, of which α1-antitrypsin is one of the most important. Therapeutic trials have even been instituted to examine the possible benefits of supplemental α1-antitrypsin. It is therefore somewhat surprising, and perhaps very important, that two studies (Mahadeva, 1998a, 1998b) have now suggested that CF patients who have alleles of the α1-antitrypsin gene rendering them deficient in α1-antitrypsin have milder lung disease than those with normal levels of α1-antitrypsin. Airway damage may also be worsened by oxidative stress. This stress is modulated by glutathione S-transferases (GST) that detoxify harmful organic hydroperoxides. In one study of 53 children with CF (Hull and Thomson, 1998), those who were homozygous for the GSTM1 null allele, that is, those who have no functional GST to detoxify those harmful hydroperoxides, had worse pulmonary disease. Finally, in this same group of children, those who had the allele that is associated with higher levels of tumor necrosis factor (TNF, an important proinflammatory cytokine) had worse lung disease than those with the allele associated with lower levels of TNF. Without question, other non-CFTR genes will be discovered that modify disease severity. It is possible that some of these genes may have protein products that will be amenable to therapeutic modification.

WORLDWIDE DISTRIBUTION OF CFTR MUTATIONS

CF appears to have originated in northern Europe but is found in nearly every ethnic and geographic group examined. It is most common in populations originating in northern Europe and least com-

TABLE 2–3. *Ethnic Groups in Which a Few Mutations Account for Most of the Cystic Fibrosis Chromosomes*

Group	Number of Mutations	Percent of CF Chromosomes
Alberta (Canada) Hutterites	2	100
Welsh	29	99.5
Brittany Celts	19	98
Ashkenazi Jews	5	97
Belgian	17	94.3

(Modified from Orenstein DM. *Cystic fibrosis: a guide for patient and family,* 2nd ed., Philadelphia: Lippincott-Raven, 1997:211; courtesy of Dr. Gary Cutting.)

mon in Asian and African populations. Table 2–2 provides data on the distribution of the most common CF mutations. The ΔF508 mutation is the most common worldwide. In populations whose origin can be traced to northern Europe, ΔF508 accounts for 70% to 75% of all CF mutations. The next most common mutation in the general European or North American population (G542X) accounts for only 3.4% of CF mutations, and taken together, the more than 800 mutations currently recognized account for fewer than 95% of all CF cases. Certain relatively isolated communities and ethnic groups (e.g., Ashkenazi Jews) can be characterized genetically much more tightly (Table 2–3).

IMPLICATIONS FOR TREATMENT

With the discovery and cloning of the CF gene came tremendous hope that gene therapy would be imminent. In fact, gene transfer via viral vectors in cell culture quickly succeeded and rendered the CF cells electrophysiologically normal. Within a few years, mice had been genetically engineered in several ways to lack CFTR or have modifications in CFTR to serve as an (so far imperfect) animal model for CF. However, despite extensive continuing efforts, transfer of the normal CFTR gene in vivo has proved difficult to accomplish with efficiency and lack of inflammatory host response. Although those efforts continue, other avenues have appeared that may be easier to accomplish. These include therapies aimed at getting around the physiologic consequences of CFTR protein malfunction and those that may even correct the protein malfunction (so-called protein repair therapy).

Examples of experimental treatments that attempt to get around the physiologic consequences of protein malfunction include the use of amiloride to decrease the overactive sodium reabsorptive channel activity and uridine triphosphate (UTP) to increase non-CFTR chloride channel activity (Fig. 2–4). It is a hallmark of the CF cellular defect that *in vivo* measurements of PD (most commonly measured in the nose) show a prompt response to perfusion of the epithelium with amiloride, with PD falling toward (but not reaching) normal

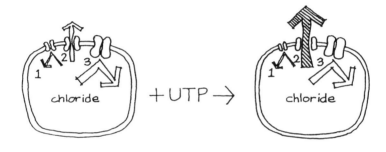

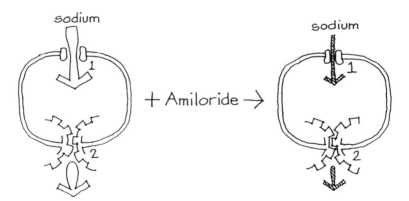

FIG. 2–4. UTP and amiloride in treating cellular defects. Channels labeled as in Figure 2–1. (From Orenstein DM. *Cystic fibrosis: a guide for patient and family, 2nd ed.* Philadelphia: Lippincott-Raven, 1997, with permission.)

(Fig. 2–2). Two studies of amiloride given by aerosol to CF patients have shown conflicting results. One study showed a promising suggestion of slowed pulmonary disease progression (Knowles et al., 1990), whereas the other study (App et al., 1990) failed to confirm these results. Further studies are ongoing or planned. UTP has been shown in cell culture to have little or no influence on CFTR channel activity itself, but it does seem to increase alternate epithelial chloride channel activity, specifically through a calcium-dependent chloride channel. *In vivo* studies with a combination of amiloride and UTP aerosols are ongoing.

Perhaps even more promising are agents that have been shown in cell culture to increase the amount of functional CFTR that reaches the cell membrane or to increase the functioning of faulty protein resident in the membrane. Several different agents have been found that perform these transformations, with the treatment being tailored for different mutations, or class of mutations (Fig. 2–5). Examples include the use of aminoglycosides for some Class 1 mutations that

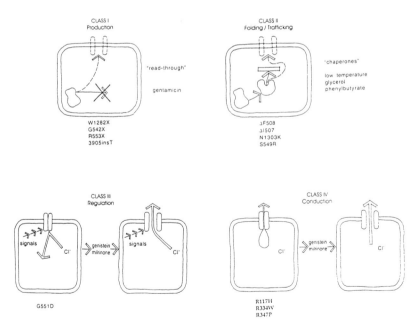

FIG. 2–5. Protein therapy for different classes.

include stop codons (wherein CFTR mRNA is terminated early and is not translated into protein). Somehow the aminoglycosides seem to enable "read-through" of these stop codons, allowing the formation of some functional protein. Class 2 mutations (including ΔF508) interfere with the folding of CFTR protein in such a way that it is not transported to the cell membrane. Several chemical "chaperones" have been discovered to enable the trafficking of CFTR protein to the cell membrane. These substances include glycerol (probably too toxic for clinical use) and phenylbutyrate. With Class 3 and 4 mutations, protein is appropriately situated at the cell membrane, but does not respond appropriately to activation signals. Milrinone, genistein (a component of tofu), and 8-cyclopentyl-1,3-dipropylxanthine (CPX) have all been shown to increase CFTR chloride conduction in cells with these mutations and are being investigated for possible therapeutic use.

REFERENCES

Alton EW, et al. Bioelectric properties of cystic fibrosis airways obtained at heart-lung transplantation. *Thorax* 1992;47:1010–1014.

Anderson M, et al. Demonstration that CFTR is a chloride channel by alteration of its anion selectivity. *Science* 1991;253:202–205.

Anonymous. Correlation between genotype and phenotype in patients with cystic fibrosis. The Cystic Fibrosis Genotype-Phenotype Consortium [see comments]. *New Engl J Med* 1993;329:1308–1313.

Anonymous. Gene therapy for cystic fibrosis utilizing a replication deficient recombinant adenovirus vector to deliver the human cystic fibrosis transmembrane conductance regulator cDNA to the airways. A phase I study. *Hum Gene Ther* 1994; 5:1019–1057.

App EM, et al. Acute and long-term amiloride inhalation in cystic fibrosis lung disease. *Am Rev Respir Dis* 1990;141:605–612.

Berger M. Inflammation in the lung in cystic fibrosis. *Clin Rev Allergy* 1991;9: 119–142.

Bernstein JM, Yankaskas JR. Increased ion transport in cultured nasal polyp epithelial cells. *Archives Otolaryngol Head Neck Surg* 1994;120:993–996.

Berul CI, et al. Lack of cystic fibrosis transmembrane regulator-type chloride current in pediatric human atrial myocytes. *Life Sci* 1997;60:189–197.

Caskey CT, et al. The American Society of Human Genetics Statement on cystic fibrosis screening. *Am J Hum Gen* 1990;46:393.

Cutting GR, et al. Two patients with cystic fibrosis, nonsense mutations in each cystic fibrosis gene, and mild pulmonary disease. *New Engl J Med* 1990;323: 1685–1689.

Davis PB, Drumm M, Konstan MW. Cystic fibrosis. State of the art. *Am J Resp Crit Care Med* 1996;154:1229–1256.

Gabriel SE, et al. Cystic fibrosis heterozygote resistance to cholera toxin in the cystic fibrosis mouse model. *Science* 1994;266:107–109.

Gan KH, et al. A cystic fibrosis mutation associated with mild lung disease. *N Engl J Med* 1995;333:95–99.

Grubb BR, et al. Inefficient gene transfer by adenovirus vector to cystic fibrosis airway epithelia of mice and humans. *Nature* 1994;371:802–806.

Harris RA, et al. Effects of various secretagogues on [Ca$_{2+}$]i in cultured human nasal epithelial cells. *Can J Physiol Pharmacol* 1991;69:1211–1216.

Hull J, Thomson AH. Contribution of genetic factors other than CFTR to disease severity in cystic fibrosis. *Thorax* 1998;53:1018–1021.

Kerem B-S, et al. Identification of the cystic fibrosis gene: Genetic analysis. *Science* 1989;345:1073–1080.

Kingdom TT, et al. Clinical characteristics and genotype analysis of patients with cystic fibrosis and nasal polyposis requiring surgery. *Arc Otolaryngol Head Neck Surg* 1996;122:1209–1213.

Knowles MR, et al. A pilot study of aerosolized amiloride for the treatment of lung disease in cystic fibrosis. *N Engl J Med* 1990;322:1189–1194.

Knowles MR, Clarke LL, Boucher RC. Activation by extracellular nucleotides of chloride secretion in the airway epithelia of patients with cystic fibrosis. *N Engl J Med* 1991;325:533–538.

Knowles M, Gatzy J, Boucher R. Increased bioelectric potential difference across respiratory epithelia in cystic fibrosis. *New Engl J Med* 1991;305:1498–1495.

Knowles MR, et al. Abnormal respiratory epithelial ion transport in cystic fibrosis. *Clin Chest Med* 1986;7:285–297.

Mahadeva R, et al. Alpha-1 antitrypsin deficiency alleles and severe cystic fibrosis lung disease. *Thorax* 1998;53:1022–1024.

Mahadeva R, et al. Alpha 1-antitrypsin deficiency alleles and the Taq-IG → A allele in cystic fibrosis lung disease. *Euro Respir* 1986;11:873–879.

Moullier P, et al. Association of 1078 del T cystic fibrosis mutation with severe disease. *J Med Genet* 1994;31:159–161.

Parad RB. Buccal cell DNA mutation analysis for diagnosis of cystic fibrosis in newborns and infants inaccessible to sweat chloride measurement. *Pediatrics* 1998;101:851–855.

Quinton PM, Bijman J. Higher bioelectric potentials due to decreased chloride absorption in the sweat glands of patients with cystic fibrosis. *N Engl J Med* 1983;308:1185.

Quinton PM. Human genetics. What is good about cystic fibrosis? [Review]. *Curr Biol* 1994;4:742–743.

Riordan JR, et al. Identification of the cystic fibrosis gene: Cloning and characterization of complementary DNA. *Science* 1989;245:1066–1073.

Rommens JM, et al. Identification of the cystic fibrosis gene: Chromosome walking and jumping. *Science* 1989;245:1059–1065.

Rosenstein BJ, Zeitlin PL. Cystic fibrosis (seminar). *Lancet* 1998;351:277–282.

Rosenstein BJ. Genotype-phenotype correlations in cystic fibrosis. *Lancet* 1994;343:746–747.

Strong TV, et al. Cystic fibrosis gene mutation in two sisters with mild disease and normal sweat electrolyte levels. *N Engl J Med* 1991;325:1630–1634.

Tsui/L-C. *International cystic fibrosis genetics consortium update.* Bethesda, MD: Cystic Fibrosis Foundation, 1991.

Tuerlings JH, et al. Mutation frequency of cystic fibrosis transmembrane regulator is not increased in oligozoospermic male candidates for intracytoplasmic sperm injection. *Fertil Steril* 1998;69:899–903.

Wallace CS, Hall M, Kuhn RJ. Pharmacologic management of cystic fibrosis. *Clin Pharmacy* 1993;12:657–674: quiz 700–1.

Zabner J, et al. Adenovirus-mediated gene transfer transiently corrects the chloride transport defect in nasal epithelia of patients with cystic fibrosis. *Cell* 1993;75: 207–216.

3

Diagnosis of Cystic Fibrosis

Cystic fibrosis (CF) is the most common profoundly life-limiting genetic disorder in whites, with an incidence of 1 in 3,200 newborns in the United States. It is less common in African-Americans (1 in 15,000) and Asian-Americans (1 in 31,000), but the diagnosis needs to be considered in patients of all racial and ethnic backgrounds. It is essential to confirm or exclude the diagnosis of CF in a timely fashion and with a high degree of accuracy to avoid inappropriate testing; provide appropriate therapies in a timely fashion; perform prognostic and genetic counseling; and ensure access to specialized medical services.

Although CF is a well-characterized genetic disorder, it remains a clinical diagnosis suggested by phenotypic (clinical) features (Table 3–1), and in most cases, it is confirmed by the demonstration of an elevated concentration of electrolytes in the sweat. It is marked by great variability in the frequency and severity of clinical manifestations and complications. The possibility of CF should never be discounted because a patient appears well. In 70% of cases, the diagnosis is established by age 1 year, often within the first several months of life. However, in 8% of patients, the diagnosis is not established until after age 10 years and the diagnosis is being made in an increasing number of adults.

Almost all patients have chronic sinopulmonary disease and, in postpubertal men, obstructive azoospermia. Approximately 85% to 90% of patients have exocrine pancreatic insufficiency, whereas the remainder are pancreatic sufficient. The subset of patients with pancreatic sufficiency is characterized by milder clinical course, better nutritional status, and better pulmonary function, and, therefore, a distinctly later age at diagnosis. In recent years, the ability to detect CF mutations and to measure transepithelial bioelectric properties

TABLE 3–1. *Phenotypic Features Consistent With a Diagnosis of Cystic Fibrosis*

1. Chronic sinopulmonary disease manifested by
   a. Persistent colonization/infection with typical CF pathogens including *Staphylococcus aureus,* nontypable *Haemophilus influenzae,* mucoid and nonmucoid *Pseudomonas aeruginosa,* and *Burkholderia cepacia*
   b. Chronic cough and sputum production
   c. Persistent chest radiograph abnormalities (e.g., bronchiectasis, atelectasis, infiltrates, hyperinflation)
   d. Airway obstruction manifested by wheezing and air trapping
   e. Nasal polyps; radiograph or CT abnormalities of all the formed paranasal sinuses
   f. Digital clubbing
2. Gastrointestinal and nutritional abnormalities, including
   a. *Intestinal:* meconium ileus; distal intestinal obstruction syndrome (DIOS); rectal prolapse
   b. *Pancreatic:* pancreatic insufficiency; recurrent pancreatitis
   c. *Hepatobiliary:* chronic hepatic disease manifested by clinical or histologic evidence of focal biliary cirrhosis or multilobular cirrhosis, cholelithiasis, microgallbladder
   d. *Nutritional:* failure to thrive (protein-calorie malnutrition); hypoproteinemia and edema; complications secondary to fat-soluble vitamin deficiency
3. Salt loss syndromes: acute salt depletion; chronic metabolic alkalosis
4. Male urogenital abnormalities resulting in obstructive azoospermia

has greatly expanded the CF clinical spectrum. In approximately 2% of patients there is an atypical phenotype in which there is chronic sinopulmonary disease, pancreatic sufficiency, and either borderline (40 to 60 mmol/L) or, rarely, normal (<40 mmol/L) sweat chloride concentrations. In addition, there are patients in whom a single clinical feature, for example, electrolyte abnormalities, pancreatitis, liver disease, sinusitis, or obstructive azoospermia, predominates.

The diagnosis of CF can also be considered in the absence of clinical features. An individual with an affected sibling has a 1 in 4 chance of having the disease. Half-siblings are also at increased risk compared with the general population (whites, 1 in 112; African-Americans, 1 in 244; and Asian-Americans, 1 in 352). These high risks justify careful clinical monitoring and, usually, testing of full and half-siblings. The risks for individuals with various family members with CF are listed in Table 3–2.

TABLE 3–2. *Risks for Individuals of North European White Background of Having a Child with Cystic Fibrosis*

One Parent	Other Parent	Risk with Each Pregnancy
No CF history	No CF history	1 in 3,200
No CF history	First cousin has CF	1 in 464
No CF history	Aunt or uncle has CF	1 in 345
No CF history	Nephew or niece has CF	1 in 232
No CF history	Sibling has CF	1 in 174
No CF history	Has CF	1 in 58
Sibling has CF	Sibling has CF	1 in 9
Sibling has CF	Has CF	1 in 3
Sibling has CF	Known carrier	1 in 6
Known carrier	Known carrier	1 in 4
Known carrier	Has CF	1 in 2

Risks are actually slightly higher than listed because the list assumes that (excluding siblings of CF patients) someone who is a carrier has *one* parent who is also a carrier; it is actually possible that *both* of this person's parents are carriers, in which case each of this person's siblings has greater than a 50-50 chance of being a carrier. Risks to other ethnic groups generally are different.

TABLE 3–3. *Presenting Features (Reasons for Testing) of 20,096 Patients Reported to the Cystic Fibrosis Foundation National Patient Registry*

	Number*	Percent*
Acute or persistent respiratory symptoms	10,141	50.5
Failure to thrive/malnutrition	8,628	42.9
Steatorrhea/abnormal stools	7,024	35.0
Meconium ileus/intestinal obstruction	3,788	18.8
Family history	3,368	16.8
Electrolyte imbalance	1,094	5.4
Rectal prolapse	677	3.4
Neonatal screening	459	2.3
Nasal polyps/sinus disease	404	2.0
Genotype	242	1.2
Hepatobiliary disease	175	0.9
Prenatal diagnosis (CVS, amniocentesis)	154	0.8
Other	236	1.2
Unknown	380	1.9

*Not mutually exclusive.

Courtesy of Stacey FitzSimmons, Cystic Fibrosis Foundation, Bethesda, Maryland.

The frequency of common presenting manifestations among patients reported to the United States Cystic Fibrosis Foundation Data Registry is shown in Table 3–3. In most cases, the family history is negative for CF.

CLINICAL PRESENTATIONS BY AGE GROUP

Prenatal

High-risk Pregnancies

The prenatal diagnosis of CF can be established in pregnancies known to be at increased risk because of a positive CF family history, or, less frequently, through routine antenatal screening programs. In cases in which the genotype status of the parents is known, the diagnosis of CF can be confirmed or excluded with a very high degree of accuracy by direct mutation analysis performed on fetal cells obtained by chorionic villus sampling (CVS; performed at 10 weeks' gestation) or cultured amniotic fluid cells (performed at 15 to 18 weeks' gestation). Prenatal testing should always be carried out in conjunction with an experienced geneticist or genetic counselor. It is mandatory to carry out postnatal sweat testing in all cases in which the diagnosis of CF has been made or excluded on the basis of prenatal DNA analysis.

An alternative for at-risk couples is the use of preimplantation genetic diagnosis to screen embryos before implantation. After *in vitro* fertilization, a cleavage stage biopsy is carried out on day 2 or 3, and one or two cells are removed for genetic analysis by nested polymerase chain reaction and heteroduplex formation. Normal or carrier embryos are then transferred to establish pregnancy. This procedure can be followed by CVS or amniocentesis to confirm the original diagnosis.

Fetal Intestinal Obstruction

In pregnancies not known to be at increased risk for CF, the diagnosis is sometimes suggested by prenatal ultrasonographic findings, including a hyperechoic bowel pattern, suggestive of intestinal obstruction. Among fetuses with this finding, approximately 1 in 10 will have CF. Hyperechoic bowel occurring as a benign variant is distinguished by spontaneous resolution, usually before the third trimester. In pregnancies in which there is evidence of fetal intestinal obstruction, carrier testing for CF gene mutations can be carried out in the parents. If both parents are carriers of a CF mutation, the diagnosis of CF in the fetus is highly likely and can be confirmed by direct mutation analysis of amniotic fluid cells.

Meconium peritonitis secondary to small bowel perforation in utero can also be detected by prenatal ultrasonography. However, only 7% of such cases are associated with CF. The presence of abdominal calcifications is significantly associated with causes of meconium peritonitis other than CF. Conversely, the absence of calcifications favors the diagnosis of CF. Parental CF carrier testing with fetal mutation analysis in at-risk couples can be useful in such cases.

Neonatal

Because of the presence of abnormal meconium (high protein concentration), newborns with CF can present with delayed passage of meconium, meconium ileus, or meconium plug syndrome.

Meconium Ileus

Approximately 18% of patients with CF present with intestinal obstruction in the immediate postnatal period secondary to inspissation of tenacious meconium in the ileum. Abdominal radiography shows dilated loops of bowel, usually without air-fluid levels, and a granular ground glass appearance in the area of the terminal ileum indicating the mixture of air bubbles with meconium (so-called soap-bubble sign); contrast enema shows a small caliber unused microcolon (see Fig. 5–12). Approximately 50% of cases are complicated by peritonitis, volvulus, atresia, necrosis, perforation, or pseudocyst formation. In rare cases, calcified scrotal masses secondary to *in utero* meconium peritonitis may be a presenting manifestation of CF. Among full-term neonates with meconium ileus, CF is confirmed in approximately 98% of cases. Patients should be presumptively treated for this diagnosis and parents appropriately counseled, pending the results of sweat testing or mutation analysis.

Meconium Plug Syndrome

Meconium plug syndrome, in which there is transient distal colonic obstruction relieved by the passage of a meconium plug, may be the presenting manifestation of CF in the neonatal period (see Fig. 5–13). The meconium plug syndrome may occur in association with prematurity, hypotonia, hypermagnesemia, sepsis, hypothyroidism, and as the earliest manifestation of Hirschsprung's disease, but its presence should also suggest the possibility of CF. It is important to distinguish meconium ileus and the meconium plug syndrome from meconium disease or inspissated meconium syndrome seen in very low birth weight infants. This entity is characterized by the development of obstructive symptoms at several days of age after the initial passage of meconium. Meconium plugs are found in the distal ileum and proximal colon. This complication often occurs in association with respiratory distress syndrome and is not associated with CF.

Jejunal Atresia

Neonatal intestinal obstruction secondary to jejunal atresia, often in association with volvulus and meconium peritonitis, may be a presenting feature of CF. A sweat test or mutation analysis is indicated.

Liver Disease

Neonates with CF may present with prolonged obstructive jaundice, presumably secondary to obstruction of extrahepatic bile ducts by thick bile along with intrahepatic bile stasis. On biopsy, there is moderate-to-severe focal fibrosis, variable portal inflammation, and some degree of ductular proliferation (see Fig. 5–8). There may be associated hepatomegaly. The clinical and laboratory features may mimic biliary atresia. Elevated serum bilirubin levels may persist for up to 6 months. Approximately 50% of cases occur in association with meconium ileus or delayed passage of meconium. The frequency with which such cases progress to liver failure or early cirrhosis is unknown. Massive hepatomegaly with steatosis (fatty replacement) may also occur, probably related to protein-calorie malnutrition or essential fatty acid deficiency.

Pulmonary Manifestations

Respiratory symptoms may begin during the first month of life. Manifestations include cough, wheezing, retractions, and tachypnea. There may be radiographic evidence of hyperinflation. Segmental or lobar atelectasis, particularly involving the right upper lobe, is highly suggestive of CF. Other infants may have severe respiratory distress associated with a bronchiolitic syndrome.

Growth Failure

Failure to regain birth weight by 2 weeks or inadequate weight gain at 4 to 6 weeks of age is common in neonates with CF. Growth failure often occurs despite normal or even increased caloric intake. Many of these infants cry after feedings, appear irritable, and are mistakenly diagnosed as having colic or milk allergy.

Infancy and Childhood

In infants and young children, the diagnosis of CF is usually suggested by respiratory tract symptoms or steatorrhea, often in association with some degree of failure to thrive.

Upper Respiratory Tract

The upper respiratory tract is usually involved secondary to abnormal mucous gland secretions and hypertrophy and edema of the mucous membranes. Nasal polyps occur frequently and may be present at a very early age. Their presence in a child is always an indication for a sweat test. Sweat testing should also be considered in a child with recurrent or chronic sinusitis refractory to antimicrobial therapy. Rarely, a patient with CF presents with unilateral proptosis secondary to a mucocele of the underlying sinus. Radiographic evidence of homogeneous opacification of the paranasal sinuses is a constant finding in almost all CF patients after infancy and may be a helpful diagnostic finding. The CT finding of bilateral medial displacement of the lateral nasal wall and uncinate process demineralization is particularly suggestive of CF. Normal radiographic and CT findings provide strong evidence against a diagnosis of CF.

Lower Respiratory Tract

In approximately 50% of CF patients, the diagnosis is first considered because of pulmonary symptoms. Although the lower respiratory tract is almost invariably involved, manifestations may not appear until months or even years after birth. CF should be considered in every patient with chronic or recurrent lower respiratory tract findings such as prolonged or recurrent pneumonia, bronchitis, bronchiectasis, atelectasis, refractory asthma, and empyema. The most prominent and consistent feature of pulmonary involvement is chronic cough. Cough is often initiated by an upper respiratory infection, after which it persists for weeks and may never resolve. At first, the cough may be dry and hacking, but with progression it becomes paroxysmal and may be associated with gagging, choking, and vomiting. It is often worse at night. Older patients may expectorate mucopurulent sputum, particularly in association with pulmonary exacerbations.

There may be crackles, rhonchi, wheezes, retractions, and tachypnea. Progressive airway obstruction leads to air trapping with an increase in the anteroposterior diameter of the chest. Digital clubbing is almost universal in symptomatic patients older than 4 years of age; its presence in a patient with chronic respiratory symptoms is always an indication for a sweat test.

Although there are no pulmonary radiographic abnormalities that are diagnostic of CF, there are findings that may be helpful in suggesting the diagnosis. Overaeration and bronchial wall thickening are the earliest radiographic findings (Fig. 3–1), and the absence of overinflation is strong evidence against CF in a child with pulmonary symptoms. In infants, segmental or lobar atelectasis, particularly involving the right upper lobe, is highly suggestive of CF. In older patients, typical findings include patchy atelectasis, bronchial

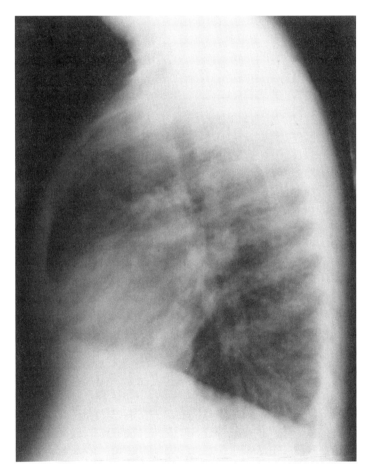

FIG. 3–1. Chest radiograph lateral view shows bronchial wall thickening, peribronchial infiltrates, flattened diaphragm, and increased anterior-posterior diameter.

wall thickening, bronchial dilatation, cysts, nonspecific linear shadows, infiltrates, hilar adenopathy and overaeration. Mucoid impaction of the bronchi is highly suggestive of CF. In CF patients with mild lung disease and a normal chest radiograph, high-resolution CT often shows evidence of mild bronchiectasis involving the upper lobes. The degree of bronchial wall thickening exceeds lumen dilatation, which is predominantly proximal.

Isolation of a mucoid variant of *Pseudomonas aeruginosa* from the respiratory tract during childhood or young adulthood is almost uniquely associated with CF and is always an indication for a sweat test. Persistent colonization with other organisms such as *Burkholderia cepacia* and *Staphylococcus aureus* may suggest or support a diagnosis of CF, although these pathogens are also found in other conditions.

Gastrointestinal Tract

In infants and young children, steatorrhea is strongly suggestive of CF. Clinical features include abdominal protuberance; crampy abdominal pain; flatulence; frequent bulky, oily, malodorous stools; and poor weight gain. Stools of infants with CF-related malabsorption frequently leak from the diaper. There may be associated rectal prolapse.

In patients with apparent steatorrhea at diagnosis, fat absorption should be assessed. During early infancy, nearly 50% of patients have substantial preservation of pancreatic function. Most of these patients develop progressive decline of pancreatic function during the first few years of life. Mutation analysis is helpful in predicting the pancreatic course of such patients. Patients who have one or two mild mutations can be expected to remain pancreatic sufficient, whereas patients who have two severe mutations can be predicted to progress to pancreatic insufficiency. (Table 3–4 lists some of the mutations associated with pancreatic sufficiency, as well as those associated with particular patient groups.) Mutations are characterized as "mild" or "severe" only in relation to pancreatic function. These classifications do not relate to pulmonary status.

The only direct quantitative assessment of exocrine pancreatic function involves duodenal intubation and measurement of pancre-

TABLE 3–4. *Cystic Fibrosis Mutations Found With Increased Frequency in Specific Patient Groups*

Ashkenazi Jewish	African- American	Pancreatic sufficiency	Normal or borderline sweat electrolytes
W1282X	405+3A→C	R117H	R117H
G542X	444delA	R334W	G551S
3849+10 kb C→T	G480C	R347P	A455E
N1303K	R553X	A455E	3849+10 kb C→T
	A559T	P574H	2789+5G→A
	2307insA	G551S	3659delC
	3120+1G→A	3849+10 kb C→T	1898+1G→T
	S1255X	Y563N	G542X
			711+1G→T
			621+1G→T

atic enzyme and bicarbonate concentrations in duodenal fluid at baseline and following stimulation with intravenous secretin and cholecystokinin. This is an invasive, expensive, and time-consuming procedure that is rarely performed except for research purposes. There are several indirect and noninvasive measurements of exocrine pancreatic status, all of which have one or more limitations. Among the indirect tests, fecal fat analysis using a timed pooled stool collection (minimum of 72 hours), although cumbersome to perform, is the most widely used and probably the most informative. Normally, stool fat output is less than 7% of fat intake (coefficient of absorption greater than 93%). An enzyme-linked immunosorbent assay (ELISA) for the detection of pancreatic elastase-1 in stool is a highly sensitive and specific marker of exocrine pancreatic function that may prove useful as an indirect measure of pancreatic function in patients with CF.

Other gastrointestinal manifestations of CF in infancy and childhood include intussusception, pancreatitis, gastroesophageal reflux, ulcer, diffuse duodenitis, and asymptomatic right lower quadrant mass, representing mucoid impaction of the appendix. The diagnosis of CF may be suggested by the histologic appearance of an appendix removed from a patient with acute or recurrent and chronic abdominal pain (see Fig. 5–11).

Miscellaneous

A variety of presentations related to a deficiency of protein, vitamins, minerals, or fat are suggestive of CF. Infants with CF may present with edema and hypoproteinemia, usually in association with breast milk or soy protein feedings. Associated findings include anemia, hepatomegaly, an elevated concentration of liver enzymes, and rash (acrodermatitis enteropathica) (see Fig. 6–4). The sweat test may initially be falsely negative in such cases, especially in the presence of edema.

An increased concentration of electrolytes in the sweat may result in a salty taste to the skin, salt crystal formation on the skin, hyponatremic or hypochloremic dehydration secondary to salt depletion, or hypokalemic metabolic alkalosis secondary to chronic salt loss. This form of hypokalemic metabolic alkalosis is particularly common in hot climates. CF should always be considered in an infant with profound hypoelectrolytemia that is not accounted for by gastrointestinal losses.

A deficiency of fat-soluble vitamins may result in a bulging fontanel (vitamin A), hemolytic anemia (vitamin E), and hemorrhagic complications (vitamin K) (see Fig. 5–5).

The incidental finding of the absence of the vas deferens at the time of an orchiopexy or herniorrhaphy may be the initial clue to the diagnosis of CF.

Adolescents and Adults

In approximately 8% to 10% of patients with CF, the diagnosis is first made during adolescence or adulthood. Many of these cases have a history of typical, although somewhat mild, respiratory tract and gastrointestinal features of CF, with onset in childhood, often associated with a poor growth pattern. In some patients, however, pulmonary symptoms may first become manifest after the age of 13 years. Chronic cough, sputum production, wheezing, recurrent pneumonia, chronic sinusitis, and chest radiograph abnormalities are common presenting features. The diagnosis of CF should be considered in patients with hemoptysis, allergic bronchopulmonary aspergillosis, poorly controlled asthma, and in those from whom *P. aeruginosa* is recovered from the respiratory tract. All adolescents and adults with unexplained chronic lung disease, malabsorption, or both, should undergo a sweat test as part of their evaluation.

Older patients may present with cirrhosis in the absence of pulmonary symptoms; CF should be considered in any patient with obscure liver disease. Other unusual presentations include pancreatitis, intussusception, night blindness, and intestinal obstruction.

One of the most consistent features of the CF phenotype in postpubertal males is obstructive azoospermia, a finding present in 98% to 99% of affected individuals. Functional sperm and fertility have been reported in males hemizygous or homozygous for the 3849+10 kb C→T mutation. In the majority of CF patients, azoospermia occurs secondary to an absent or atretic vas deferens. The evaluation of postpubertal males with atypical presentations should include a careful evaluation of urogenital status by urologic examination, semen analysis, ultrasound study of the urogenital structures, and rarely, scrotal exploration.

Of particular interest are individuals with congenital bilateral absence of the vas deferens (CBAVD) and other forms of obstructive azoospermia, many of whom have CF mutations of one or both CF transmembrane conductance regulator (CFTR) genes, or an incompletely penetrant mutation (5T) in a noncoding region (intron 8) of the CFTR gene. They usually have no evidence of respiratory tract or pancreatic abnormalities and may have normal, intermediate, or elevated sweat chloride concentrations. They should be assigned a diagnosis of CF only if there is evidence of CFTR dysfunction, as documented by elevated sweat chloride concentrations, identification of two CF mutations, or the in vivo demonstration of abnormal ion transport across the nasal epithelium (see later). The prognosis for such patients assigned a diagnosis of CF appears to be excellent, but they should be closely monitored for the development of other CF-related complications. Their relatives should receive appropriate genetic counseling.

Clinical manifestations that should prompt a sweat test are summarized in Table 3–5.

TABLE 3–5. *Indications for Sweat Testing*

Pulmonary and Upper Respiratory Tract	Gastrointestinal	Metabolic and Miscellaneous
Chronic cough	Meconium ileus	Acrodermatitis enteropathica
Recurrent or chronic pneumonia	Meconium plug syndrome	Family history of CF
Wheezing*	Prolonged neonatal jaundice	Failure to thrive
Hyperinflation*	Steatorrhea	Salty taste to skin
Tachypnea*	Rectal prolapse	Salt crystals on skin
Retractions*	Mucoid impacted appendix	Salt-depletion syndrome
Atelectasis (especially of the right upper lobe)	Late intestinal obstruction	Metabolic alkalosis
Bronchiectasis	Intussusception, recurrent or at an atypical age	Vitamin K deficiency (hypoprothrombinemia and bleeding)
Hemoptysis	Cirrhosis	Vitamin A deficiency (bulging fontanel, night blindness)
Pseudomonas colonization, especially with a mucoid strain	Portal hypertension	Vitamin E deficiency (hemolytic anemia)
Nasal polyps	Recurrent pancreatitis	Obstructive azoospermia
		Absent vas deferens
Pansinusitis		Scrotal calcification
Digital clubbing		Hypoproteinemia and edema

*If persistent or refractory to usual therapy.

CRITERIA FOR THE DIAGNOSIS OF CYSTIC FIBROSIS

The diagnosis of CF should be based on the presence of one or more characteristic phenotypic features (Table 3–1), a history of CF in a sibling, or a positive newborn screening test, plus laboratory evidence of a CFTR abnormality, as documented by elevated sweat chloride concentrations, or identification of mutations known to cause CF in each CFTR gene, or *in vivo* demonstration of characteristic abnormalities in ion transport across the nasal epithelium.

Diagnostic Testing

Sweat Test

The sweat test remains the gold standard for the confirmation or exclusion of the diagnosis of CF. During the first 24 hours after birth, sweat electrolyte values may be transiently elevated in normal infants. After the first 2 days of life, there is a rapid decline in sweat electrolyte concentrations and an elevated value can be used to confirm the diagnosis of CF. It may be difficult to obtain an adequate sweat sample during the first 2 to 3 weeks after birth, especially among preterm infants. Ideally, sweat testing should be carried out at a time when the patient is clinically stable, well hydrated, free of acute illness, and not receiving mineralocorticoids.

Methodology

Sweat testing should be carried out in accordance with the guidelines of the National Committee for Clinical Laboratory Standards. It is crucial that testing be carried out by experienced personnel using standardized methodologies in facilities in which adequate numbers of tests are performed to maintain laboratory proficiency and quality control. The only acceptable procedure is the quantitative pilocarpine iontophoresis sweat test. When a physician orders a sweat test, he or she must ensure that the methodology is acceptable.

Sample Collection

The methods of sample collection approved by the United States Cystic Fibrosis Foundation are the Gibson-Cooke procedure and the Macroduct Sweat Collection System (Wescor, Inc., Logan, Utah). In both methods, localized sweating is stimulated by the iontophoresis of pilocarpine into the skin of the flexor surface of the forearm or thigh. Sweat is then collected on filter paper or gauze (Gibson-Cooke), or in microbore tubing (Macroduct), the amount of sweat quantitated, and the sample then analyzed for chloride concentration, sodium concentration, or both. The minimum acceptable sweat volume for the Gibson-Cooke procedure is 75 mg and for the Macroduct system 15 μL. When an adequate sweat sample cannot be obtained from one site, collection can be repeated at another site, but inadequate samples from several sites must never be pooled for analysis.

Sweat should not be stimulated or collected from the head (including forehead), trunk, or any area of diffuse inflammation (e.g., eczema), or serous or bloody discharge. Sweat can be collected from a site receiving intravenous fluids as long as good contact between the skin and electrode is possible and the collection technique does not interfere with venous flow. Sweat testing can be carried out if a patient is receiving oxygen by a closed delivery system (e.g., nasal cannula) but not if the patient is receiving oxygen by an open system.

When performed properly, pilocarpine iontophoresis sweat testing has an excellent safety profile, but localized complications can occur. There can be temporary reddening of the skin, reflecting sensitivity to the pilocarpine solution, or blistering, with or without scarring, probably due to acid generated electrolytically during iontophoresis. Frank electrical burns may be produced by high current density over a small skin area, usually as a result of metal contact with the skin. Wescor estimates one burn for every 15,000 to 20,000 iontophoresis procedures with their equipment. Operator training, use of power units with automatic cut-off features, a moist interface between electrode and skin, and adherence to standardized operating procedures should reduce the risk of injury.

Sample Analysis

Electrolytes. Although either sodium or chloride can be measured, chloride provides better discrimination between CF patients and unaffected individuals, and is usually the analyte of choice. Among adults, there may be overlap in sweat sodium concentration between CF patients and unaffected individuals, leading to diagnostic confusion. In cases in which there is a borderline sweat sodium concentration, the percentage suppression after administration of a mineralocorticoid has been used to improve diagnostic accuracy; the sweat sodium concentration of CF patients does not decrease, whereas it does decrease in unaffected individuals. However, there is too much overlap between CF and unaffected individuals for this to be useful. For quality control, it may be helpful to measure the concentration of both sodium and chloride, which should be proportionately increased or decreased. Discordant values can indicate problems with collection or analysis. Sweat chloride or sodium concentrations greater than 160 mmol/L are not physiologically possible, and the patient should be retested.

Conductivity. Conductivity represents a nonselective measurement of ions. Sweat conductivity is increased in patients with CF, and its measurement has been proposed as a diagnostic test. A conductivity analyzer (Wescor Sweat-Chek) designed specifically for use with the Wescor Macroduct sweat collector has been approved by the Cystic Fibrosis Foundation as a screening method. There is excellent correlation between the results of sweat sodium and chloride concentrations and sweat conductivity. A conductivity result greater than 50 mmol/L (equivalent NaCl) is considered positive and should be followed up by a quantitative sweat test.

Osmolality. Osmolality of sweat reflects the total solute concentration in millimoles per kilogram of sweat. It is necessary to use an osmometer capable of measuring undiluted microsamples of sweat. The reference interval for sweat osmolality in children is approximately 50 to 150 mmol/kg. Children with CF have sweat osmolality values greater than 200 mmol/kg; values between 150 and 200 mmol/kg are equivocal. Positive and equivocal results should always be followed up by a quantitative sweat test.

Alternative Sweat Methodology

Alternative sweat test procedures such as direct-reading conductivity measurements or a paper-patch indicator system are associated with an increased incidence of false-positive and false-negative results and should never be used either as the basis of a definitive CF diagnosis or to rule out the disease.

Results Reporting

The results of quantitative analysis of sweat chloride in patients with CF, unaffected siblings, and controls are shown in Figure 3–2. A chloride concentration greater than 60 mmol/L is consistent with the diagnosis of CF. The results should be interpreted with regard to the patient's age. There are data to suggest that in infants younger than 3 months of age, a sweat chloride concentration greater than 40 mmol/L is highly suggestive of a diagnosis of CF. Some unaffected adults can have values higher than 60 mmol/L, but the sweat test

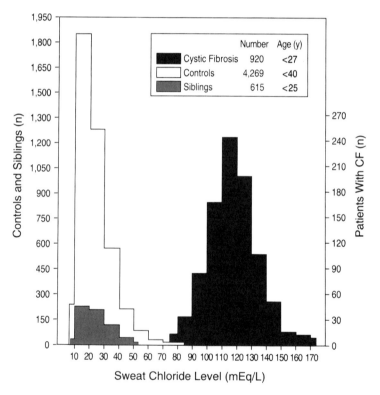

FIG. 3–2. Chloride concentrations in patients with CF, healthy persons, and healthy siblings of patients with CF. (From Shwachman H, Mahmoodian A. *Pilocarpine iontophoresis sweat testing: results of seven years' experience.* In: Rose E, Stoll E, eds. *Modern problems in pediatric.* S. Karger, Basel (Switzerland), New York: 1967:158–182; with permission.)

remains the gold standard confirmatory test in adults. Borderline sweat chloride concentrations in the range of 40 to 60 mmol/L occur in approximately 4% to 5% of all sweat tests. In such cases, repeat testing may yield results that clearly fall in the normal or abnormal range. Analysis of the ratio of sodium to chloride also may be helpful. In patients with CF, the chloride concentration is usually higher than the sodium concentration, whereas in normal subjects, the reverse usually occurs. An exception may be patients who carry less common CF mutations associated with pancreatic sufficiency, in which case the sweat sodium concentration is often higher than the sweat chloride.

Diagnostic Criteria

Sweat test results should be interpreted in relation to the patient's clinical picture by a physician knowledgeable about CF. The test results need to be consistent with the clinical picture; no single laboratory result is sufficient to establish or rule out the diagnosis of CF. The diagnosis usually cannot be made unless there is an elevated sweat chloride concentration on two separate occasions in a patient with one or more typical phenotypic features, a history of CF in a sibling, or a positive newborn screening test. In 0.1 to 1.0% of cases, the diagnosis of CF is established (nasal potential difference measurement, histopathology, mutation analysis) in patients with borderline or normal electrolyte concentrations. As more information becomes available concerning the phenotypic expressions of the CF genotype, this number may increase.

Sources of Error

The incidence of erroneous sweat test results is probably in the range of 10% to 15%. Although most errors represent false-positive results, false-negative results are also a problem. Most errors are caused by the use of unreliable methodology, inadequate sweat collection, technical errors, and misinterpretation of results.

Technical problems include contamination by salt-containing materials; failure to dry the skin adequately before sweat collection;

evaporation of the sweat sample during collection, transfer, and transport; failure to include condensate in the sweat sample when using gauze or filter paper; and errors in sample weighing, dilution, elution, electrolyte analysis, and result computation.

Duplicate sweat collection (e.g., right and left arms) and analysis may be useful for quality assurance. There is generally a good correlation between the electrolyte concentrations of sweat collected at different sites. Chloride values from two different sites usually agree within 10 mmol/L for values less than 60 mmol/L and within 15 mmol/L for values greater than 60 mmol/L.

Errors in interpretation include the establishment of a diagnosis of CF on the basis of a single positive test; failure to repeat a borderline test result; and failure to repeat a negative test in a patient with a clinical picture highly suggestive of CF. Transiently negative sweat electrolyte results have been reported in the presence of edema and hypoproteinemia. The test should be repeated after resolution of the edema.

Other Diseases Associated With Elevated Sweat Electrolyte Concentrations

A variety of diseases other than CF may be associated with moderately elevated concentrations of sodium and chloride in sweat (Table 3–6). However, with few exceptions, these conditions do not represent a problem in differential diagnosis.

There is evidence that there may be physiologic variability of sweat electrolyte concentrations over time and that there may be transient elevation of sweat electrolyte values in unaffected persons. Transient elevations in electrolyte concentrations have also been reported in infants and young children with environmental deprivation (nonorganic failure to thrive) and in adolescents with anorexia nervosa. Repeat testing after medical stabilization is indicated.

When an elevated sweat electrolyte concentration is not consistent with the patient's clinical picture, there is marked variability in electrolyte concentrations on repeat testing, the sweat electrolyte concentration is above a physiologically possible level, or there is a discrepancy among the medical history, examination, laboratory results

TABLE 3–6. *Conditions Other Than Cystic Fibrosis Associated With an Elevated Sweat Electrolyte Concentration*

*Adrenal insufficiency	*Hypoparathyroidism, familial
*Anorexia nervosa	*Hypothyroidism (untreated)
*Atopic dermatitis	Klinefelter's syndrome
Autonomic dysfunction	Mauriac's syndrome
*Celiac disease	Mucopolysaccharidosis type I
Ectodermal dysplasia	*Malnutrition
*Environmental deprivation	*Nephrogenic diabetes insipidus
Familial cholestasis (Byler's disease)	*Nephrosis
Fucosidosis	*Prostaglandin E_1 infusion,
Glucose-6-phosphate	long-term
dehydrogenase deficiency	*Protein-calorie malnutrition
Glycogen storage disease type 1	*Pseudohypoaldosteronism
Hypogammaglobulinemia	*Psychosocial failure to thrive

*Sweat test reverts to normal with resolution of underlying condition.

and response to treatment, it is important to consider the possibility of Munchausen syndrome by proxy.

Indications for Repeat Sweat Testing

1. All positive sweat test results must be repeated or confirmed by mutation analysis. The diagnosis of CF should never be based on a single positive sweat test.
2. All borderline sweat test results (chloride or sodium concentration of 40 to 60 mmol/L) should be repeated; if results remain in an indeterminate range, additional ancillary tests may be helpful.
3. Sweat testing should be repeated in patients thought to have CF but who do not follow an expected clinical course.

As patients are followed, the clinical, laboratory and chest radiograph findings should be consistent with the diagnosis of CF. It is especially important to reevaluate those patients in whom the diagnosis was suggested primarily on the basis of failure to thrive or a positive family history; the clinical features prompting the initial sweat test disappear; the patient's course is consistent with asthma without evidence of suppurative lung disease; or there is a normal growth pattern without evidence of digital clubbing, pseudomonas colonization, or typical chest radiograph findings.

Indeterminate Sweat Test Results

Patients who have persistent borderline sweat chloride or sodium concentrations present a diagnostic challenge. In such cases, it is important to carry out a comprehensive clinical, radiographic, and laboratory evaluation for features known to be consistent with the CF phenotype or for alternative diagnoses (Table 3–7). Mutation analysis and measurement of nasal potential difference (PD) may be helpful.

Mutation Analysis

In most patients with CF the diagnosis will be confirmed by a positive sweat test result, but cloning of the gene responsible for CF and identification of disease-producing mutations has raised the possibility that DNA testing may substitute for the sweat test in certain circumstances. The presence of mutations known to cause CF in each CFTR gene predicts with a high degree of certainty that an individual has CF. To date, more than 800 putative CF mutations have been described. In white populations, the ΔF508 mutation is

TABLE 3–7. *Clinical Evaluation of Atypical Cases*

Respiratory tract microbiology
Assessment for bronchiectasis
  Plain radiography
  CT
Evaluation of paranasal sinuses
  Plain radiography
  CT
Assessment of pancreatic function and structure
Male genital tract evaluation
  Semen analysis
  Urologic examination
  Ultrasound
  Scrotal exploration
Exclusion of other diagnoses
  Ciliary structure and function
  Immunologic status
  Allergy
  Infection

found in 68% of CF alleles. No other mutation accounts for more than 2% of CF alleles.

Alterations in the CFTR gene designated as CF-causing mutations should fulfill at least one of the following criteria. The mutation has been shown to (a) cause a change in the amino acid sequence that severely affects CFTR synthesis and/or function; (b) introduce a premature termination signal (insertion, deletion or nonsense mutations); (c) alter the so-called invariant nucleotides of intron splice sites (the first two or last two nucleotides); or (d) cause a novel amino acid sequence that does not occur in the normal CFTR genes from at least 100 carriers of CF mutations from the patient's ethnic group. Mutations that are included in currently available CF mutation tests and that meet one or more of these criteria are shown in Table 3–8. Improvement in DNA technology indicates that CF mutation tests in the future will include a larger panel of mutant alleles than that shown in Table 3–8. Each additional mutation should meet one or more of the four criteria listed earlier to provide a reasonable degree of certainty that it is disease producing.

A more complicated situation is presented by the R117H and 5T mutations. Presence of both mutations in the same gene (R117H-5T) is associated with CF. However, neither the R117H mutation alone (i.e., R117H with the common splice variant 7T) nor the 5T mutation alone meets the criteria for a CF mutation. Although these mutations have been associated with male infertility due to CBAVD, diagnosis of CF in patients carrying R117H-7T or 5T requires demonstration of a CFTR abnormality by sweat testing or nasal PD testing.

Confirming the diagnosis of CF based on the presence of two CF-producing mutations is highly specific but not very sensitive. Sensitivity is decreased due to the large number of CF alleles. Current commercially available mutation screening panels detect at most only 80% to 85% of CF alleles. In the United States, variability in the mutation detection rate reflects the ethnic origin of individuals in various regions of the country. However, there are CF mutations that occur with increased frequency, or even uniquely, in specific population groups, for example, Ashkenazi Jews, African-Americans, and in patients with specific clinical features such as pancreatic sufficiency or normal or borderline sweat electrolyte concentrations (Table 3–4). By customizing mutation panels to match the patient's

TABLE 3–8. *Mutations that Cause Cystic Fibrosis and How They Change the CFTR Gene*

Mutation	Frequency (in Whites)	How Gene is Altered
ΔF508	66%	1,2
G542X	2.4%	3
G551D	1.6%	1,4
N1303K	1.3%	1,4
W1282X	1.2%	2
621+1G→T	0.7%	1,3
R553X	0.7%	2
1717-1G→T	0.6%	2
R117H	0.3%	1
R1162X	0.3%	2
3849+10 kb C→T	0.2%	1,4
G85E	0.2%	4
R347P	0.2%	1
ΔI507	0.2%	4
1078delT	0.1%	2
R334W	0.1%	1
711+1G→T	0.1%	1,3
A455E	0.1%	1
S549N	0.1%	4
R560T	0.1%	4
A455E	0.1%	1
1898+1G→T	0.1%	3
2184delA	0.1%	2
2789+5G→T	0.1%	1,4
3659delC	0.1%	3

*Gene alteration.

1 causes a change in the amino acid sequence that severely affects CFTR synthesis and/or function.

2 introduces a premature termination signal.

3 alters the invariant nucleotides of spliced sites.

4 causes a change in the amino acid sequence that does not occur in the normal genes from at least 100 carriers of CF mutation from the same ethnic group.

ethnic background and phenotype, the sensitivity of DNA testing may be enhanced, although this is not routine clinical practice. Increasing test sensitivity increases the fraction of patients with CF with two mutations identified. However, some patients with CF will carry an unidentified mutation, even when test sensitivity approaches 95%. Among 9,391 genotyped patients in the CF Foundation Data Registry, in 25.1%, only one CF mutation was identified, and in

7.7%, no CF mutations were identified. These patients have to be diagnosed using other measures of CFTR dysfunction (sweat test or nasal PD testing). Even among patients diagnosed by a positive sweat test result, mutation analysis is indicated, because it can confirm a diagnosis and may provide useful information regarding genetic counseling, pancreatic function status, prognostic counseling, and appropriateness for enrollment in trials of new therapeutic agents.

Perhaps the most difficult diagnostic situation facing the clinician is the patient with clinical features consistent with CF but also with a nondiagnostic sweat test and only one identified CF mutation. In such cases, evaluation involves weighing the possibility that the individual is a carrier of a single CF mutation against the possibility that the patient has atypical CF. The situation is further complicated by the possibility that heterozygotes for a CF mutation may be predisposed to certain CF phenotypic features such as pancreatitis and CBAVD. Nasal PD testing and ancillary laboratory tests may be particularly helpful in this group of patients. If CFTR dysfunction cannot be demonstrated by any method (sweat test, mutation analysis, or nasal PD), a definitive diagnosis cannot be made and the decision to monitor or treat the patient rests on the strength of that individual's clinical presentation.

Nasal Potential Difference Measurements

Sinopulmonary, including nasal, epithelia regulate the composition of fluids that bathe airway surfaces by controlling transport of ions such as sodium (Na^+) and chloride (Cl^-). This active transport of ions generates a transepithelial electrical potential difference (PD), which can be measured *in vivo*. Abnormalities of ion transport in respiratory epithelia of patients with CF are associated with a different pattern of nasal PD compared with normal epithelia (Fig. 3–3). This provides a rationale for the use of nasal PD as a diagnostic aid. Specifically, there are three features that distinguish CF: (a) more negative basal PD, which reflects enhanced Na^+ transport across a relatively Cl^- impermeable barrier; (b) larger inhibition of PD after nasal perfusion with the Na^+ channel inhibitor, amiloride,

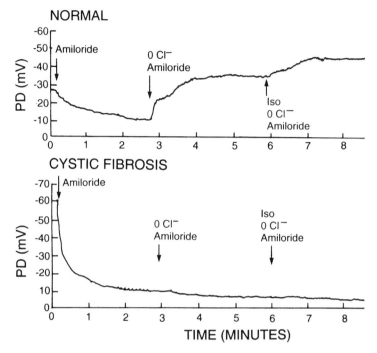

FIG. 3–3. Nasal bioelectric potential difference (PD). The tracings illustrate the response of the PD to perfusion with amiloride (10^{-4} M), the addition of a Cl⁻-free solution to amiloride, and the addition of isoproterenol (10^{-5} M) to the Cl⁻-free solution containing amiloride. **Top:** In a healthy (non-CF) subject. **Bottom:** In a patient with CF (see text for explanation). (Adapted from Knowles MR, Paradiso AM, Boucher RC. In vivo nasal potential difference: techniques and protocols for assessing efficacy of gene transfer in cystic fibrosis. *Hum Gene Ther* 1995;6:445, with permission.)

which reflects inhibition of accelerated Na⁺ transport; and (c) little or no change in PD in response to perfusion of the nasal epithelial surface with a Cl⁻-free solution in conjunction with isoproterenol, which reflects an absence of CFTR-mediated Cl⁻ secretion. Although the measurement of nasal PD may assist in the diagnosis or exclusion of CF, there are important variables that need to be rigorously addressed to ensure the safety and accuracy of testing. The technique is safe, provided the PD equipment (high impedance voltmeter) meets appropriate clinical electrical engineering standards and subcutaneous skin bridges are prepared in an aseptic manner.

Technical considerations mandate that nasal anatomy be clearly understood, because the sites of PD measurements are critical to the accuracy of the measurement. Equipment must be rigorously validated, and the protocol should be well-defined and standardized. These technical considerations have been described in great detail. Methodologies should be validated and reproducible at any facility that employs this technique for diagnostic purposes. Nasal PD can be measured in infants as young as a few hours of life; young children (2 to 5 years of age) may require modest sedation. The presence of nasal polyps or inflamed mucosa alters bioelectric properties and may yield a false-negative result.

Interpretation of PD measurements requires understanding of the ion transport characteristics of the nasal epithelium and the PD responses to perfusion with different agonists and antagonists of ion transport (Fig. 3–3). For example, a raised (more negative) basal nasal PD is strong evidence for the diagnosis of CF. However, the absence of a raised PD does not rule out CF because a false-negative result may occur in the presence of inflamed epithelium. As with any laboratory test that is used to confirm a diagnosis, an abnormal PD must be duplicated on more than one occasion to be valid as a diagnostic adjunct. It should be emphasized that the absence of a large CFTR-mediated Cl^- conductance (voltage change) in response to perfusion with a low (or zero) Cl^- solution and a beta agonist does not establish the diagnosis of CF, because there are nonspecific effects that inhibit the CFTR-mediated Cl^- conductance. However, the presence of a large response to Cl^--free perfusion is strong evidence against CF. Any laboratory planning to establish nasal PD as a clinical diagnostic tool must carry out a large enough number of studies in CF patients with defined mutations, normal subjects, and disease control subjects to establish reference values and to ensure adequate rigor of the technique. Each individual test is labor intensive.

General Caveats Concerning the Diagnosis of CF

The most commonly encountered errors regarding the diagnosis of CF are

1. Failure to consider the diagnosis because the patient is not white, the patient looks too healthy, or pancreatic function is normal.
2. Use of unacceptable sweat test methodology.
3. Misinterpretation of sweat test result because of inadequate sweat sample; confusing values for sweat weight, osmolality, and electrolyte concentration; failure to repeat positive and borderline results; and failure to repeat a negative sweat test in a patient with a highly suggestive clinical picture.
4. Failure to reconsider the diagnosis in a patient who does not follow the usual or expected clinical course.

CARRIER SCREENING

The identification of the CF gene and its most common mutations has introduced the possibility of widespread population screening for CF carrier status. In the United States, it has been recommended that such screening should not be undertaken until approximately 95% of mutations can be detected. At this detection rate, 90% of couples at risk of having a child with CF would be identified. This is currently possible in only a few populations (Ashkenazi Jewish; Saguenay-Lac St. Jean), in which CF is probably the result of founder effect. Several screening strategies are currently being evaluated. In the United Kingdom, a screening program has been successfully implemented in antenatal clinics using a so-called couple model in which both partners must agree to participate before testing begins. In most cases, only one of the partners needs to be tested because a negative result means that the couple is not at high risk. This strategy had an acceptance rate of 70% and significantly decreased the demand for counseling services. Successful implementation of carrier screening will require an extensive commitment to public education and genetic counseling.

NEWBORN SCREENING

Because of well-documented delays in diagnosis, and because earlier diagnosis may improve prognosis, there has been considerable interest in establishing a satisfactory method for the detection of CF

in newborns. The goals of newborn screening include the presymptomatic identification and early treatment of patients with CF and
the identification and counseling of at-risk families.

Since 1979, effective newborn screening for CF has been possible,
based on the observation that newborns with CF (including those

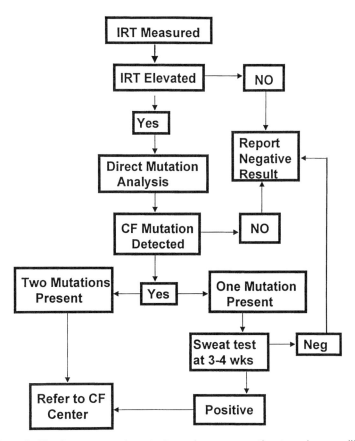

FIG. 3–4. Newborn screening strategy: Immunoreactive trypsinogen (IRT)
is measured in dried blood spots followed by direct gene analysis for ΔF508
or a panel of common mutations on those samples with an IRT value above
a predetermined cut-off level (typically the 99th percentile). Infants with two
CF mutations are referred to a CF center, and those with one identified
mutation are referred for sweat testing. (Adapted from Ranieri E, Lewis BD,
Gerace RL, et al. Neonatal screening for cystic fibrosis using immunoreactive trypsinogen and direct gene analysis: four years' experience. *Br Med J*
1994;308:1469.)

without steatorrhea) have persistently elevated concentrations of immunoreactive cationic trypsinogen (IRT), a pancreatic enzyme precursor, in their blood, probably secondary to pancreatic ductular blockage and leakage of enzyme into the circulation. Screening was initially carried out using a two-tier protocol in which IRT was measured in dried blood spots, followed by a sweat test in patients with persistently elevated values. More recently, IRT/DNA protocols (Fig. 3–4) have been used in which an IRT assay is performed on all samples, followed by direct gene analysis for ΔF508 or a panel of common mutations on those samples with an IRT value above a predetermined cut-off level (typically the 99th percentile). Infants with two CF mutations are referred to a CF center, and those with one identified mutation are referred for sweat testing and further evaluation. Timely access to reliable quantitative pilocarpine iontophoresis sweat testing is a crucial component of the screening program.

Both protocols have acceptable sensitivity in the range of 91% to 100%. The IRT/DNA strategy has the advantage of fewer false-positive results (higher specificity), thereby reducing the number of infants recalled for a second IRT sample, the number of infants requiring a sweat test, and parental anxiety. The positive predictive value is in the range of 15.2% to 37.4%. The disadvantage of this strategy is the unwanted detection of healthy carriers and the attendant requirements for parental education and counseling. Another disadvantage is that some infants without identified CF mutations will later be found to have CF. It is important for physicians to understand that this is only a screening strategy and that newborns with a negative screen might still have CF. It is of interest that in most IRT/DNA screening programs, the detection of apparent CF carriers among newborns with elevated IRT levels is significantly higher than expected. The reason is not clear, but one explanation is that some of these infants have a mild form of CF. Because of better efficiency, equal or better detection rates, higher positive predictive values, more rapid diagnosis and minimal additional cost, most screening programs are now using an IRT/DNA protocol.

Measurement of IRT is only a screening procedure and should never be used as laboratory confirmation of a CF diagnosis. Also, physicians need to remain alert to the possibility of CF in infants and children with suggestive symptoms and a history of a negative newborn screening test.

The role of population-based newborn screening remains contro-versial. Nonrandomized, noncontrolled studies have demonstrated fewer hospitalizations, decreased morbidity, and better nutritional status in the first 2 years among patients diagnosed by screening (Wilcken and Chalmers, 1985). Also, a randomized trial carried out over 10 years in Wisconsin has demonstrated a long-term benefit in height and weight among the group diagnosed by newborn screen-ing (Farrell et al., 1997). Other potential benefits are earlier genetic counseling and a reduction in the anxiety associated with delayed diagnosis. However, improved survival has not been demonstrated among patients diagnosed by newborn screening, and it is possible that a presymptomatic diagnosis might lead to inappropriate and expensive therapy with untoward consequences.

Newborn screening programs have been successfully imple-mented in many parts of the world and may be of particular benefit in areas where cases of CF are usually diagnosed late or not at all. Pending demonstration of a long-term benefit, newborn screening has not been recommended in the United States and, at present, is carried out statewide only in Colorado and, as part of a research pro-tocol, in Wisconsin. It is also being evaluated in several regional and statewide pilot programs elsewhere.

POSTMORTEM DIAGNOSIS

A patient may die before the diagnosis of CF can be confirmed or ruled out. Making the diagnosis remains important for family knowl-edge and family planning. Postmortem diagnosis can sometimes be strongly suggested by the typical histologic pattern of the pancreas and intestines, particularly the appendix and ileum, with hypere-osinophilic secretions overfilling mucous glands.

A 1-g section of fresh tissue from any organ, but particularly the liver, can be used for DNA analysis. The tissue is best obtained within hours of death but may suffice even within 72 hours. If the tissue is cut, wrapped in foil, and put in dry ice, it should be usable. DNA analysis can, on occasion, be carried out on paraffin-embed-ded biopsy or autopsy tissue from years before and, in extenuating circumstances, even from autopsy slides. The limitations previously discussed for DNA diagnosis also apply. Finding two CF alleles makes the diagnosis likely; finding one or none may modify the estimated likelihood of CF but does not rule it out.

REFERENCES

Alton EW, Currie D, Logan-Sinclair R, et al. Nasal potential difference: A clinical diagnosis test for cystic fibrosis. *Eur Respir J* 1990;3:922–926.

Ao A, Ray P, Harper J, et al. Clinical experience with preimplantation genetic diagnosis of cystic fibrosis (delta F508). *Prenat Diagn* 1996;16:137–142.

Brock DJ. Prenatal screening for cystic fibrosis; 5 years' experience reviewed. *Lancet* 1996;347:148–150.

Christoffel KS, Lloyd-Still JD, Brown G, et al. Environmental deprivation and transient elevation of sweat electrolytes. *J Pediatr* 1985;107:231–234.

Corteville JE, Gray DL, Langer JC. Bowel abnormalities in the fetus—correlation of prenatal ultrasonographic findings with outcome. *Am J Obstet Gynecol* 1996; 175:724–729.

Cystic Fibrosis Genetic Analysis Consortium. Population variation of common cystic fibrosis mutations. *Hum Mutat* 1994;4:167–177.

Farrell PM, Kosorok MR, Laxova A, et al. Nutritional benefits of neonatal screening for cystic fibrosis. *N Engl J Med* 1997;337:963–969.

Farrell PM, Koscik RE. Sweat chloride concentrations in infants homozygous or heterozygous for F508 cystic fibrosis. *Pediatrics* 1996;97:524–528.

Farrell PM, Mischler EH. Newborn screening for cystic fibrosis. The Cystic Fibrosis Neonatal Screening Study Group. *Adv Pediatr* 1992;39:35–70.

Gregg RG, Simantel A, Farrell PM, et al. Newborn screening for cystic fibrosis in Wisconsin: Comparison of biochemical and molecular methods. *Pediatrics* 1997; 99:819–824.

Hall SK, Stableforth DE, Green A. Sweat sodium and chloride concentrations— essential criteria for the diagnosis of cystic fibrosis in adults. *Ann Clin Biochem* 1990;27:318–320.

Hammond KB, Turcios NL, Gibson LE. Clinical evaluation of the macroduct sweat collection system and conductivity analyzer in the diagnosis of cystic fibrosis. *J Pediatr* 1994;124:255–260.

Knowles MR, Paradiso AM, Boucher RC. In vivo nasal potential difference: Techniques and protocols for assessing efficacy of gene transfer in cystic fibrosis. *Hum Gene Ther* 1995;6:445–455.

LeGrys VA. Sweat testing for the diagnosis of cystic fibrosis: practical considerations. *J Pediatr* 1996;129:892–897.

Macek MJ, Mackova A, Hamosh A, et al. Identification of common cystic fibrosis mutations in African-Americans with cystic fibrosis increases the detection rate to 75%. *Am J Hum Genet* 1997;60:1122–1127.

National Committee for Clinical Laboratory Standards. Sweat testing: sample collection and quantitative analysis-approved guideline [Document C34-A]. Wayne, PA: The Committee, 1994:1.

Rosenstein BJ. What is a cystic fibrosis diagnosis? *Clin Chest Med* 1998;19: 423–441.

Rosenstein BJ, Cutting GR for the Cystic Fibrosis Foundation Consensus Panel. The diagnosis of cystic fibrosis: A consensus statement. *J Pediatr* 1998;132:589–595.

Stern RC, Boat TF, Abramowsky CR, et al. Intermediate-range sweat chloride concentration and *Pseudomonas* bronchitis. A cystic fibrosis variant with preservation of exocrine pancreatic function. *JAMA* 1978;239:2676–2680.

Stewart B, Zabner J, Shuber AP, et al. Normal sweat chloride values do not exclude the diagnosis of cystic fibrosis. *Am J Respir Crit Care Med* 1995;151:899–903.

Wiatrak BJ, Myer CM, Cotton RT. Cystic fibrosis presenting with sinus disease in children. *Am J Dis Child* 1993;147:258–260.

Wilcken B, Chalmers G. Reduced morbidity in cystic fibrosis patients detected by neonatal screening. *Lancet* 1985;2:1319–1321.

Wilcken B, Wiley V, Sherry G, et al. Neonatal screening for cystic fibrosis: A comparison of two strategies for case detection in 1.2 million babies. *J Pediatr* 1995;127:965–970.

Wilfond BS, Fost N. The cystic fibrosis gene: medical and social implications for heterozygote detection. *JAMA* 1990;263:2777–2783.

4
The Respiratory System

OVERVIEW OF TREATMENT

Chronic pulmonary inflammation and infection (and associated complications) account for much of the morbidity and almost all the mortality of cystic fibrosis (CF). Considerable improvement in pulmonary treatment has occurred in the 60 years since the introduction of pancreatic enzyme treatment essentially eliminated malnutrition as a primary cause of death. Improved pulmonary treatment has resulted in spectacular improvement in median survival (now greater than 30 years), but considerably better pulmonary treatment is needed before lung disease no longer presents a continuing threat to health and life. In the absence of successful gene-based or protein repair therapies, which would completely prevent CF-related pulmonary disease, a comprehensive prevention and treatment approach is essential. It is not unreasonable to speculate that, as more is known of the pathophysiology of the pulmonary disease, a successful multipronged attack could be formulated. Some of these measures are available now and should be implemented. Others can be expected soon.

INFECTION

Introduction

Chronic bacterial infection is an important characteristic of the disease and is directly or indirectly involved in the pathophysiologic sequence that is responsible for death in the vast majority of patients. The dominant organisms are usually *Staphylococcus aureus* or *Pseudomonas aeruginosa,* or both. Occasionally, *Burk-*

55

*holderia cepacia, Stenotrophomas maltophilia, Alcaligenes
xylosoxidans, Escherichia coli,* and others are involved. Intermittent periods of increased respiratory symptoms (so-called pulmonary exacerbations), the causes of which are only partially understood, cause considerable morbidity and probably play an important role in causing the progressive parenchymal destruction and fibrosis that ultimately kills the patient. Treatment of bacterial infection is addressed later. However, there is no doubt that intercurrent community-acquired viral respiratory infections are important triggers of these exacerbations, and preventive and therapeutic measures for these illnesses are also important.

The importance of bacterial pathogens, which commonly colonize CF airways, and the increasing evidence that early treatment is beneficial, suggest that surveillance cultures should be done. CF is one of the few diseases in which easily obtained throat and sputum cultures have sufficiently high correlation to lower respiratory tract cultures (bronchoalveolar lavage fluid, direct lung aspirates, and lung tissue specimens) to be clinically useful. Patients who are not yet colonized with potential pathogens have the most to gain by regular surveillance and prompt treatment aimed at eradication. Deep throat cultures should be done on asymptomatic patients. For symptomatic patients, particularly infants, bronchoscopically obtained specimens can be very useful if routine throat cultures do not reveal pathogens or if the pathogens found on throat cultures merit antibiotic treatment (how to make that decision is discussed later).

Preventive Measures

Immunizations

All routine infant immunizations should be given at the usually recommended intervals. Intercurrent illnesses, even if they are associated with low-grade fever, are not a valid reason for delay. Of particular importance is the prevention of those illnesses that have primarily or occasionally severe pulmonary manifestations; these illnesses include pertussis, measles, varicella, and *Haemophilus influenzae* type b. Treatment with systemic and, possibly, aerosolized corticosteroids is a valid reason to delay use of live virus vaccine (e.g., varicella).

Influenza vaccine should be given as well. Influenza can be an extremely serious illness in CF patients. Although the vaccine must be given each year and it is not always completely effective, this vaccine is clearly worthwhile. Because the influenza vaccine is not always completely protective, most experts recommend vaccinating the entire family to reduce the CF patient's risk of being exposed to someone with active infection.

Pneumococcal vaccine is more controversial, but its use is not unreasonable in CF patients. Pneumococcal pneumonia is not a common complication of CF (which is the reason many centers have not advocated routine use of this vaccine), but the recent rapidly increasing incidence of very resistant organisms argues for giving this vaccine. Furthermore, it need not be given every year. The combination of greater threat than in the past and an improved vaccine suggest that it probably should be given.

Although considerable effort has been made to develop antistaphylococcal and antipseudomonas vaccines, there are theoretical arguments against their efficacy (e.g., failure of IgG antibodies to be present in sufficient amounts in the airways to be effective). In any case, the vaccines that have been tested experimentally thus far do not appear to have had much clinical success in CF.

Respiratory syncytial virus infection is a major problem in CF patients, especially during infancy, when it can initiate a series of pathophysiologic events that can lead to substantial irreversible lung damage or even death. Unfortunately, there is as yet no effective and safe vaccine. Passive immunization with intravenous (IV) immunoglobulin (e.g., RespiGam) or monoclonal antibody (Synagis) has not yet been shown to be sufficiently effective in CF to warrant widespread use; also, the safety (e.g., RespiGam is a blood product) of these formulations has not been unequivocally established. Furthermore, they are extremely expensive and must be given every 4 weeks for several months during each of the first 2 years.

Other vaccines that are effective against adenovirus or even against some milder viral respiratory diseases (e.g., even those caused by rhinovirus), for example, would be desirable but do not appear imminent.

Other Preventive Measures

1. Limiting exposure to viral respiratory illnesses. Avoidance of day care for infants and young children is probably desirable, but this is one of many areas where the reality of modern life often prevails over the medical ideal. Similarly, restriction of access of sick family members and friends is theoretically desirable but often not logistically feasible. Nonetheless, for families who want to do everything possible, reasonable precautions regarding contagion could probably be helpful, at least for some preschoolers.

2. Limiting exposure to traditional CF bacterial pathogens. The fact that patient-to-patient transmission of CF pathogens (e.g., *B. cepacia*) occurs is now widely accepted. Most centers use some form of isolation for *B. cepacia* infection (ranging from separate rooms to separate wards; and from different clinic rooms to different clinic days), whereas other centers use complex isolation measures to protect subgroups of patients (those with multiresistant as opposed to susceptible strains of *P. aeruginosa*). Patients and families should be knowledgeable about the potential risks of exposure to other CF patients (ranging from no effect [i.e., no transmission of organisms] to generally worsened health [e.g., a worsened antibiotic susceptibility pattern] to rapid and severe worsening, ending with death [e.g., after acquisition of *B. cepacia* infection]) so they can make informed decisions about allowing or limiting social exposures.

Pharmacologic Prophylaxis

Amantadine/ramantidine is effective prophylaxis for type A influenza and is reasonably effective treatment for early infection with this virus. All patients should have a sufficient amount of drug on hand to begin empiric treatment promptly (within a couple of hours, if possible, but optimally within minutes) for otherwise unexplained high fever and cough during the peak influenza season (e.g., December through early April). The drug should also be considered during the peak epidemic period for patients who cannot tolerate the vaccine (egg allergy; other reactions) or refuse to get it.

Continuous antibiotic treatment for *S. aureus* was not effective in preventing chronic staphylococcal carriage or in delaying or preventing progressive pulmonary disease in the one long-term multicenter trial (the cephalexin trial) in which it was tested; there was increased acquisition of *P. aeruginosa* in the patients who received cephalexin.

Therapy

Eradication of Bacterial Pathogens

Eradication of *P. aeruginosa* from the respiratory tract is an achievable goal in some patients. This is particularly true in newly colonized patients, particularly if the patient is young and if the mucoid strain is not present. Three to six weeks of combined oral ciprofloxacin and aerosolized colistin is a reasonable treatment approach.

For patients who have required antipseudomonal treatment in the preceding 6 months (or perhaps those whose first positive culture reveals a mucoid strain, which also suggests an infection of longer duration), a more prolonged course is indicated. A 3-month course of oral ciprofloxacin and aerosolized colistin has been shown to be effective. Alternatively, IV (e.g., tobramycin and ceftazidime) or aerosolized antibiotics (e.g,. tobramycin) can be used for either patient group. The IV route obviously has considerable logistic and economic disadvantages, as well as being uncomfortable for the patient.

Early eradication may not be worthwhile in younger siblings of chronically infected patients. Frequent reinfection occurs, and the risk of emergence of resistant organisms, which would then threaten both patients, is probably high.

S. aureus is so commonly found in upper airway cultures that routine antibiotics aimed at eradication in asymptomatic patients is probably not warranted. A fail-safe nonbronchoscopic method of distinguishing clinically significant pulmonary infection from benign upper airway carriage in the asymptomatic patient is not available. When treatment is needed, high-dose treatment with a single agent (with proven *in vitro* efficacy) is sufficient. However, a 4-week course (or longer) is often necessary. Even if the criteria for diagnosis of a pulmonary exacerbation are not met, the patient with deterioration of pulmonary function, prolonged respiratory symptoms in the wake of an upper respiratory infection (URI), new onset of cough without preceding nasal symptoms, and other indications of progression of pulmonary infection often warrant treatment as described later.

Treatment of a Pulmonary Exacerbation

Diagnosis of Exacerbation

The most widely accepted diagnostic scheme is the following: An exacerbation is present if the patient has four or more of the following 12 findings: (a) a change in sputum; (b) new or increased hemoptysis; (c) increased cough; (d) increased dyspnea; (e) onset or worsening of malaise, fatigue, or lethargy; (f) temperature greater than 38°C; (g) anorexia or weight loss; (h) sinus pain or tenderness; (i) a change in sinus discharge; (j) increased abnormality on chest physical examination; (k) a decrease in pulmonary function by 10% or more from a previously recorded value; (l) radiographic changes indicative of pulmonary infection.

Treatment of Exacerbation

Treatment should always include antibiotics and airway clearance, and often includes other approaches (e.g., bronchodilators, mucolytic agents) tailored to the individual patient's needs. These treatment modalities are discussed later in this chapter. Hospitalization is often appropriate to initiate treatment and, in some cases, for the entire duration of treatment.

Antibiotic treatment should include the safest systemic or aerosolized agent, or combination of agents, that offers a reasonable chance of therapeutic success. Examples of antibiotic doses are given in Table 4–1. Treatment is needed for a minimum of 2 weeks and often longer. The duration of treatment should be guided by the patient's subjective response as well as quantitative outcome measures, such as pulmonary function results, arterial blood gas analyses, and overall clinical scores. Exacerbations often require IV antibiotic treatment. The principles for selecting antibiotic combinations are given in Table 4–2.

TABLE 4-1. *(Doses for Systemic Drugs) Antibiotic Doses (Assuming Normal Renal Function)*

Antibiotic	Daily Dose Calculation	Dosage Interval
Azithromycin	10 mg/kg/d up to 500 first day 5 mg/kg up to 250 q.d. next 4 days	24 hours
Aztreonam	100–150 mg/kg/d	8 hours
Ceftazidime	200–300 mg/kg/d (maximum 12 g.d.)	8 hours*
Cephalexin	50–100 mg/kg/d	q.i.d.
Cefipime	Insufficient data and not recommended for use in children Standard dose of 2 g q 8 h for adults	8 hours
Ciprofloxacin, oral	20–50 mg/kg/d	b.i.d.
Ciprofloxacin, IV	10–15 mg/kg/d	12 hours
Clindamycin	20–40 mg/kg/d	8 hours
Clarithromycin	15 mg/kg/d	b.i.d.
Colistin	5–7 mg/kg/d (max dose 100 mg q8h)	8 hours
Doxycycline oral	4–6 mg/kg/d	b.i.d.
Imipenem	60–100 mg/kg/d (children); 2–4 g/d (adults)	6 hours
Meropenem	120 mg/kg/d (children); 1.5–4 g/d (adults)	8 hours
Piperacillin	300–500 mg/kg/d	6 hours*
Nafcillin	100–200 mg/kg/d	6 hours*
Ticarcillin	300–500 mg/kg/d	6 hours*
Trimethoprim/ sulfamethoxazole, oral	trimethoprim 8–10 mg/kg/d	b.i.d.
IV	trimethoprim 10–20 mg/kg/d	6 hours*
Tobramycin	8–15 mg/kg/d	8 hours† or 24 hours
Vancomycin	30–60 mg/kg/d up to 2 g/d	12 hours
Metronidazole, oral	30–40 mg/kg/d	t.i.d.
IV	30 mg/kg/d	6
Chloramphenicol	50–100 mg/kg/d	6 hours
Levofloxacin, oral	Insufficient data and not recommended for use in children Adults: 500 mg/d	8 hours q.d.
IV	500 mg	q.d.
Amphotericin IV	2.5 mg/kg	q.d.
Itraconazole	Maximum adult dose 400 mg	b.i.d.
Ketoconazole	Maximum adult dose 400 mg	b.i.d.
Dicloxacillin	Children: 4–7 mg/kg/d Adults: 2000 mg/d	b.i.d. 6 hours

*Maximum dosage interval; other considerations may justify shorter intervals.
†Use either one of these dosage intervals in patients with normal renal function. Blood levels can be used to guide treatment for the q8h regimen. No blood levels necessary for the q.d. dosing regimen.

TABLE 4–2. *Principles of Antibiotic Combinations*

1. Use the minimum number of antibiotics to cover each recovered gram-negative pathogen with two agents.
2. If possible, use only one antibiotic from any given family of drugs.
3. Try to avoid giving two systemic antibiotics whose principal toxicity affects the same organ.
4. If possible, use systemic agents only if they have demonstrated *in vitro* efficacy, but if this is not possible, use an agent that has been shown to be effective empirically in the patient (or is often effective in CF patients).
5. Use of an aerosolized antibiotic should be considered if (a) it is effective *in vitro* or is thought to be effective *in vivo* at the concentrations achieveable in sputum; (b) the aerosolized drug is not likely to be toxic to other people (e.g., do not use chloramphenicol by aerosol); (c) the chosen drug can be aerosolized and is not overly noxious because of smell; (d) the patient does not have an idiosyncratic reaction (e.g., allergy or wheezing); (e) the patient's pulmonary status suggests that he or she is capable of adequate distribution of the drug by inhalation.
6. Use the highest possible dose of each antibiotic, based on official recommendations, personal experience with other patients, and the individual patient's prior course.

Chronic Suppression of Long-standing Bacterial Infection

Patients with advanced disease often need virtually continuous antibiotic treatment. These patients include those who deteriorate shortly after finishing each course of antibiotics. They should not be required to fail antibiotic-free periods time after time but rather should be treated. The choice of antimicrobials is based on *in vitro* susceptibility studies, but *in vitro* resistance should not preclude use of a drug because some therapeutic benefit may still be possible if (a) the drug is effective against organisms (including anaerobes) that were not identified on the culture; (b) the drug acts synergistically with other antibiotics the patient is receiving; or (c) the drug has a therapeutic effect that is not based on antimicrobial action at all (e.g., if it has an antiinflammatory effect).

Intermittent Suppression of Long-standing Bacterial Infection

Some patients are benefitted by intermittent (e.g., 2 to 4 weeks out of every 6 to 12 weeks) treatment with either nonspecific wide-spectrum antibiotics (e.g., a fluoroquinolone, tetracycline, trimethoprim-sulfamethoxazole, or chloramphenicol [the latter drug is not easily obtained for oral use in the United States]) or with a specific agent (e.g., a fluoroquinolone) based on *in vitro* susceptibility studies.

Continuous or Frequent Intravenous Antibiotic Treatment

Some patients with very severe disease improve during IV treatment but then relapse almost immediately after it is discontinued. These patients occasionally can stabilize when they are given virtually continuous IV antibiotics at home (9 to 12 months per year).

AIRWAY CLEARANCE

Introduction

Retained secretions play at least two key roles in the pathophysiology of CF pulmonary disease. First, they physically obstruct the airway, aggravating infection (by causing stagnation of secretions), and directly cause overinflation and suboptimal ventilation/perfusion adjustment regulation. Second, they contain high concentrations of injurious inflammatory mediators (e.g., cytokines and leukotrienes), which can cause bronchospasm and, more important, are the main cause of progressive parenchymal injury, destruction, and subsequent fibrosis.

Physical Removal of Secretions

Many techniques for airway clearance have been developed since postural drainage with percussion was introduced early in this century for the treatment of chronic bronchitis in adults. Effective removal of secretions requires three distinct steps: (a) loosening of secretions from the airway walls; (b) mobilization of secretions within the airways so they can be moved toward the trachea; and (c) clearance from the trachea and upper airway so that the material can be expectorated or swallowed.

Loosening of Secretions From the Airway Walls

Loosening of secretions can be facilitated with mucolytic agents or by mechanical devices that physically separate secretions from the airways by some form of vibratory energy. The idea of expectorants is old, but there are no systemically administered drugs with proven effectiveness as expectorants. For example, saturated solution of potassium iodide (SSKI), although widely prescribed, has never been shown to be an effective expectorant. Excess water (e.g., IV fluid in excess of that necessary to maintain hydration) has not been shown to liquefy secretions. Guaifenesin, also widely used in both nonprescription and prescription formulations, does not have proven efficacy.

However, locally active drugs that can be given by inhalation can be effective. *N*-acetylcysteine, the first chemical mucolytic agent to gain widespread acceptance, is definitely effective *in vitro,* but its usefulness *in vivo* is compromised by the fact that it is often irritating and thus capable of inducing a self-defeating hypersecretory state or bronchoconstriction, or both. Nonetheless, when the drug is judiciously used in selected patients, it can be helpful. Human recombinant DNase, a much more potent mucolytic agent, has other advantages (e.g., better patient acceptance because it is odorless), and has largely replaced *N*-acetylcysteine. However, acute toxicity, for example, due to excess liquification of voluminous secretions with dissemination of infection peripherally, may occur in the occasional patient, especially in someone with severe pulmonary disease. Finally, it is possible that the present dosing recommendations are not optimal for every patient. Some patients may need substantially less or more than one dose a day.

Mobilization of Secretions

Mobilization of secretions can be accomplished by a variety of techniques and devices. Postural drainage with clapping is effective for some patients and is virtually all that is available for infants and very young children. However, Flutter, active cycle of breathing, positive end-expiratory pressure (PEP) mask, and other techniques that use forced expiration and various percussion devices, including a chest vest with pulsating percussion (ThAIRapy Vest) are all effective in some patients. For very sick patients who do not have the energy (or the lung capacity) for techniques that depend on forced expiration, only postural drainage with clapping and the ThAIRapy Vest are worth trying.

Removal of Secretions From the Respiratory Tract and Expectoration of Sputum

Removal of secretions from the respiratory tract can be aided by many of the techniques noted earlier. In addition, physical removal with tracheal suctioning (or bronchoscopic suctioning) is occasionally done, especially if secretions are very tenacious.

Other Techniques

Bronchoscopic Lavage

Bronchoscopic lavage (also called wash-outs) was an attractive idea but has proven to be a disappointing treatment in practice. There may, however, be isolated instances in which it can be effective. Bronchoscopic lavage with saline appears to remove so much surface-active material that, over the long term, the prolonged adverse effects of the resultant microatelectasis outweigh the benefit of the short-lived removal of secretions. Furthermore, improving ventilation to underperfused areas of lung may worsen, at least transiently, already compromised ventilation/perfusion matching. Whether success with bronchoscopic lavage can be improved substantially if it is done with perflubron is not known, but one inevitable problem with such a technique is that standard radiographs of the chest will not be useful for a prolonged period (perhaps a year or more) after the procedure.

Exercise

There is no doubt that exercise can indirectly benefit patients with obstructive pulmonary disease by forcing deep breathing and, for many people, bronchodilatation, thus facilitating cough and airway clearance. Becoming active and exercising also makes patients feel more in control and virtuous. Overall, exercise is beneficial, and should be encouraged, but there are no data to support the view (optimistically held by many patients and occasionally by their physicians) that exercise can obviate the need for rigorous airway clearance.

Detoxification of Secretions

There are a great many potentially injurious inflammatory mediators in CF respiratory secretions, and it is unclear if inactivation or inhibition of synthesis of any one (or even a group) of these substances would substantially slow the progression of CF lung disease. However, while waiting for the final proof, it is reasonable to use present knowledge of pathophysiology both experimentally and therapeutically to the extent safety considerations will allow. Thus, as they become available, inhibitors of synthesis of and blockers of receptors for leukocyte elastase, inflammatory interleukins, destructive leukotrienes, and similar mediators should be seriously considered. These drugs are discussed in somewhat more detail later.

PREVENTION AND TREATMENT OF COEXISTING UNRELATED NONINFECTIOUS PULMONARY DISEASES

Examples of conditions that threaten the lung itself (or pulmonary function) of CF patients but that may not be directly related to CF are scoliosis, asthma and reactive airways disease (discussed under Complication below), cigarette or marijuana smoking, IV substance abuse with talc emboli to pulmonary vessels, and occupational exposures (e.g., hair spray [cosmetology]).

Recreational drug use, ranging from cigarette and marijuana smoking to IV drug abuse is not infrequent in teenage and young adult patients. The only effective treatment is prevention (or cessation). Although first-hand tobacco smoke has not been proven to affect CF patients' pulmonary course adversely, it is reasonable to presume that it does. Preteens should be warned about the additional risk they incur by smoking. Teenage smokers should be explicitly told that smoking is a more imminent threat to their health and life than it is for their peers. All smokers should be educated about their options for obtaining help with smoking cessation. Similarly, second-hand cigarette smoke is almost certainly capable of aggravating CF lung disease, and all families should be warned of this problem when the diagnosis is made and, if appropriate, occasionally thereafter.

Idiopathic adolescent scoliosis occurs with equal frequency as in the general population. Scoliosis may also result from asymmetric CF-related lung disease. When scoliosis is severe enough to warrant treatment (e.g., with brace or surgery), it can obviously add to or aggravate CF-pulmonary disease. Patients with scoliosis present difficult management problems. Scoliosis braces themselves cause restriction of chest expansion, and fusion surgery, with its severe postoperative pain and prolonged need for a body cast, also causes restriction. CF patients with marginal pulmonary status can be driven to frank respiratory failure, which may require mechanical ventilation. These patients often do not tolerate braces, and as a practical matter in most cases, surgery is the only option.

IV drug abuse is usually associated with the embolization of inactive filler, often talc, into the pulmonary arterioles. This factor produces gradual obliteration of the pulmonary arterial bed, potentially aggravating hypoxia-induced pulmonary hypertension. Again, education is the only answer.

Occupational exposures are common in teenagers (e.g., teenagers who pump gasoline; factory jobs with exposure to industrial fumes). More important, potentially, however, is career choice. A career of auto painting or cosmetology results in far more exposure to toxins than does a summer job at the gas station. However, some patients may be so psychologically devastated at having to give up their main career goal that pursuit of their life dream may be less dangerous and therefore preferable to the depression that would ensue if they were forced to give it up.

INFLAMMATION

Introduction

Chronic inflammation is now widely acknowledged to play a pivotal role in the pathophysiologic sequence leading to parenchymal lung destruction and fibrosis. It is increasingly clear that inflammation can occur in the absence of infection and, in fact, may be the initial event, at least in some patients, that facilitates the onset of chronic infection. Furthermore, the main role of inflammation (i.e., overcoming infection and helping restore the lungs to their preinfection state) does not seem to apply in CF. The invading microorganisms are rarely cleared, and the inflammatory mediators, which are present in unusually high concentrations, become the primary threat to the integrity of the lung parenchyma. The overall theoretical strategies for the medical treatment of inflammation are shown in Table 4–3. Some specific antiinflammatory agents now in use, in development, or proposed that are directed at these goals are presented in the following sections.

Systemic Corticosteroids

Long-term alternate-day systemic corticosteroid treatment (e.g., 1 or 2 mg/kg of prednisone) slows the progression of the pulmonary

TABLE 4–3. *Some Theoretical Strategies for Suppression, Prevention, and Treatment of Pulmonary Inflammation in Cystic Fibrosis*

1. Control infection
2. Decrease the production/concentration/effect of potentially proinflammatory substances
   A. Decrease synthesis of potentially toxic mediators of inflammation (including oxygen radicals)
   B. Interfere with receptors of inflammatory stimuli
   C. Interfere with receptors of inflammatory mediators
   D. Decrease cellular response to inflammatory mediators
   E. Decrease inflammatory cell access to lung/airways
   F. Inactivate toxic antibacterial substances (e.g., protease)
   G. Deplete body reserves of proinflammatory cells (e.g., neutrophils)
   H. Provide protection against oxygen radicals (e.g., aerosolized or systemic antioxidants, such as pycnoic acid, glutathione, vitamin C, and vitamin E)
   I. Institute environmental measures directed at reducing exposure to oxygen radicals and related substances
3. Increase the production, concentration, effect of potentially antiinflammatory substances
   A. Stimulate production of naturally occurring antiinflammatory substances (e.g., IL-10)
   B. Receptor agonists of naturally occurring antiinflammatory substances
   C. Administer synthetic antiinflammatory drugs

lesion of CF. However, after a few years, the costs of toxicity (i.e., glucose intolerance and diabetes, growth retardation, cataract) may outweigh the benefits in most patients, and therefore, this approach is rarely used for more than a few weeks to months. Patients with certain CF complications discussed later (e.g., allergic bronchopulmonary aspergillosis, severe asthma, severe bronchiolitis) and some other ill-defined severe steroid responsive or steroid-dependent airways obstruction may require prolonged treatment. In addition, patients who are taking high-dose corticosteroids for an unrelated disease would, theoretically, be treating their CF lung disease at the same time.

Aerosolized Corticosteroid

The demonstrated beneficial effect of systemic corticosteroids has led to renewed interest in using aerosolized corticosteroids to achieve at least some benefit while drastically reducing toxicity. Aerosolized steroids are widely and justifiably used in CF patients for specific indications (e.g., hyperreactive airways disease). However, it has been difficult to assess their impact on primary CF pathology, and there are no published data on their prolonged use in unselected CF patients. Some toxicity from these agents, comparable with that seen in non-CF patients, would be inevitable, and there are some unpublished data suggesting that their use in infants with CF may hasten the advent of infection with *P. aeruginosa.*

Systemic Ibuprofen

Although perhaps not as potent as corticosteroids, chronic high-dose ibuprofen therapy does result in substantial slowing of the progression of the pulmonary lesion in most, but by no means all, patients (e.g., reduction in the rate of decline of FEV_1 from 4% to 0.5% per year in school-age CF patients with mild pulmonary disease).

Inhaled Cromolyn or Nedocromil

These agents inhibit mast cell degranulation after exposure to specific antigens, but are also thought to prevent or ameliorate bronchospasm caused by triggers other than classic allergens (e.g., cold air, exercise, and pollutants). Theoretically, therefore, they may attenuate inflammation in CF patients with asthma and those whose airways are hyperreactive to infection, but they have not yet been shown to do so.

Systemically Administered Leukotriene Receptor Antagonists (e.g., Zafirlukast [Accolate] and Montelukast [Singulair])

These agents are competitive leukotriene C_4 (LTC$_4$), LTD$_4$, or LTE$_4$ receptor antagonists, approved initially for the treatment of asthma. Levels of these mediators are also increased in CF pulmonary secretions, and these agents could theoretically be helpful. However, there are many other inflammatory mediators in CF secretions, and the effect of these agents on the action of only two or three of them may be offset by the others.

Systemically Administered Inhibitors of Neutrophil Elastase Synthesis

Neutrophil elastase is one of the most (if not the most) important destructive cell products in CF secretions. In CF patients, the concentrations of elastase in the airway greatly exceeds the amount that can be neutralized by naturally produced antiproteases. Drugs in this class, such as dimethyl phthalate (DMP), block the synthesis of elastase in the neutrophil, so that even if neutrophils are attracted to (and subsequently die in) the airways, they contain no elastase.

Aerosolized Antiproteases

Some experimental work has focused on recombinant human antiproteases (produced, for example, in the milk of genetically altered and then cloned sheep). Although preliminary data indicate that aerosolized plasma-derived α_1-antitrypsin suppresses airway elastase in humans, there are no comparable data (and certainly no data on clinical usefulness) on recombinant antiprotease.

Aerosolized or Systemic Antioxidants, Including Picnoic Acid, Glutathione, Vitamin C, and Vitamin E

There is considerable interest in this area among both physicians and patients, but very little useful data have been generated.

Fish Oil and Other Membrane Stabilizers

Very large doses of fish oil and other membrane stabilizers would be needed, making compliance a major problem for the majority of patients. No efficacy data for use of this treatment in CF have been generated to date.

CORRECTION AND AMELIORATION OF THE BASIC (INTRACELLULAR) DEFECT CAUSED BY THE ABNORMAL CFTR PROTEIN

Introduction

The complete pathophysiologic sequence from the abnormal gene to the typical progressive lung disease is not known. In general, therapeutic approaches using gene therapy assume that supplying a normally functioning CFTR gene (or correcting the defect in electrolyte transport caused by an abnormal CFTR protein) would be sufficient to avert health-threatening and life-threatening lung disease. Although this assumption is likely to be true, it is not a certainty (e.g., the abnormal gene product could act as a receptor to which bacteria could attach; or as a receptor for an inflammatory mediator). The following treatment strategies assume that restoring normal (or perhaps partial) CFTR function in the airways would be sufficient to treat or even cure the pulmonary disease.

Insertion of the Normal CFTR Gene Into Pulmonary Airway (and Perhaps Mucous Gland) Epithelium

Although gene transfer has been demonstrated *in vitro,* and transient gene insertion and function has been accomplished *in vivo,* clinical improvement or even sustained function has not been demonstrated as yet.

Improving Function of the Abnormal CFTR Gene

A wide variety of theoretical approaches to improving gene function have been proposed (see also Chapter 2). Unlike insertion of a normal gene, strategies for improving gene function may vary, depending on the patient's exact CFTR mutation. Splice mutations, which have a markedly reduced production of normal gene product (and a large production of faulty protein), may be treatable by increasing overall gene activity so that a small but adequate percentage of the product would be functional CFTR. Trafficking mutations may be approached with a view toward shepherding the gene product toward and eventually into the cell surface. Human studies using this approach (e.g., with β-hydroxybutyrate), are now entering clinical trials.

UPPER RESPIRATORY TRACT MANIFESTATIONS

Colds and Upper Respiratory Infections

Uncomplicated URIs in CF patients (after infancy) follow the same course as they do in unaffected persons: slight (scratchy) sore throat for less than 2 days (which may not be noticed or remembered by children); coryza or sinus pressure for several days, but peaking on the third or fourth day of the illness; cough, which is dry at first but eventually minimally productive, beginning after 3 to 4 days, and lasting about 3 days before gradually resolving over the subsequent 3 to 4 days. The total duration of the illness is about 10 days. For relatively healthy CF patients, little more than careful surveillance is needed. As long as the course is uncomplicated, no antibiotic changes are indicated. Intensification of airway clearance may be prudent, particularly when the symptoms seem to be localized to the chest. However, if the clinical picture deviates from the normal course (e.g., total course longer than 11 days, or the patient's pulmonary symptoms start resolving and then get worse), it is no longer an uncomplicated cold, and more aggressive antibiotic or other treatment should be seriously considered. At that point, the illness should be treated as an early pulmonary exacerbation.

For patients who are more seriously ill at their initial presentation, intensified treatment (both airway clearance and antibiotics) should be considered early in the course of the URI. It is not unreasonable for all patients to have a plan for dealing with URIs (and the medications to carry it out) available to them before these illnesses occur. For example, the parents could be instructed to institute cephalexin promptly when their baby (with *S. aureus* previously recovered from cultures) develops a cold.

URIs in CF infants often do not follow the usual course described earlier. Patients may develop acute bronchiolitis with every URI (the most common pulmonary presenting symptom that leads to the diagnosis of CF during infancy) and may need hospitalization, aerosolized or systemic corticosteroids, bronchodilators, and antibiotics. Occasional patients need mechanical ventilation.

Identification of the specific virus responsible for a URI (e.g., influenza virus, adenovirus, or respiratory syncytial virus [RSV] versus rhinovirus) could be useful in predicting which URIs are likely to precipitate pulmonary exacerbations. Although routine viral studies on all URIs on all CF patients is not a practical option at present, viral studies on selected patients could be useful. If different viruses were shown to have different implications for precipitating CF-related pulmonary exacerbations or if specific antiviral agents become available, rapid cheap tests for viral agents, if available, could greatly simplify the management of URIs in patients with CF. (Also, note the possibility of pharmacologic treatment of influenza virus discussed earlier.)

Sinus Disease

That sinus disease occurs in patients with CF is not at all surprising. Abnormally thick or viscid secretions may result from abnormal electrolyte content or underhydration, or both. In addition, various pathogens (including *P. aeruginosa* and other gram-negative organisms) have been recovered from sinuses of patients with CF, and as in the lung, it seems likely that infection contributes to sinus inflammation and disease. There may also be a primary tendency toward chronic inflammation (even in the absence of infection) in the respiratory mucosa perhaps due to an imbalance of proinflammatory and antiinflammatory mediators. In patients with advanced pulmonary disease, chronic hypoxemia (or acidosis, or both) may adversely affect ciliary function, impairing mucus clearance. If nasal polyps are present, they can physically block sinus drainage. Aeration of the sinuses is delayed, and in many patients, the frontal sinuses are very small or absent.

Despite the extremely high prevalence (almost 100% for classic CF; somewhat lower for some milder variants) of radiologically demonstrable sinus abnormalities, usually complete opacification of all the paranasal sinuses, it is not clear if the prevalence of the traditional symptoms of chronic sinusitis (Table 4–4) is any higher in CF patients than it is in the general population. In fact, most CF patients never develop symptomatic chronic sinusitis at all, and except for rare patients whose mucoceles erode a sinus wall, the peculiar lack of correlation between symptoms and radiologic findings limits the usefulness of routine radiologic imaging in guiding therapeutic decisions. In essence, if sinus symptoms are not present, imaging is unlikely to show a severe complication of sinus disease, and the patient does not require treatment. Furthermore, it is important to note that, even in the absence of symptomatic sinusitis, CF patients often have erythematous and swollen (from mucosal edema) nasal turbinates.

Patients with transient sinus symptoms, which occur in the normal course of URIs (and which can be expected to resolve without specific treatment), often recover without antibiotic treatment, but it is not unreasonable to treat these patients with antibiotics in anticipation of a virus-induced pulmonary exacerbation. On the other hand, however, although it is not common, chronic symptomatic sinusitis is often difficult to treat in CF patients. Systemic and local antibiotics are the cornerstones of medical treatment. Local antibiotics are delivered either by aerosol (e.g., tobramycin) or by indwelling surgically inserted catheters (see later). Antibiotic therapy should cover the organisms previously recovered from respiratory cultures, and if the patient does not respond, the more classic sinus pathogens should be treated as well. Doses should be the same as would be given for

TABLE 4–4. *Classic Symptoms of Chronic Sinus Disease*

1. Chronic frontal headache or pain in upper jaw
2. Persistent nasal obstruction, mouth breathing, or snoring
3. Facial pain, swelling, or tenderness in the absence of an acute URI
4. Chronic halitosis
5. Persistent purulent nasal discharge or postnasal drip
6. Anosmia or dysosmia
7. Ophthalmologic symptoms or signs (e.g., diplopia; proptosis)

URI, upper respiratory infection.

CF pulmonary disease. Local decongestants (e.g., phenylephrine) and nasal hygiene (nasal spray or Water Pic with saline) can be very helpful. Recently, some physicians have proposed using rhDNase (Pulmozyme) to liquify sinus secretions, but controlled studies with direct instillation (e.g., as described later) or sprays have not been reported.

Chronic symptomatic sinusitis that does not respond adequately to medical treatment may justify surgical intervention. Drainage procedures (clearing secretions, removing polyps, or enlarging or creating drainage pathways) are often successful, especially over the short term, but the addition of direct instillation of antibiotics (usually tobramycin) appears to be considerably more effective. Considerable success has been reported with one such procedure, in which a combined surgical and pharmacologic approach is used. Endoscopic maxillary antrostomies are performed, and a flexible catheter is then inserted into each maxillary sinus via the antrostomy. The other end of the catheter is taped to the patient's cheek. Tobramycin (40 mg in 1 mL saline) is then instilled into each sinus three times a day. During the instillation, the irrigated sinus is in the dependent position. This procedure is continued for 7 to 10 days, after which the catheters are removed. Repeat tobramycin instillations, under local anesthesia, are then continued at monthly intervals. This procedure has not been evaluated in any controlled studies.

CF patients develop mucoceles, and these lesions occasionally cause erosion of one of the sinus walls (usually the frontal sinus), either posteriorly (toward the brain) or medially (toward the orbit). At that point, with only soft tissue separating the infected sinus cavity from the central nervous system or the eye, surgical treatment is essential and may be urgent. The most common approach is to attempt obliteration by transplanting fat into the sinus. Success is not ensured with this method. The procedure is often complicated by the lack of sufficient subcutaneous fat for the transplant (due to the cachexia of chronic illness) or by graft failure, perhaps due to the generally inhospitable environment of the sinus (infection, hypoxemia, or acidosis).

Nasal Polyps

There is no question that inflammatory nasal polyps (but not allergic polyps) are associated with CF. The incidence of polyps is probably less than 15%. Symptoms and signs associated with nasal polyps are shown in Table 4–5. Diagnosis can often be made by direct visual inspection, especially if phenylephrine spray is used to shrink the nasal mucosa first. However, some polyps can be diagnosed only by computed tomographic (CT) sinus studies; such studies are desirable before surgery.

Surgical removal of polyps, usually combined with a sinus drainage procedure, has been the traditional and, until recently, the only treatment with proven efficacy. Nasal obstruction and many of the other symptoms are immediately relieved or ameliorated. However, some symptoms (e.g., dysosmia and anosmia, epistaxis, change in voice, and widening of the nasal bridge) may be unaffected, possibly because the polyps have already caused irreversible anatomic change or because the symptom was not due to the polyps. Because a significant percentage of patients never experience a recurrence, surgical excision, with an endoscopic sinus drainage procedure, seems reasonable as initial treatment. Unfortunately, polyps recur in the majority of patients, and subsequent excisions become more difficult (because of synechiae and bleeding) and riskier (because of progressive thinning of the cribiform plate). Patients and families should be warned of these potential problems before surgery.

The results of medical treatment are less clear cut. Control of allergic nasal symptoms may allow delay of surgical treatment of the polyps. Corticosteroid nasal spray and intrapolyp injections of corticosteroid may help some patients (whether allergic disease is suspected or not). After high-dose ibuprofen treatment for preventing

TABLE 4–5. *Clinical Manifestations and Presenting Symptoms of Nasal Polyps in Patients with Cystic Fibrosis*

1. Symptoms due to obstruction of air flow
   Stuffy nose
   Mouth breathing
   Snoring
2. Symptoms due to increased mucus secretion
   Rhinorrhea
   Purulent discharge
3. Symptoms due to mass effects
   Nasal pain
   Change in voice
   Polyp visible protruding out of the nose
   Distortion of facial features and spreading of nasal bridge
   Polyp or polyp tissue sneezed or blown out of nose
4. Miscellaneous
   Epistaxis
   Halitosis
   Dysosmia or anosmia
   Aggravation of pulmonary disease

progression of CF lung disease was introduced in some centers in 1996, anecdotal reports have suggested some improvement in nasal polyps. This finding may be supported by data from the National CF Registry, but the results are preliminary.

LOWER RESPIRATORY TRACT

Standard Daily Care

Routine Treatment

Airway Clearance

All CF patients, even those with minimal or no ongoing pulmonary symptoms, deserve some daily treatment and regular surveillance to optimize the chance that health can be maintained. This includes, at a minimum, one airway clearance treatment session, the goal of which is to ensure that the airways are functionally cleared at least once a day. This involves the performance of one or a combination of airway clearance techniques (discussed earlier) to completion, that is, to the point at which the patient cannot, even with maximal effort, raise any more sputum. Depending on the individual patient and what is then thought to be optimal, this approach may include aerosolized bronchodilators or mucolytics, or both. The head-down position for traditional postural drainage probably worsens gastroesophageal reflux in infants; it may therefore be prudent to avoid that position in patients younger than one year old. Performance of airway clearance procedures at least daily, even in asymptomatic patients, also incorporates these treatments into the patient's and family's everyday routine so that they become second nature, and if symptoms increase and treatments are needed more frequently, both patient and family are prepared.

Intermittent Antibiotic Treatment

For patients who are not yet infected with gram-negative pathogens, especially *P. aeruginosa*, regular surveillance cultures should be done (at 6- to 12-week intervals) to detect the onset of infection early. When such an organism is recovered, aggressive antibiotic treatment (e.g., an oral fluoroquinolone plus inhaled colistin, or inhaled tobramycin) should be instituted (at present, the recommended duration of this treatment is 6 weeks for the initial episode and 3 months for any recurrence within 6 months).

For symptomatic patients who are chronically infected with *S. aureus* or one or more gram-negative pathogens, particularly *P. aeruginosa* (but also *B. cepacia, S. maltophilia, A. xylosoxidans,* and *Klebsiella pneumoniae*) ongoing treatment with antibiotics with *in vitro* efficacy (or occasionally antibiotics without demonstrable *in vitro* efficacy but seemingly reliable empiric effectiveness, such as tetracycline, trimethoprim-sulfamethoxazole, and various quinolones) is appropriate.

Antiinflammatory Agents

Alternate-day administration of corticosteroids (prednisone at 1 or 2 mg/kg q.o.d.) has been demonstrated to delay the progression of

CF lung disease. At 2 mg/kg q.o.d., toxicity was unacceptable. However, although there is corticosteroid toxicity at 1 mg/kg q.o.d., some physicians believe the risk/benefit ratio favors its use.

Ibuprofen is the only other antiinflammatory agent that has both proven efficacy as a prophylactic agent and acceptable safety. Although, thus far, efficacy has been shown only for patients who are 5 to 13 years old and have mild lung disease, it seems likely that the real age range for which the drug is useful is wider. Pharmacokinetic studies are necessary before treatment (there is substantial patient-to-patient variability) to ensure that an adequate dose is given (i.e., one that achieves peak blood levels of 50 to 100 µg/L); an inadequate dose may actually increase inflammation. The possibility of combination antiinflammatory therapy is totally unexplored, and it is not known whether two or more drugs will have additive, synergistic (or no) beneficial effect.

Routine Center Visits

Although it seems obvious that intermittent visits to a CF center (to update the patient's history, physical examination, respiratory culture, reinstruction in airway clearance or other treatment modality, nutrition assessment, and financial and insurance advice and counseling) are important, the optimal frequency of such visits is a subject of considerable debate. Intervals of less than 6 weeks are probably too short to be practical; intervals of more than 4 months are probably too long (for one thing, that would be enough time for a gram-negative infection to become firmly established). Similarly, the ideal frequency for pulmonary function tests, chest roentgenograms, and other diagnostic imaging studies is also not firmly established. In addition, as a practical matter, both the timing of interval visits and the performance of routine laboratory studies (including pulmonary function studies) are increasingly influenced by restrictions made by the patients' insurance carriers.

Visits to a physician at 6- to 12-week intervals, depending on the baseline health of the patient, would be reasonable. Ideally, pulmonary function studies (including the FEV_1) should be done at every visit. Cultures should be obtained every 3 to 6 months.

The intervals between visits, cultures, and pulmonary function studies for patients who have no acute increase in symptoms should be shorter for healthier patients. Initial worsening is likely to involve more subtle symptoms and often requires FEV_1 measurement to detect. Early deterioration is probably the most important time to intervene, because that period offers the greatest chance to prevent progressive airway damage. The absence of symptoms (or lack of change in symptoms) and an unchanging FEV_1 is reasonable evidence of clinical stability. However, the proper approach to an isolated fall in FEV_1 (without accompanying increased symptoms and without change in the respiratory flora) is not clear. At the least, however, such a fall would indicate the need for even more careful follow-up (e.g., repeat visit and pulmonary function tests [PFTs] within a few weeks; or, for some patients, bronchoscopy with bronchoalveolar lavage [BAL] to detect potential pathogens early).

Bronchiolitis

Introduction

Infection and inflammation of the smallest airways is one of the earliest pathologic changes in CF, and it is not surprising therefore that recurrent bronchiolitis is the most common pulmonary presentation of the disease in infancy. Recurrent wheezing, occasionally severe, due to inflammatory obstruction (with or without bronchospasm) is extremely common after diagnosis as well. In some patients, the primary pathophysiology (small airway inflammation and infection) is aggravated by allergy or gastroesophageal (GE) reflux (which, in turn, may be exacerbated by positioning for airway clearance treatments).

Treatment of Persistent or Severe Wheezing in Infancy

Some CF infants wheeze virtually continuously during their first year but are not in any overt distress. It is usually futile to attempt to eliminate wheezing in these babies. Antibiotic treatment should be used as indicated by *in vitro* susceptibility studies on pathogens recovered from throat or BAL cultures.

Patients who are in more distress or who are failing to thrive despite the use of antibiotics and conventional bronchodilators deserve more aggressive treatment. They usually show some response to systemic corticosteroids, and they often respond and stabilize when placed on an inhaled corticosteroid. Standard preparations (fluticasone and beclomethasone) can be tried first, but if these drugs are not adequate, nebulization of nasal preparations (e.g., Nasolide), or of the intravenous (IV) form of dexamethasone (e.g., Decadron or Hexadrol, 4 mg/mL at doses of 0.5 mL down to 0.05 mL) can be used, and the dose tapered (e.g., from 0.5 b.i.d. down to [for some patients] minute amounts [e.g., 0.05 mL q.d.]). This approach is usually effective, but there is some unpublished evidence that any inhaled corticosteroid facilitates the acquisition and permanent establishment of *P. aeruginosa* infection. Overall, however, despite this risk, such treatment is still worthwhile for many of these patients. The physician must keep in mind that systemic absorption of nebulized dexamethasone is probably greater than it is for beclomethasone or fluticasone.

Severe or Life-Threatening Bronchiolitis

Babies with severe bronchiolitis should be treated with high-dose systemic corticosteroids, nebulized corticosteroids, and antibiotics that cover both *S. aureus* and *P. aeruginosa*. This treatment should be guided by culture, if possible, but if the patient is culture negative, empiric tobramycin and ceftazidime should be given. Mechanical ventilation may be needed.

Asthma

Because inflammatory obstruction of the small airways (i.e., bronchiolitis) is one of the earliest pathologic changes in CF lung disease, it should not be surprising that wheezing occurs in many infants with the disease, and that this wheezing (because it is due to inflammatory obstruction rather than bronchospasm) is often unresponsive to bronchodilators. On the other hand, reducing inflammation, as with corticosteroids, may ameliorate this problem whether it is inflammatory obstruction or bronchospasm. Most of these infants, despite definite wheezing, do not necessarily have asthma, and bronchodilators may not be helpful. However, in some infants and many older patients, true bronchospasm is present and easily documented by pulmonary function studies before and after the use of aerosolized bronchodilators. Whether these patients would have had true asthma even if they did not have CF, or just bronchospasm secondary to the CF infection is impossible to know. This may be a "distinction without a difference" because much of the treatment is identical.

It is important to remember that some CF patients with severe (and widespread) disease and very damaged airways depend on smooth muscle tone to maintain the integrity of the lumen. These patients may have a paradoxical (and clinically important) worsening in response to aerosolized bronchodilator (more wheezing and a greater fall in FEV_1).

Other Complications

Pneumothorax and Pneumomediastinum

Superficial thin-walled cysts (blebs), usually in an upper lobe, are virtually universal in patients with advanced CF pulmonary disease. Rupture of such a bleb results in an air leak that causes either a pneumothorax or a pneumomediastinum (often with subcutaneous emphysema), or both. Air leaks can also occur as a complication of a medical procedure (e.g., percutaneous insertion of a central catheter, insertion of a central venous access device, or thoracentesis). A unilateral pneumothorax that has sufficient tension to cause a life-threatening progressive accumulation of extrapulmonary air and that restricts expansion of both lungs (or simultaneous bilateral pneumothoraces with the same functional result) is a medical emergency and requires immediate action (rapid tube thoracostomy or needle thoracentesis followed by chest tube insertion). Fortunately, this condition is relatively uncommon in CF patients.

Pneumothorax, itself, is fairly common in CF patients. The cardinal symptoms are abrupt onset of unilateral chest pain and simultaneous onset of (or increase in) dyspnea. However, either or both symptoms may be absent with either small or large collections of extrapulmonary air. When the volume of extrapulmonary air is large, pleural surfaces are less likely to rub against each other, and pain is minimal or absent. The leak often occurs on the patient's worse side. Previous ventilation/perfusion adjustments may have already directed most of the blood flow to the other lung (minimizing the physiologic impact of the loss of functioning lung), and the pre-existing parenchymal overinflation (so-called stiff lung) may prevent the lung from collapsing completely. The surprising lack of symp-toms of pneumothorax may delay diagnosis and underscore the need to have a high index of suspicion about suggestive symptoms (see also the section entitled Chest Pain).

Treatment. Small air leaks may not require anything more than symptomatic treatment. A small extrapulmonary air collection dis-covered on a routine chest film of an asymptomatic patient or in a patient who presents with mild chest pain but little or no dyspnea can be observed, usually in hospital, until it is clear that the leak has stopped. Low-flow oxygen (or a slightly increased FiO_2 from the patient's baseline) may be all that is necessary. However, in many cases, the pneumothorax will occur during an exacerbation of pul-monary disease, in which case, institution of IV antibiotic treatment (see Treatment of a Pulmonary Exacerbation, page 60) should be considered.

Patients with larger (or longer lasting or recurrent) air leaks require more definitive treatment. The goals are to achieve resolution of the leak and reexpansion of the lung, and to prevent recurrence. These goals can be accomplished either by open thoracotomy (or perhaps with a thoracoscope) with upper lobe pleural stripping and over-sewing of visible blebs (under direct vision), and pleural abrasion elsewhere, or by tube thoracostomy with chemical pleurodesis. The pleurodesis approach has a slightly higher percentage of nonresolu-tion and a moderately higher risk of recurrence. The choice depends on the individual experience of the CF center, the preference of the patient and the family, and other factors (e.g., previous experience of the thoracic surgeon or the type of anaesthesia coverage available).

The treatment of pneumothorax in CF patients has been compli-cated in recent years by the advent of the double lung transplant as a treatment for end-stage lung disease. Most transplant centers accept patients who have had previous chest surgery or chemical pleurodesis (with the possible exception of talc, which can injure or freeze the diaphragm). However, there is no question that a previous sclerosing procedure does make removing the native lungs more difficult and increases the chance that postoperative bleeding will necessitate a return to the operating room. The desire to preserve ideal transplant status has led many physicians to return to a more conservative approach for many patients, especially with the initial episode of pneumothorax. This more conservative approach begins with simple tube thoracostomy and suction. If the leak resolves and the lung expands, and stays expanded after discontinuation of suction, the tube can be removed. If this approach fails, open or thoracoscopic blebectomy, without pleural stripping or pleurodesis, could be considered.

The treatment of iatrogenic pneumothorax is similar in principle to a spontaneous pneumothorax. However, the prognosis for resolution after tube thoracostomy may be better, and the recurrence rate is very low.

Hemoptysis

CF patients bleed into an airway when infection erodes through a blood vessel wall. Although other factors may be involved, the characteristics of the bleeding, including its severity, depend mainly on the severity of the infection, the competence of the clotting pathways, and the size of the eroded vessel and the pressure of the blood within it. Bleeding from vessels within the airway walls (so-called feeders) usually results in the expectoration of small amounts of blood (streaks or spots) mixed with sputum. Although bleeding is always a frightening symptom for most patients, bleeding from these feeder vessels rarely progresses to health-threatening or life-threatening blood loss. The patient can usually be reassured and managed at home often by simply intensifying antiinfection measures, ensuring that vitamin K deficiency is not present, and advising the patient to discontinue or avoid drugs that interfere with platelet function (e.g., nonsteroidal antiinflammatory drugs [NSAIDS]). Airway clearance measures, including chest percussion, can continue. There is neither a theoretical reason nor clinical data to support the need to discontinue aerosolized DNase because of hemoptysis. However, in some patients, DNase may aggravate cough, and that could interfere with hemostasis.

More serious bleeding arises from larger vessels, often those with systemic blood pressure (bronchial arteries and their tributaries) and, infrequently, from pulmonary arterioles in patients with substantial pulmonary hypertension. CF patients often have large and tortuous bronchial arteries that are particularly vulnerable to erosion and injury. Bleeding can range from episodic, low volume, and short duration (and not recurrent) to rapid, explosive bleeding with exsanguination or suffocation. The common feature of this type of bleeding is the expectoration of so-called pure blood. Actually the expectorated blood is not really pure but is usually diluted with thin secretions or saliva; nonetheless, it looks pure to the patient, family, and medical personnel.

Patients with hemoptysis always present difficult management problems. Even the decision to admit or observe at home is seldom straightforward. It depends on the actual details of the bleeding episode or episodes and the physician's rapport with and knowledge of the patient, as well as the distance of the patient's home from the CF center or from any major medical center. CF patients often develop a consistent pattern with respect to hemoptysis. For some, the initial bleed invariably presages continued episodes that ultimately result in considerable blood loss; these patients should be admitted immediately. Others rarely continue even though the first bleeding episode may have been quite voluminous. Many factors other than the estimated volume of blood lost (including whether the patient is clearly in the midst of a pulmonary exacerbation [and its severity], present pulmonary status, microbiology, whether the patient lives alone, and the patient's and family's level of anxiety), must be considered in the decision to admit. However, either substantial blood loss, especially over a short period of time, or clinical suspicion of orthostatic blood pressure changes clearly necessitates admission.

Whatever the decision about admission, antiinfectious measures should be optimized (often including IV antibiotics), NSAIDS discontinued, activity minimized, and the patient positioned to minimize bleeding based on the physician's best guess as to the location of the bleeding vessel. In the absence of specific knowledge of the bleeding site, it is reasonable to assume that it is coming from an upper lobe and, more specifically, the right upper lobe. The patient should be positioned so that the suspected area of bleeding is upper-most to reduce blood flow to that area (e.g., for a patient with a bleeder that is suspected to be in the right upper lobe, he or she should lie with the apex up and leaning toward the left).

Vitamin K (5 mg) should be given by intramuscular (IM) injec-tion, and then continued with daily oral doses. Antibiotics that are known to interfere with platelet function (e.g., some synthetic peni-cillins) should be avoided, if possible, but not if they are the only agents with *in vitro* efficacy. If the patient is hospitalized, blood should be obtained for type and cross match, but volume expanders (including blood transfusion) should be avoided unless absolutely necessary, because they may perpetuate bleeding. Chest physiother-apy (airway clearance procedures) can be resumed slowly beginning about 12 to 18 hours after the last episode of frank (new) bleeding.

Most bleeding episodes, including those that involve substantial blood loss, can be managed conservatively. However, the physician (and CF center) should have a general plan regarding the sequence of therapeutic maneuvers to be undertaken for those few patients whose dangerous bleeding continues. Patients who require transfu-sion (and some who do not but whose bleeding has been steady and fairly brisk) and those with severe hypotension or shock should be treated emergently (i.e., even before transfer to the intensive care unit) with IV vasopressin (Pitressin; for adults, 20 units in 15 min-utes followed by 0.2 U/minute). Once Pitressin is given, the patient should be transferred to an intensive care unit even if bleeding stops. IV Pitressin is usually effective in immediately terminating the bleeding episode, but its use also implies the need to proceed (pref-erably when the acute bleeding has been controlled) with bronchial artery embolization. More drastic measures, including bronchoscopy with balloon tamponade (e.g., with Swan-Ganz or Foley catheter) or lobectomy, are rarely necessary.

Chest Pain

The differential diagnosis of chest pain in a CF patient is shown in Table 4–6. These entities can usually be readily differentiated with only a few questions and radiologic examinations. For example, bilateral symmetric pain almost never originates in the lung or pleura. This is because it is extremely unlikely for an acute painful lesion of the lung or pleura, by coincidence, to arise symmetrically (in both hemithoraces) and simultaneously. Bilateral pain is almost always the result of the sudden increased work of breathing with stress of the respiratory muscles and rib cage. Similarly, with the exception of tracheitis (in which burning or searing pain occurs with each cough) or pneumomediastinum, midline pain is unlikely to be pulmonary in origin. In the absence of subcutaneous emphysema or radiographic evidence of pneumomediastinum, anterior or deep pain, which is present even without cough, is most likely caused by esophagitis. Vertebral pain (from kyphoscoliosis or vertebral fracture) is usually easily localized by the patient to the posterior midline.

TABLE 4–6. *Differential Diagnosis of Chest Pain in Cystic Fibrosis*

Related to Cystic Fibrosis
  Pulmonary Causes
    1. Pneumothorax
    2. Pleurisy without effusion
    3. Pleurisy with effusion
    4. Lobar or segmental atelectasis
    5. Acute tracheal pain and coughing paroxysms
    6. Lung abscess
    7. Acute lobar pneumonia
  Muscle/Bone
    1. Muscular pain (accessory muscles)
    2. Kyphosis
    3. Rib fracture secondary to cough
    4. Compression vertebral fracture
  Other
    1. Iatrogenic (bronchial artery embolization)
    2. Esophagitis
Unrelated to Cystic Fibrosis Intrathoracic Disease
    1. Costochondritis
    2. Trauma
    3. Pericarditis
    4. Herpes zoster
    5. Cardiac origin (very rare)
    6. Referred pain from abdomen
    7. Pleural catch syndrome

Unilateral pleuritic pain in CF patients is usually caused by pleurisy without effusion. In general, these patients prefer to lie on the side affected by the pain (to restrict excursion of the lung on that side), whereas in spontaneous rib fracture, the patient lies on the contralateral side and there is point tenderness on physical examination. Lung abscess pain usually is nonpleuritic and deep within the thorax. Many patients have recurrent miniabscesses with each exacerbation, and for them, the pain is just another symptom of exacerbation. The pain with a pneumothorax usually has an abrupt onset and is often associated with immediate increase in dyspnea. Classic lobar pneumonia is uncommon in patients with CF, and therefore, pleural effusion is not encountered very often. However, it can occur with acute staphylococcal disease in infancy and with mycoplasma disease in older patients. Clearly, new onset unilateral chest pain, unless it is trivial or frequently recurring, requires a chest film to rule out pneumothorax (which often requires specific treatment), and to distinguish among the other entities.

Allergic Bronchopulmonary Aspergillosis

Allergic bronchopulmonary aspergillosis (ABPA) should be suspected in any CF patient whose pulmonary disease deteriorates precipitously, suddenly, or unexpectedly. There appears to be considerable geographic variability in the frequency of this complication, but no area is completely safe. All inpatients should be screened for ABPA on admission with quantitative IgE and sputum fungus culture, unless the patient does not have suggestive clinical findings and has had these tests performed as an inpatient or outpatient within the previous 12 months. Outpatients with substantial pulmonary symptoms should have a total serum IgE measured yearly. Patients with very high IgE levels (normal values vary geographically and from laboratory to laboratory) should be investigated further (aspergillus skin test; fungal hypersensitivity pneumonitis panel; and, perhaps, measurements of aspergillus-specific IgG and IgE). The diagnosis of ABPA in CF patients is often difficult because many of the clinical findings usually used as criteria for this diagnosis (fleeting infiltrates and wheezing) are also common in CF patients. In some areas, elevated aspergillus-specific IgE can be documented in 50% of the patients, suggesting that this test is not as specific as its name suggests (or that ABPA is extremely common). Each CF center must develop its own criteria for making a presumptive diagnosis of ABPA. For example, one reasonable approach is to treat patients as if they had ABPA if the serum IgE is more than five times the normal value and the aspergillus skin test is positive. Failure to treat ABPA may result in considerable additional morbidity and, ultimately, in ABPA-related central bronchiectasis superimposed on the pathology of CF.

Once ABPA is diagnosed, the treatment in CF patients is the same as it is for other patient populations. In the standard approach to treatment, a systemic corticosteroid, for example, oral prednisone (0.5 to 1.0 mg/kg/day is the usual starting dose) is given until the IgE returns to normal (or plateaus far below the initial level). Prednisone can then be tapered and eventually discontinued. However, the patient should then be followed with regular measurement of IgE levels, for example, at 3- to 6-month intervals. Aerosolized corticosteroids are frequently considered in patients who refuse systemic treatment or who do not tolerate it (because it aggravates diabetes or causes pseudotumor cerebri), but there is no good evidence of efficacy. Systemic antifungal agents (e.g., amphotericin B) have long been thought to be ineffective because according to theory, the aspergillus cannot be eradicated and sufficient antigen would remain to continue the stimulus to make IgE. However, with the advent of less toxic antifungal agents, some anecdotal success has been reported (e.g., with prolonged use of itraconazole either without corticosteroids or with a very abbreviated course of corticosteroids). Similarly, some CF physicians believe that aerosolized amphotericin B can be helpful.

Respiratory Failure

Acute Respiratory Failure. Because hyperventilation by relatively uninvolved areas of lung can compensate for the failure of severely affected areas to excrete carbon dioxide, the arterial P_{CO_2} does not begin to rise until substantial loss of functional lung has occurred. Thus, some patients who are barely able to maintain normal Pa_{CO_2} levels when pulmonary disease is relatively quiescent can manifest overt hypercapnic respiratory failure during acute CF exacerbations or superimposed respiratory illnesses (e.g., influenza or acute pneumonia). The symptoms presented by the patient are those of the CF exacerbation (e.g., increased cough and sputum production, dyspnea, and anorexia), plus those caused specifically by the derangement in arterial blood gases (e.g., headache and somnolence due to either hypoxemia or hypercapnia).

Treatment must include measures aimed at the exacerbation itself (e.g., appropriate antibiotics, airway clearance, and possibly, bronchodilators and corticosteroids) and, depending on the gravity of the situation, may require aggressive management of other complications (e.g., treatment of right-sided heart failure), or the blood gas abnormalities themselves (supplemental oxygen, ventilatory muscle stimulants [e.g., theophylline or progesterone], parenteral nutrition, transfer to an intensive care unit, and if appropriate, mechanical ventilation, including bilevel positive airway pressure [BiPAP]). The majority of patients with acute superimposed illnesses (e.g., influenza) will regain baseline status if treated only with nonspecific (i.e., antiexacerbation) measures, including supplemental oxygen. In general, the chance for recovery is greatest in those patients who have experienced the most rapid deterioration in pulmonary status. Considerable experience is needed to guide therapeutic decisions and to ensure recovery with the least invasive, least uncomfortable, and least risky treatment necessary. This approach also increases the probability that the patient will have had the most efficient and economically sound treatment.

Many very sick patients who are no longer deteriorating rapidly have already made extreme physiologic adjustments and can appear clinically stable despite laboratory values that would indicate extremis when encountered in clinical situations other than CF. For example, stability can exist with arterial P_{CO_2} values in excess of 100 mm Hg, arterial oxygen values below 40 mm Hg, serum bicarbonate values in excess of 55 mEq/L, and serum chloride values below 55 mEq/L. These patients are often best served by the slow introduction of therapeutic agents, a gradual increase of oxygen dose, and the cautious delay in the institution of mechanical ventilation, rather than by an all-out effort to correct all abnormalities at once.

Chronic Respiratory Failure. Chronic respiratory failure (referring here to long-standing chronic hypercapnia with stable renal compensation for acidosis) eventually occurs in almost all CF patients who have pulmonary involvement. Symptoms of hypercapnia and hypoxemia, many of which overlap with those of the chronic pulmonary disease, include the following: headache (especially severe on awakening), fatigue, sleepiness and confusion, dyspnea and air hunger, irritability, and anorexia.

Chronic respiratory failure (e.g., P_{CO_2} levels in the 50- to 70-mm Hg range with compensated acidosis) can remain stable for years, particularly in adults. Patients should receive their ongoing CF pulmonary treatment, with intensification during exacerbations, but specific treatment (e.g., oxygen and mechanical ventilation) may not be needed. However, if symptomatic hypoxemia develops, nocturnal or continuous supplemental oxygen should be offered.

An occasional patient with severe chronic respiratory failure (P_{CO_2} greater than 75 mm Hg and, rarely, greater than 100 mm Hg) achieves long-term stability, but these patients almost always require supplemental oxygen. However, even these patients often do not require nocturnal BiPAP or other type of mechanical ventilation.

REFERENCES

Brinson GM, Noone PG, Mauro MA, et al. Bronchial artery embolization for the treatment of hemoptysis in patients with cystic fibrosis. *Am J Respir Crit Care Med* 1998;157:1951–1958.

Eigen H, Rosenstein BJ, FitzSimmons S, Schidlow DV. A multicenter study of alternate-day prednisone therapy in patients with cystic fibrosis. *J Pediatr* 1995;126:515–523.

Frederiksen B, Koch C, Hoiby N. Antibiotic treatment of initial colonization with *Pseudomonas aeruginosa* postpones chronic infection and prevents deterioration of pulmonary function in cystic fibrosis. *Pediatr Pulmonol* 1997;23:330–335.

Govan JRW, Brown PH, Maddison J, et al. Evidence for transmission of *Pseudomonas cepacia* by social contact in cystic fibrosis. *Lancet* 1993;342:15–19.

Hardy KA. A review of airway clearance: new techniques, indications, and recommendations. *Respir Care* 1994;39:440–455.

Harms HK, Matouk E, Tournier G, et al. (on behalf of DNase International Study Group): Multicenter, open-label study of recombinant human DNase in cystic fibrosis patients with moderate lung disease. *Pediatr Pulmonol* 1998;26:155–161.

Kerem E, Reisman J, Corey M, et al. Wheezing in infants with cystic fibrosis: Clinical course, pulmonary function, and survival analysis. *Pediatrics* 1992;90: 703–706.

Konstan MW, Byard PJ, Hoppel CL, Davis PB. Effect of high-dose ibuprofen in patients with cystic fibrosis. *N Engl J Med* 1995;332:848–854.

Nepomuceno IB, Esrig S, Moss RB. Allergic bronchopulmonary aspergillosis in cystic fibrosis. Role of atopy and response to itraconazole. *Chest* 1999;115: 364–370.

Nishioka GJ, Barbero GJ, Konig P, et al. Symptom outcome after functional endoscopic sinus surgery in patients with cystic fibrosis: a prospective study. *Otolaryngol Head Neck Surg* 1995;113:440–445.

Ramsey B, Richardson MA. Impact of sinusitis in cystic fibrosis. *J Allergy Clin Immunol* 1992;90:547–552.

Ramsey BW. Management of pulmonary disease in patients with cystic fibrosis. *N Engl J Med* 1996;335:179–188.

Ramsey BW, Pepe MS, Quan JM, et al. Intermittent administration of inhaled tobramycin in patients with cystic fibrosis. *N Engl J Med* 1999;340:23–30.

Spector ML, Stern RC. Pneumothorax in cystic fibrosis: A 26 year experience. *Ann Thorac Surg* 1989;47:204–207.

Wang EEL, Prober CG, Manson B, et al. Association of respiratory viral infections with pulmonary deterioration in patients with cystic fibrosis. *N Engl J Med* 1984; 311:1653–1658.

5

Gastrointestinal System and Pancreas

PANCREATIC EXOCRINE INSUFFICIENCY

Pathophysiology

Exocrine pancreatic insufficiency occurs in 85% to 90% of patients with cystic fibrosis (CF). There is striking concordance for pancreatic status within CF families, and CF genotype is strongly predictive of pancreatic status. Mutations can be classified as "mild" (predictive of pancreatic sufficiency) or "severe" (predictive of pancreatic insufficiency). Patients carrying one or two mild mutations are almost always pancreatic sufficient. Among patients homozygous for the common ΔF508 mutation, 99% are—or will become—pancreatic insufficient. Mutations associated with pancreatic sufficiency are generally Class IV or V CF transmembrane conductance regulator (CFTR) defects (see Chapter 2), and include R117H, R334W, R347P, A455E, 3489 + 10 kb C→T, and P574H. In patients with pancreatic insufficiency, the pancreas is shrunken and shows marked fibrosis, fatty replacement, and cyst formation. Stenosis and atresia of large pancreatic ducts have been reported, but in general, pancreatic lesions are caused by obstruction of small ducts by inspissated secretions and cellular debris. Hypoplasia and eventually necrosis of ductular and centroacinar cells, together with inspissated secretions, block pancreatic ductules and can cause atrophy of the lining epithelium. Cystic spaces filled with eosinophilic concretions are embedded in a fibrous stroma. A mild inflammatory reaction may be present around obliterated acini, and progressive fibrosis gradually separates and replaces the pancreatic lobules.

Ultrasonography of the pancreas shows a small and echo-dense pancreatic body relative to a large pancreatic head. Multiple diffuse granular calcifications may be present inside the pancreatic ducts and can be detected by radiography (with gastric insufflation) and computed tomography. Multiple macroscopic cysts of the pancreas have been diagnosed at autopsy, or antemortem by computed tomography, ultrasound, and radionuclide imaging. Rarely, severe abdominal pain has been associated with diffuse, microcystic pancreatic enlargement.

It is postulated that abnormal CFTR processing leads to a defect in epithelial electrolyte permeability within the pancreatic ducts. This problem leads to reduced ductular flow and hyperconcentrated proteinaceous secretions that precipitate and block pancreatic ductules. Eventually, there is acinar atrophy. As a result of ductular obstruction, volume and bicarbonate secretion (ductular activity) are greatly reduced irrespective of pancreatic enzyme output. This leads to a consistently lower fasting and postprandial duodenal pH. In patients with steatorrhea, enzyme secretion (acinar activity) is virtually absent. Only 1% to 2% of residual colipase and lipase secretion is required to prevent steatorrhea. There can be a progressive decline in pancreatic function with advancing age. Among infants identified as having CF in a neonatal screening program, 37% were found to have substantial preservation of pancreatic function, but most of these patients developed pancreatic failure by 3 years of age. The majority of older pancreatic sufficient patients with enzyme secretion within the normal range show no deterioration of function over an extended period of time. However, a small percentage of older pancreatic-sufficient patients, especially those with reduced enzyme, fluid, and electrolyte secretion, are at risk of progression to pancreatic failure. In patients with pancreatic sufficiency (especially in those not carrying a mild mutation) fat absorption should be monitored periodically. Patients with pancreatic sufficiency also are at risk of developing acute pancreatitis.

Pancreatic Function Testing

Assessment of pancreatic function may be useful in newly diagnosed patients to determine if malabsorption is present. If the presence of steatorrhea is not clear-cut, an assessment of fat absorption is mandatory. When the diagnosis of CF is in doubt, specific tests of pancreatic function may be of value in supporting a diagnosis. Direct testing of pancreatic function involves exogenous hormonal (secretin or cholecystokinin) or endogenous nutrient (Lundh test meal) pancreatic stimulation, collection of pancreatic secretions via duodenal intubation, and analysis of enzyme (e.g., lipase, colipase) output. This is the best method for accurately measuring pancreatic exocrine function over its entire range, but it is invasive, expensive, technically difficult to perform, and usually performed only in the context of research studies.

As an alternative, a number of noninvasive indirect tests of pancreatic function are available. Random stool samples can be examined for the presence of fat globules or trypsin, chymotrypsin, or pancreatic elastase-1 concentrations. Of these tests, an enzyme-linked immunosorbent assay (ELISA) for pancreatic elastase-1 appears to be the most sensitive and specific assay for exocrine pancreatic function. A 72-hour stool collection for measurement of fat output is cumbersome but is probably the most commonly used quantitative test of pancreatic function in patients with CF. It should be carried out in collaboration with a dietitian in order to ensure adequate fat intake during the collection period and to calculate total fat intake. Normally stool fat output is less than 7% of fat intake (coefficient of fat absorption more than 93%) in children and adults and less than 15% of fat intake in infants.

There are several tests of pancreatic function that involve the oral administration of a measurable tracer bound to a peptide that is specifically cleaved by one of the pancreatic enzymes. The synthetic peptide *N*-benzoyl-*l*-tyrosyl-*p*-amino-benzoic acid (bentiromide or PABA) is cleaved by chymotrypsin. The liberated PABA is absorbed and excreted in the urine. Accordingly, PABA recovery reflects intraluminal chymotrypsin activity. The sensitivity and specificity of the test can be improved by measuring PABA in plasma 90 minutes after the administration of a large (500-mg) dose of PABA, as well as by administration of a test meal to stimulate enzyme secretion. It should be noted that the bentiromide test has not always been available in the United States.

The pancreolauryl test consists of the administration of fluorescein dilaurate. The substrate is hydrolyzed by cholesterol ester hydrolase of pancreatic origin in the upper small intestine and releases fluorescein, which is absorbed and excreted in the urine, where it can be quantitated. Stimulation of enzyme secretion with a test meal and measurement of plasma fluorescein have been used to increase the sensitivity and specificity of the test. Pancreolauryl and PABA test results correlate well with other measures of pancreatic exocrine function, but abnormal results are also seen in patients with malabsorption unrelated to CF.

There are several methods for direct measurement of various pancreatic enzymes in serum or plasma after infancy. Patients with CF have low serum concentrations of pancreas-specific isoenzymes of amylase (isoamylases), immunoreactive cationic trypsinogen, and

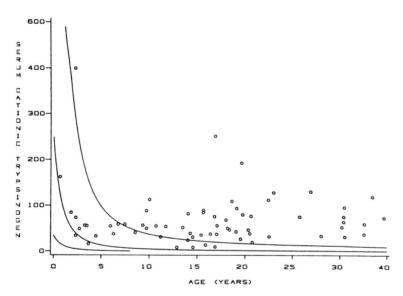

FIG. 5–1. Individual serum trypsinogen values (milligrams per liter) plotted against age for 67 patients with pancreatic sufficiency, superimposed on a mathematically derived equation for cystic fibrosis patients with pancreatic insufficiency. After 7 years of age, only six patients with pancreatic sufficiency had values within the 95% confidence limits of the values for those with pancreatic insufficiency. (From Durie PR, Fostner GG, Gaskin KJ, et al. Age-related alterations of immunoreactive pancreatic cationic trypsinogen in sera from cystic fibrosis patients with and without pancreatic insufficiency. *Pediatr Res* 1986;20:209.)

pancreatic lipase. In infants younger than 2 years of age, there is elevation of serum trypsinogen and pancreatic lipase values secondary to pancreatic ductular obstruction and reflux of pancreatic enzymes into the circulation. With advancing age, however, there is a progressive decline in serum levels of these enzymes, and after the age of 7 years, most patients with pancreatic insufficiency have undetectable or low levels. Enzyme assays are of value in discriminating older CF patients with or without pancreatic insufficiency (Fig. 5–1) and for the monitoring of longitudinal changes in pancreatic function, particularly in patients with pancreatic sufficiency. Between 2 and 7 years of age, serum enzyme assays are of little diagnostic value unless levels are distinctly low.

Clinical Manifestations

Exocrine pancreatic insufficiency leads to intestinal malabsorption of fats, proteins, and to a lesser extent, carbohydrates. Steatorrhea and azotorrhea can be pronounced (Fig. 5–2). Mean fecal fat excretion is 38% of intake but may range as high as 80% in some patients. Clinical consequences include poor or absent weight gain; abdominal distention; crampy abdominal pain; flatulence; deficiency of subcutaneous fat and muscle tissue; frequent passage of pale, bulky, malodorous and often oily stools; and rectal prolapse. Biochemical consequences include deficiencies of fat-soluble vitamins (A, D, K, E), essential fatty acids, and albumin. Patients with preservation of exocrine pancreatic function (pancreatic sufficiency)—as a group—are diagnosed at a later age, have lower mean sweat chloride values, maintain better pulmonary function over time, are less likely to be colonized by pseudomonas, and have a better overall prognosis than those with pancreatic insufficiency. There is significant individual variation, however, and pancreatic sufficiency should not be used as a reason for less aggressive overall care, nor pancreatic insufficiency for despair.

Pancreatic Enzyme Therapy

Patients with exocrine pancreatic insufficiency require life-long replacement therapy with pancreatic enzyme supplements. In young

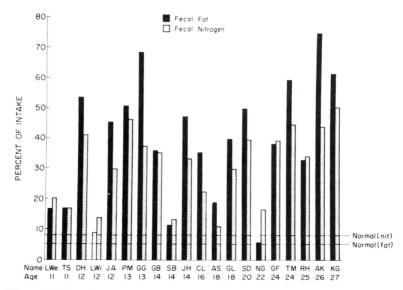

FIG. 5–2. Fecal fat and nitrogen excretion in 20 patients with cystic fibrosis not receiving pancreatic supplements. (From Lapey A, Kattwinkel J, Di Sant'Agnese PA, Lester L. Steatorrhea and azotorrhea and their relation to growth and nutrition in adolescents and young adults with cystic fibrosis. *J Pediatr* 1974;84:328–334.)

infants, this may be given as a powdered pancreatic extract. Beyond early infancy, enzyme supplements are given in the form of gelatin capsules containing pH-sensitive, enteric-coated microspheres or microtablets of pancrelipase. The capsule can be swallowed or it can be opened and the microspheres or microtablets can be placed in a soft nonalkaline food such as applesauce. When given this way, the tablets or spheres should be swallowed with food and not crushed or chewed. These preparations are formulated so that the enzymes are protected against gastric acid inactivation; release of enzyme is delayed until the pH is above 5.5. In infants, enzyme dosing can be based on food intake starting with 2,000 to 4,000 lipase units/120 mL of formula or breast feeding. Beyond infancy, weight-based dosing is more practical. It should begin with 1,000 lipase units/kg of body weight per meal for children younger than 4 years of age and at 500 lipase units/kg of body weight for those older than 4 years of age. Enzyme dose expressed as lipase units per kilogram of body weight per meal should be lower in older patients because they tend to ingest less fat per kilogram of body weight. Usually, half the standard dose is given with snacks.

There is great variation in response to enzymes; thus, a range of doses is recommended, based on stool pattern and weight gain. Doses greater than 2,500 lipase units/kg of body weight per meal or 10,000 lipase units/kg of body weight per day should be used with caution and only if they are documented to be effective by 3-day fecal fat measure. Doses greater than 6,000 lipase units/kg of body weight per meal have been associated with the development of fibrosing colonopathy in patients younger than 12 years regardless of enzyme strength or brand. High enzyme doses are not needed to achieve adequate nutrient absorption and growth. In patients receiving high-dose enzyme replacement, the dosage can be drastically reduced over a short period of time without an adverse effect on abdominal symptoms or growth. After initiation of enzyme therapy, there should be almost immediate reduction in stool frequency and degree of steatorrhea, improvement in abdominal symptoms, and decrease in appetite. Most patients are able to achieve a coefficient of fat absorption of greater than 85%.

Variations in enzyme requirements and patient response may be related to endogenous enzyme output, type of diet, microsphere size, gastric emptying time of microspheres, postprandial duodenal pH, bile salt concentrations, and prior intestinal resection. Failure of enzyme release secondary to a low postprandial duodenal pH is probably the major factor leading to inefficient enzyme function. In patients who have persistent steatorrhea (greater than 10% fecal fat loss) in spite of what should be adequate enzyme dosage, the addition of an acid-reducing agent such as ranitidine, famotidine, misoprostol, or omeprazole may lead to significant enhancement of fat absorption. Some patients on high-dosage enzyme therapy have ongoing abdominal symptoms that may be unrelated to exocrine pancreatic deficiency. In such cases, 72-hour fecal fat measurement and evaluation for concurrent gastrointestinal disorders (lactose malabsorption, giardiasis, bacterial overgrowth, celiac disease, and Crohn's disease) are indicated. Parents and patients should be cautioned not to increase enzyme dosage on their own in an attempt to treat symptoms that may not be related to malabsorption. The development of constipation in a patient who is taking enzymes may be an indication for more, not less, enzymes. A misguided reduction in enzyme dosage in this situation may precipitate an episode of distal intestinal obstruction syndrome (DIOS).

The most serious complication of pancreatic enzyme therapy is fibrosing colonopathy, a condition associated with the use of high daily doses of enzyme (Fig. 5–3). This diagnosis should be considered in patients who have symptoms of obstruction, bloody diarrhea, chylous ascites, or the combination of abdominal pain with ongoing diarrhea or poor weight gain. Patients at highest risk are those who are younger than 12 years, have taken more than 6,000 lipase units/kg of body weight per meal for more than 6 months, or have had gastrointestinal surgery or complications. Most cases involve the ascending colon, but pancolonic involvement can occur. A barium enema is the most reliable diagnostic measure. Colonic shortening, focal or extensive narrowing, and a lack of distensibility are highly suggestive of fibrosing colonopathy. The diagnosis is confirmed by biopsy. In patients with CF, colonic abnormalities consisting of proximal wall thickening, mesenteric infiltration, increased pericolonic fat and mural striation may be detected by CT, even in the absence of fibrosing colonopathy. Most cases of fibrosing colonopathy require hemicolectomy.

Skin and mucous membrane irritation secondary to pancreatic extract may be seen in infants. Before the advent of enteric-coated microsphere preparations, hyperuricosemia and hyperuricosuria occurred secondary to the high purine content of powdered preparations. Immunoglobulin E–mediated nasal and bronchial immediate hypersensitivity reactions and anaphylaxis may occur in caretakers exposed to powdered pancreatic extracts, but clinical hypersensitivity is extremely rare in patients themselves.

Nutrition

Chronic undernutrition with significant weight retardation, linear growth failure, and pubertal delay is a major problem in patients with CF. Nutritional deficiencies including decreased body fat stores and decreased serum levels of essential fatty acids, prealbumin,

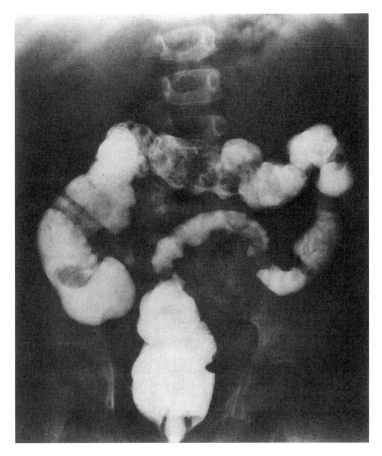

FIG. 5–3. Barium enema showing loss of haustration throughout the colon, with severe narrowing of the transverse and proximal descending colon in a patient with fibrosing colonopathy. (From Schwartzenberg SJ, et al. Cystic fibrosis-associated colitis and fibrosing colonopathy. *J Pediatr* 1995;127:565.)

albumin, cholesterol, retinol, retinol-binding protein, 25-hydroxy-vitamin D, and α-tocopherol have been well documented and may be evident as early as 2 months of age in presymptomatic infants with CF detected by newborn screening. Growth retardation and wasting often accelerate before and during adolescence, and patients often fail to achieve their genetic growth potential. Among patients in the United States Cystic Fibrosis Registry, 28% are below the 10th percentile for height for age and 34% are below the 10th percentile for weight for age. There is a correlation among degree of malnutrition, pulmonary function, clinical status, and survival.

Most growth problems in patients with CF are due to unfavorable energy balance rather than to an inherent factor of the disease itself (Fig. 5–4). Energy imbalance is related to the combination of increased energy losses, suboptimal energy intake, and increased energy expenditure. Increased energy loss is primarily due to impaired nutrient absorption secondary to pancreatic exocrine insufficiency, but a reduced bile salt pool and increased intestinal mucus may play a role. Supplementation with pancreatic enzymes improves, but does not normalize, fat absorption. Patients may still lose 5% or more of total calories consumed.

Patients are recommended to receive 120% to 140% of daily energy requirements. Yet, in spite of anecdotal reports of a voracious appetite in patients with CF, energy intake is frequently 80% to 100% of recommended daily allowances (RDA) for age, weight, and gender. This may be a particular problem among adolescent girls,

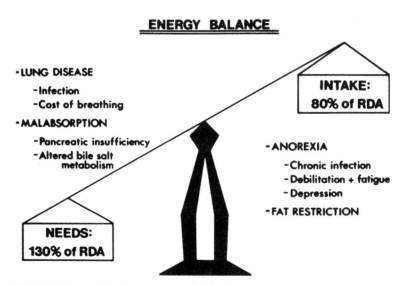

FIG. 5–4. Factors leading to energy imbalance in patients with cystic fibrosis. (From Roy C, et al. A rational approach to meeting macro- and micronutrient needs in cystic fibrosis. *J Pediatr Gastroenterol Nutr* [Suppl] 1984;3:154.)

some of whom may be trying to limit weight gain. Appetite and oral intake may be limited by esophagitis, postprandial abdominal pain, depression, fatigue, and acute and chronic respiratory tract infection. There are data that suggest that there is increased resting energy expenditure and total energy expenditure in patients with CF. These increases appear to be independent of the degree of pulmonary disease but may be related to genotype.

Edema and Hypoproteinemia

Secondary to proteolytic enzyme deficiency and malabsorption, infants with CF may develop severe protein-calorie malnutrition and edema, often as the presenting manifestation of their disease. Features include severe hypoalbuminemia, hepatomegaly, elevation of liver enzyme values, anemia and a characteristic dermatitis (acrodermatitis enteropathica) secondary to deficiencies of protein, zinc, and essential fatty acids. Infants fed breast milk or soy protein–based formula may be at increased risk of developing this syndrome. A false-negative sweat test result may occur in the presence of edema, probably secondary to a low sweat secretory rate. Infants with this syndrome need intensive therapy including adequate calories, essential fatty acids, protein, zinc, and vitamins, along with pancreatic enzyme supplementation. A prolonged course of parenteral nutrition or enteral supplementation often is required. Patients who present with this syndrome have been shown to be at high risk for early pulmonary complications, prolonged hospitalization, and death.

Vitamins and Trace Metals

Water-soluble Vitamins. All water-soluble vitamins, except vitamin B_{12}, appear to be well absorbed, and there is no evidence of clinically significant deficiency in well-nourished patients. With pancreatic enzyme supplementation, vitamin B absorption normalizes and supplementation is not necessary.

Fat-Soluble Vitamins. Biochemical deficiencies of vitamins A, D, E, and K have been repeatedly demonstrated in CF patients at diagnosis. Serum vitamin levels may be low even in patients receiving pancreatic enzyme and vitamin supplementation.

Vitamin A. Serum concentrations of vitamin A (retinol), α-carotene and β-carotene are often low in spite of apparently adequate supplementation and significantly increased hepatic stores of vitamin A. Decreased serum vitamin A levels correlate with decreased levels of retinol-binding protein. These abnormalities may be due to a marked decrease in vitamin A absorption from the digestive tract, defective synthesis of retinol-binding protein, or defective release of vitamin A stores from the liver. Infants may rarely present with a bulging fontanel and symptoms of increased intracranial pressure. Conjunctival xerosis is uncommon, but night blindness and subnormal dark adaptation are surprisingly common in adolescents and young adult patients, especially those with liver disease and noncompliance with enzyme and vitamin supplementation. Serum vitamin A levels should be monitored, especially in patients with poor nutritional status.

Vitamin D. Although overt rickets is rare in patients with CF, they often have a significant reduction in vitamin D activity manifested by secondary hyperparathyroidism, reduced bone mineral content, delayed bone maturation, and an increased risk of atraumatic fractures (especially vertebral fractures). Low bone mass before lung transplantation may place patients at increased risk for fractures after transplantation. The degree of demineralization correlates with disease severity. Despite oral vitamin D supplementation, serum 25-hydroxyvitamin D levels tend to be at the low end of normal or frankly low. Consequently, it is important to monitor serum 25-hydroxyvitamin D levels. Vitamin D supplementation may need to be individualized to ensure normal vitamin D stores.

Vitamin E. Biochemical evidence of vitamin E deficiency is present in virtually all untreated CF patients who have pancreatic exocrine insufficiency. Erythrocyte survival is shortened and may lead to hemolytic anemia in infancy. Other manifestations include ophthalmoplegia, diminished deep tendon reflexes, decreased vibratory and proprioceptive sensation, ataxia, and muscle weakness. Axonal dystrophy and degenerative changes within the posterior columns have been demonstrated postmortem.

Vitamin K. Although severe bleeding in association with hypoprothrombinemia and deficiency of clotting factors II, VII, IX, and

X may occur in infants secondary to vitamin K deficiency (Fig. 5–5), in patients who are adequately supplemented with pancreatic enzymes, vitamin K deficiency is very infrequent. Patients with liver disease and those on prolonged antibiotic therapy appear to be at greatest risk.

Trace Metals. Plasma zinc levels are low in CF patients who are moderately to severely malnourished, but there is no recognized defect in zinc absorption or metabolism in patients treated with pan-

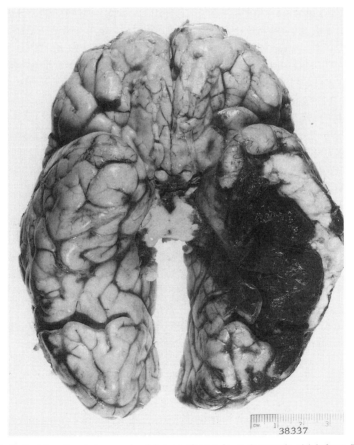

FIG. 5–5. Massive intracerebral hemorrhage in a 6-month-old infant. The diagnosis of cystic fibrosis was established just before death.

creatic enzymes. Plasma levels of copper and ceruloplasmin may be elevated, possibly because ceruloplasmin is an acute-phase reactant. Plasma or whole-blood selenium levels may be low, probably related to geography and selenium levels in the soil. There is no evidence that selenium deficiency is clinically significant. Chronic hypomagnesemia may occur, usually in the absence of symptoms. Symptomatic hypomagnesemia (paresthesias, weakness, tremulousness, muscle cramps, and carpopedal spasm) has been reported in patients treated with repeated courses of intravenous (IV) aminoglycoside therapy and in those treated for the DIOS with *N*-acetylcysteine or sodium diatrizoate orally or by enema. Malabsorption may also play a role. Magnesium replacement is indicated in symptomatic patients and in any patient with serum Mg^{2+} concentration below 1.2 mEq/L. Because serum magnesium is but a small portion of total body magnesium, replacement requires large doses (e.g., magnesium sulfate, 4 to 5 g, given IV over 24 hours and repeated daily until serum magnesium levels exceed 1.5 mEq/L). Iron deficiency anemia occurs in 33% to 66% of patients and is probably related to inadequate dietary iron intake, blood loss, iron malabsorption, and chronic infection.

It is recommended that patients with CF receive daily supplementation with a water-soluble vitamin-mineral preparation that includes B vitamins, vitamin C, vitamin A (5,000 units), vitamin D (400 units), zinc, and iron. Patients should also receive a water-soluble preparation of vitamin E (α-tocopherol) at a dose of 5 to 10 units/kg of body weight per day (to a maximum of 400 units). Vitamin K supplementation at a dose of 5 mg twice weekly is indicated for patients with liver disease, abnormal clotting study results, and those on prolonged antibiotic therapy. Routine supplementation with vitamin K is not recommended. Documented vitamin A deficiency is treated with 25,000 units vitamin A daily for 1 week, followed by supplementation with 5,000 units/day.

Essential Fatty Acids

In CF patients with pancreatic insufficiency, all four plasma lipid factors (triglycerides, phospholipids, free fatty acids, cholesterol esters) are abnormal. In the plasma, linoleic acid is decreased, whereas palmitoleic and oleic acids are increased. Linoleic acid levels are decreased in various tissues. Deficiency of fatty acids is probably related to malabsorption because essential fatty acid levels are normal in CF patients with pancreatic sufficiency. However, essential fatty acid deficiency is also present in young patients in the absence of protein-energy malnutrition, suggesting that there may be specific defects in fatty acid metabolism. Untreated infants may present with dermatitis, growth failure, and thrombocytopenia secondary to linoleic acid deficiency, but in older patients, clinical manifestations of fatty acid deficiency are rare. Plasma fatty acid profiles can be normalized by the oral (corn oil, safflower oil) or IV (Intralipid) administration of fatty acids, but there is no evidence that this approach results in any major clinical benefit. It is possible that fatty acid deficiency might lead to a subtle alteration in cellular metabolism or in the composition of membranes that could lead to cellular dysfunction.

ELECTROLYTE ABNORMALITIES

Increased electrolyte loss in sweat may cause patients with CF to have a salty taste to the skin or salt crystals on the skin, either of which may be the initial clue to the diagnosis.

Metabolic Alkalosis

Increased electrolyte loss in the sweat over a prolonged period may lead to electrolyte depletion and chronic metabolic alkalosis either as the initial presentation or as a complication of CF. Contributory factors include increased gastrointestinal losses, acute intercurrent illness, thermal stress, and limited electrolyte intake. Although current feeding recommendations satisfy sodium requirements for the growth of healthy infants, they are inadequate to compensate for the increased electrolyte losses present in infants with CF. During a period of profuse sweating, an infant with CF may lose 80 mEq of sodium, 100 mEq of chloride, and 40 mEq of potassium per day, depending on body surface area and sweating rate. There may be a higher incidence of this complication in arid climates, but there have been reports of cases in the absence of environmental or endogenous thermal stress.

Patients present with anorexia, irritability, vomiting, and failure to thrive, usually in the absence of dehydration or cardiovascular instability. Laboratory abnormalities include elevation of blood pH, P_{CO_2} and bicarbonate, base excess, and low serum concentrations of sodium, chloride, and potassium. Urinary excretion of sodium and chloride is markedly decreased, probably related to secondary hyperaldosteronism in an appropriate, but insufficient, response to compensate for sweat losses of these electrolytes. Preventive measures include avoidance of thermal stress, along with provision of adequate salt in the diet. This can be accomplished by adding 1/4 teaspoon table salt (23 mEq of sodium) to each liter of infant formula or liberal amounts of salt to solid foods. Most patients older than toddlers adjust their own salt intake adequately to prevent hypoelectrolytemia. CF patients should almost always be allowed to use as much salt as they choose. Treatment consists of the replacement of calculated fluid and electrolyte losses.

Acute Salt Depletion

In 1951, it was first reported that patients with CF are susceptible to dehydration and vasomotor collapse during periods of environmental thermal stress (Kessler, 1951). This observation led di Sant'Agnese and colleagues to elucidate the sweat gland defect in CF (di Sant'Agnese, et al., 1953). Subsequently, there have been a number of reports of acute hypoelectrolytemia and dehydration as a presenting manifestation or complication of CF (Beckerman, 1979; Ruddy, et al., 1982). Patients present with anorexia, decreased oral intake, lethargy, and signs of dehydration. Laboratory findings include low serum electrolyte concentrations and metabolic (contraction) alkalosis. Serum chloride concentrations can be strikingly low (40–50 mEq/L). Episodes may be precipitated by acute intercurrent illness, gastrointestinal losses, fever, decreased oral intake, and environmental thermal stress. However, cases have been reported in the absence of thermal stress (Nussbaum, 1979).

It is important to consider the possibility of CF in any child who presents with dehydration and severe hypoelectrolytemia, especially in the absence of obvious gastrointestinal losses. Management consists of replacement of fluid and electrolyte losses. Preventive measures include avoidance of thermal stress, along with maintenance of adequate fluid and electrolyte intake during periods of stress. Salt needs should be met through increased dietary salt intake. Supplementation with salt tablets is not generally recommended.

Heat Acclimation

Patients with CF have normal thermal, renal, and cardiac responses to exercise and heat and can acclimate to heat. In response to salt and fluid losses, they maintain normal sweat volumes and show significant increases in renin and aldosterone, resulting in normal renal salt conservation. However, during exposure to exercise and heat stress, CF patients lose significantly more electrolyte in sweat than controls, with a concomitant fall in serum sodium and chloride concentrations and serum osmolality. During extended exposure to heat and exercise, patients may underestimate their fluid needs and place themselves at risk of dehydration. This probably results from absence of hyperosmolality of body fluids as a stimulus to thirst. During vigorous exercise, patients should be encouraged to drink electrolyte-containing solutions at regular intervals.

Response to Salt Restriction

In response to salt restriction, patients with CF can maintain blood pressure, body fluid compartments, and weight, probably owing to an endocrine adaptation involving secondary hyperreninism, hyperaldosteronism, sympathetic activation, and vasopressin effects. Increased activity of angiotensin and vasopressin mechanisms may preserve capillary perfusion and increase orthostatic mechanisms. As a consequence, the degree of salt depletion and dehydration may be underestimated using routine clinical measurements such as capillary refill, serum sodium levels, and tachycardia, and patients may underestimate their salt and fluid needs. With chronic salt depletion, these protective mechanisms may not function effectively. Thus, in the absence of a specific contraindication (e.g., congestive heart failure or liver disease with ascites) generous supplementation of dietary salt intake is warranted for all patients with CF.

NUTRITION MANAGEMENT

Attention to nutrition should be an integral part of the overall care of the patient with CF. Nutrition assessment requires close clinical evaluation, monitoring of growth rates and nutrition, and appropriate dietary counseling. This is best accomplished in collaboration with an experienced dietitian who can assess the patient's energy requirements and eating habits, collect and interpret anthropometric data, evaluate nutritional adequacy, and provide anticipatory guidance and recommendations regarding nutrition interventions. The goal is to optimize growth and nutrition. The diet should be tailored to meet individual energy needs and should be consistent with food preferences and life style. If possible, it should provide 120% to 140% of the recommended daily allowance for calories. This can be accomplished by a well-balanced diet with increased fat (35% to 40%) as a source of energy. Fat restriction is not recommended. Complex carbohydrates are well tolerated and are another good energy source.

Infants can be breast fed, but they require pancreatic enzyme supplements, sodium chloride supplementation (1/8 to 1/4 teaspoon of table salt per day), especially during the summer, and close monitoring of nutrition. Most infants show adequate growth on standard formula feedings, which can be concentrated to maximize caloric intake. Predigested formulas containing medium chain triglycerides (MCTs) may be advantageous in infants with liver involvement, persistent steatorrhea, or short gut syndrome. Contrary to common belief, MCTs require pancreatic enzymes for optimal digestion and absorption. Soy-based formulas are not recommended. Nutrition intervention options for patients who have inadequate caloric intake and poor growth in spite of nutritional counseling include behavioral treatment, oral supplementation, enteral nutrition, and parenteral nutrition. All have been shown to be effective in producing weight gain in some patients with CF.

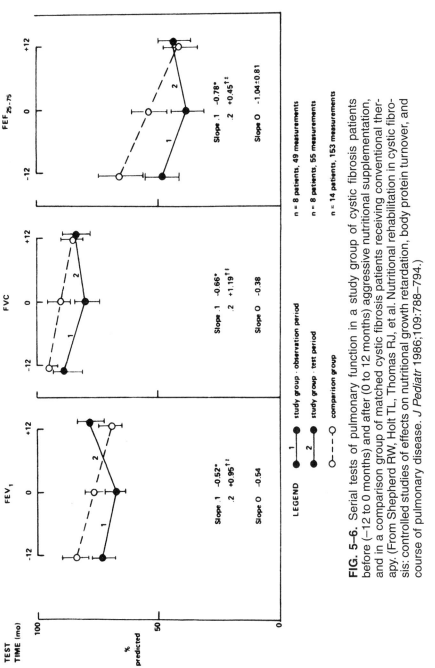

FIG. 5–6. Serial tests of pulmonary function in a study group of cystic fibrosis patients before (−12 to 0 months) and after (0 to 12 months) aggressive nutritional supplementation, and in a comparison group of matched cystic fibrosis patients receiving conventional therapy. (From Shepherd RW, Holt TL, Thomas RJ, et al. Nutritional rehabilitation in cystic fibrosis: controlled studies of effects on nutritional growth retardation, body protein turnover, and course of pulmonary disease. *J Pediatr* 1986;109:788–794.)

Behavioral treatment consists of providing nutrition education for the patient and his or her family, positive reinforcement of appropriate eating, and parent training in behavioral child management skills to modify problematic mealtime interactions. In older patients, caloric intake can be boosted by encouraging the use of nutrient dense foods, homemade oral supplements, or commercially available high-energy liquid dietary supplements. This approach, however, may be difficult to maintain over an extended period of time. In patients who continue to show poor growth in spite of counseling and attempts at oral supplementation, enteral feeding techniques may be useful. This is accomplished by the nocturnal infusion of a high-calorie formula through a nasogastric, gastrostomy, or jejunostomy tube to provide 40% to 50% of total energy needs. Although elemental or semielemental formulas are often used, they may not offer any advantage over an infant formula. This approach, when carried out over an extended period of time, can improve growth velocity, body composition, and patient well-being, and may stabilize or even improve pulmonary function (Fig. 5–6). Parenteral nutrition may be indicated for short-term use in patients with specific problems such as short-gut syndrome and pancreatitis, and in the postoperative period. Long-term use is not indicated because of cost, inconvenience, and potential complications. It is doubtful that any of these nutrition measures has any impact during the terminal stage of a patient's course, and they should be discouraged.

There is no strong evidence to support the use of artificial elemental diets or supplements with essential fatty acids. Taurine supplementation may improve fat absorption in patients with poorly controlled steatorrhea. The effect on overall growth is questionable.

PANCREATIC ENDOCRINE DEFICIENCY AND CYSTIC FIBROSIS–RELATED DIABETES MELLITUS

Pathology

With advancing age, there is acinar atrophy, fatty infiltration, and fibrosis of the pancreas, with a decrease in the number of pancreatic islets in CF patients with and without diabetes mellitus (DM). Islet cells exist in disorganized clusters separated by broad bands of fibrous tissue. Pancreatic neoislet formation (nesidioblastosis) is present and may be protective against DM. The proportions of glucagon-secreting alpha cells and insulin-secreting beta cells are decreased

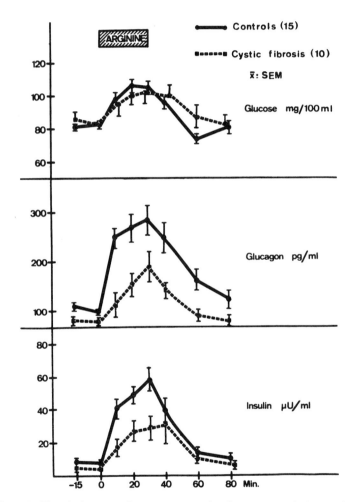

FIG. 5–7. Blood glucose, plasma pancreatic glucagon, and plasma insulin during arginine infusion in 15 controls and 10 children with cystic fibrosis. (From Stahl M, Girard J, Rutishauser M, et al. Endocrine function of the pancreas in cystic fibrosis: evidence for an impaired glucagon and insulin response following arginine infusion. *J Pediatr* 1974;84:821–824.)

(although with marked variation), and somatostatin-containing cells are moderately increased. The decrease in the proportion of beta cells is more pronounced in patients with DM. Secondary to a decrease in the proportion of beta cells and reduction in total pancreatic mass, the number of beta cells may be decreased by 90% or more. Because somatostatin inhibits both insulin and glucagon release, it is postulated that both decreased insulin production and increased somatostatin production contribute to DM in patients with CF. In contrast to type 1 DM, however, in CF patients with DM, there is relative insulin preservation and decreased glucagon secretion (Fig. 5–7).

Pathophysiology

The clinical course and metabolic responses seen in CF-related DM (CFRDM) differ from both type 1 (juvenile-onset DM) and type 2 (adult-onset, nonketotic diabetes). Although CFRDM begins during the juvenile or early adult period, it is characterized by an insidious onset, a mild clinical course, rarity of ketoacidosis, and intermittent periods of hyperglycemia between periods of normoglycemia. It differs from type 2 DM in that it is associated with underweight, hypoinsulinemia, and onset in early life. The HLA-related genes that confer susceptibility to type 1 DM are not necessary for the development of glucose intolerance in CF patients. Unlike type 1 diabetes, CFRDM is not an autoimmune process, but islet cell antibodies may play a role in some patients. Patients are modestly resistant to insulin, probably as a result of hyperglycemia.

From a biochemical standpoint, CFRDM is characterized by (a) reduction in serum levels of insulin, glucagon, and pancreatic polypeptide; (b) normal levels of gastric inhibitory polypeptide (GIP); (c) diminished GIP and pancreatic polypeptide responses after ingestion of a meal; (d) reduction and delay in insulin secretion in response to oral or IV glucose, IV arginine, and IV tolbutamide; and (e) impaired glucagon release following an arginine infusion. Insulin and GIP responses may be improved after an elemental meal, suggesting that insulin deficiency may arise through deficient GIP release secondary to malabsorption. The loss of carbohydrate tolerance in patients with CF, like that seen with classic chronic pancreatitis, parallels the loss of pancreatic exocrine function; an increased risk for CFRDM is seen only in patients with pancreatic exocrine insufficiency. There is evidence that there is some loss of pancreatic endocrine and exocrine reserve in CF heterozygotes.

Clinical Features

CFRDM is associated with a variety of adverse consequences, including loss of calories secondary to glycosuria, muscle wasting, fatigue, impaired ability to respond to infection, and renal insufficiency. Microvascular complications such as retinopathy, nephropathy, and neuropathy probably occur as frequently in CFRDM as in other forms of diabetes, but the risk of macrovascular complications (e.g., coronary artery disease) does not appear to be significant. Other potential adverse metabolic effects relate to the role of insulin as an anabolic hormone involved in cellular amino acid uptake and as stimulator of other growth factors. There is evidence that when DM develops in CF patients, an insidious decline in overall clinical status occurs over several years before its diagnosis. Body weight and body mass index begin to deviate about 4 years before the diagnosis of DM, whereas deviation in pulmonary function appears 1 to 3 years before the diagnosis of DM.

The milder clinical course of DM in CF patients may be accounted for by relative insulin preservation, impaired glucagon secretion, and enhanced sensitivity of peripheral tissues to insulin. However, in most (but not all) studies, CFRDM is associated with worse growth, worse pulmonary function, and earlier death.

Diagnosis and Screening

There is a spectrum of glucose tolerance in CF ranging from normal to varying degrees of impaired tolerance and overt diabetes. Patients can be classified based on the results of fasting blood glucose (FBG) and oral glucose tolerance test (OGTT) results (Table 5–1). CFRDM, with or without fasting hyperglycemia, may be chronic or intermittent. In addition to OGTT categories, acceptable criteria for the diagnosis of CFRDM include FBG greater than 126

TABLE 5–1. *Glucose Tolerance Categories in Cystic Fibrosis*

Category	Fasting Blood Glucose (mg/dL)	Oral Glucose Tolerance Test (OGTT) (mg/dL at 2 h)
Normal glucose tolerance (NGT)	<126	<140
Impaired glucose tolerance (IGT)	<126	140–200
Cystic fibrosis–related diabetes mellitus (CFRDM) without fasting hyperglycemia	<126	≥200
CFRDM with fasting hyperglycemia	≥126	OGTT not necessary

The OGTT is performed by giving a 1.75 mg/kg of body weight (max 75 g) oral glucose load to a fasting patient who has consumed at least 150 g/d of carbohydrate during the 3 days before testing. Fasting and 2-hour glucose levels are measured. (From *Diagnosis, Screening and Management of Cystic Fibrosis Related Diabetes Mellitus: A Consensus Conference Report.* Bethesda, Maryland, Cystic Fibrosis Foundation, 1998.)

mg/dL on two or more occasions; FBG greater than 126, plus random glucose levels greater than 200 mg/dL or random glucose levels greater than 200 mg/dL on two or more occasions, with symptoms.

In order to make a timely diagnosis of CFRDM, random glucose levels should be measured annually as part of routine management. If the level is less than 126 mg/dL, there is no need for further evaluation unless symptoms are present; if the level is greater than 126 mg/dL, fasting blood glucose levels should be checked. In order to identify patients with impaired or abnormal glucose tolerance in the absence of fasting hyperglycemia, an OGTT should be considered in the following circumstances: unexplained polyuria or polydipsia; failure to gain or maintain weight despite appropriate intervention; delayed puberty; or unexplained decline in pulmonary function. There is no reliable way to predict which patients with impaired glucose tolerance will progress to CFRDM. They may have normal fasting and premeal glucose levels, normal hemoglobin A1c levels, and minimal glucosuria despite relative insulin deficiency. Such patients should be monitored with home blood glucose testing, especially at times of stress (infection, glucocorticoid therapy, pregnancy, enteral or parenteral nutrition). Women with CF are particularly prone to develop gestational diabetes.

An acute illness such as an intercurrent pulmonary infection can be associated with severe insulin resistance. Therefore, all CF patients who have pancreatic insufficiency should be screened with at least two random blood glucose levels at times of pulmonary exacerbations that require intravenous antibiotic therapy.

Measurement of hemoglobin A1c is not a useful screening procedure for CFRDM, because Hg A1c may be normal in those with CFRDM; however, an elevated Hg A1c is associated with abnormal glucose tolerance.

Although CFRDM can occur at any age, it is rare in children younger than 10 years of age; average age of onset is between 18 and 21 years. Among all CF patients, approximately 5% require chronic insulin therapy, 5% require intermittent insulin during periods of stress and 30% have impaired glucose tolerance. After 30 years of age, 40% to 50% have CFRDM.

Management

The standard medical therapy for patients with CFRDM is insulin. The goal of treatment is to achieve glucose homeostasis and good nutritional status with minimal hypoglycemia. It is important to promote optimal psychological, social, and emotional adaptation to living with diabetes. Physical activity and a regular exercise program should be encouraged. Blood glucose goals include levels of 80 to 120 mg/dL before meals and 100 to 140 mg/dL at bedtime. In most patients, this can be achieved with split-dose NPH or regular insulin, or regular insulin before meals with or without nighttime NPH. Oral hypoglycemic agents have not been found to be helpful in patients with CFRDM. Patients may develop hypoglycemia on low-dose sulfonylurea therapy while still experiencing postprandial hyperglycemia. Hyperglycemia seen in association with parenteral nutrition can be managed by adding regular insulin to the total parenteral nutrition solution or into the infusion line. Patients with hyperglycemia with nighttime enteral supplementation should receive regular and NPH insulin before the start of feedings. Short-term insulin therapy is recommended for patients with impaired glucose tolerance at times of stress-induced hyperglycemia.

Nutrition management of CFRDM should focus on consistent timing and carbohydrate content of meals and snacks. This is usually accomplished with three meals and three snacks that are synchronized with the time of action of the insulin regimen. Carbohydrate counting is a useful way of managing the dietary requirements of both CF and diabetes. Fat (40% of total daily calories) is emphasized as an important energy source. Simple carbohydrates are not limited, but patients are discouraged from ingesting highly absorbable sugars such as cola drinks. Caloric restriction is not an appropriate method of controlling blood glucose levels, and protein intake should not be reduced. Patients and families should be instructed in the use of sucrose for mild hypoglycemia and glucagon for severe hypoglycemia. They should be counseled as to the danger of severe hypoglycemia in association with alcohol, especially when it is consumed on an empty stomach.

Patients with CFRDM should monitor blood glucose levels 3 to 4 times each day with a home glucose meter. Early morning (1 to 3 AM) glucose levels should be checked at least monthly to exclude nocturnal hypoglycemia. Hemoglobin A1C should be measured every 3 months. The patient should be taught to recognize glucose patterns related to insulin dose, diet, activity, and intercurrent illnesses. Patients should be screened for chronic diabetes-related complications with a blood pressure measurement at each visit, an annual eye exam, and annual evaluation for microalbuminuria.

HEPATOBILIARY DISEASE

Liver Pathology

Nonspecific hepatic lesions consisting of periportal inflammation, focal fibrosis, bile duct proliferation, and cholestasis are present in approximately one-third of infants with CF (Fig. 5–8). In approximately 10% of young infants and 20% of older patients, there is focal biliary fibrosis, which is characterized by inspissation of gran-

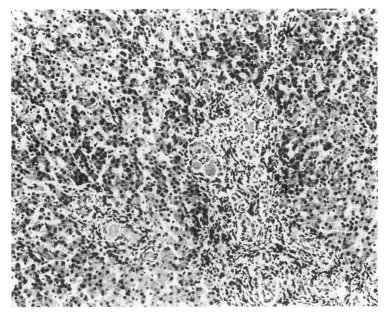

FIG. 5–8. Typical focal biliary cirrhosis in the liver of a 2-month-old infant with cystic fibrosis. There are dilated bile ducts filled with solid secretions. The proliferated ducts are in a sparse stroma containing a few mononuclear inflammatory cells.

ular eosinophilic material in the portal ducts, bile duct proliferation, chronic inflammatory infiltration, and a variable degree of fibrosis. This lesion is considered pathognomonic of CF. With increasing age, the percentage of cases with excessive intrahepatic mucus decreases; cholestasis is not a prominent feature in older patients. In approximately 2% to 5% of patients, periportal fibrosis progresses to a destructive type of multilobular biliary cirrhosis with concretions, in which there are large irregular nodules with regenerative microscopic nodules, massive foci of fibrosis, and bile duct proliferation adjacent to preserved hepatic lobular architecture.

Clinically, patients may manifest prolonged neonatal jaundice, steatosis (fatty liver), cirrhosis with portal hypertension, or hepatocellular failure.

Prolonged Neonatal Jaundice

Although it is a rare occurrence, neonates with CF may present with prolonged obstructive jaundice, presumably secondary to obstruction of extrahepatic bile ducts by thick bile, along with intrahepatic bile stasis (inspissated bile syndrome). In most cases, liver histology shows features compatible with bile obstruction. Jaundice is present during the first 48 hours after birth. The presence of persistently acholic stools and firm hepatomegaly can lead to confusion with extrahepatic biliary atresia. Approximately 50% of cases occur in association with meconium ileus (MI) or delayed passage of meconium. The prognosis for patients with neonatal cholestasis is generally good. However, elevated bilirubin values may persist for up to 7 months, and early-onset liver failure or cirrhosis may develop. In some patients, the biliary obstruction can be relieved by intraoperative irrigation of the biliary tree with saline and *N*-acetylcysteine.

Other causes of prolonged jaundice in neonates and young infants with CF include extrinsic biliary obstruction, extrahepatic atresia or obstruction of bile ducts, giant cell hepatitis, intrauterine cytomegalovirus infection, and paucity of intralobular bile ducts.

Fatty Replacement of the Liver

Massive hepatomegaly with steatosis (fatty replacement) has been reported in infants with CF, possibly related to protein-calorie malnutrition or essential fatty acid deficiency (Wilroy, et al., 1966). In one such case, there was evidence that carnitine deficiency may have been a contributory factor (Treem, 1989).

Cirrhosis and Portal Hypertension

Clinically apparent liver disease is present in 2% to 4% of patients with CF. At times, liver disease can be the predominant and, in some instances, the presenting manifestation of CF. There is a progressive rise in prevalence from 0.3% in patients from birth to 5 years of age to a peak of 8.7% among patients 16 to 20 years of age. The male-to-female ratio of affected patients is 2:1 to 3:1. There are conflicting data as to familial concordance. Almost all patients with liver disease have evidence of pancreatic exocrine deficiency. There is no association between specific CF mutations and the development of liver disease. The pathogenesis of cirrhosis in CF is not well understood. Initially, it was thought that cholestasis was an important predisposing factor, but recent evidence suggests that toxic liver injury, perhaps related to oxidative injury or the accumulation of potentially cytotoxic bile acids such as lithocholic and chenodeoxycholic acids, is the actual cause. Metabolic and nutritional deficiencies may play a role. Hypoproteinemia in infancy and MI have been implicated as predictors of subsequent liver disease.

The diagnosis of liver disease is based on enlargement of the liver or spleen, or both; abnormal liver enzyme values; abnormal hepatobiliary scintigraphy; evidence of portal hypertension and esophageal varices; and liver histology. Among patients with liver disease, at least 20% have esophageal varices. Splenomegaly predicts those patients at risk for variceal bleeding. Hepatosplenomegaly on physical examination is as useful as any biochemical parameter in demonstrating significant hepatic involvement.

Hepatic aminotransferases are frequently elevated as a result of injury to the liver parenchyma. In CF, these enzymes may be moderately elevated and may fluctuate over time. However, they also may be normal, even in the presence of liver disease. Elevated serum alkaline phosphatase and γ-glutamyltransferase (GGT) reflect injury to biliary epithelial cells and are sensitive indicators of biliary cholestasis. Likewise, thrombocytopenia and leukopenia may reflect hypersplenism.

There is an inconsistent relationship between hepatosplenomegaly and liver enzyme activity; 10% to 20% of patients have elevated liver enzyme values in the absence of other evidence of liver disease, whereas patients with hepatomegaly may have normal enzyme values. In patients with elevated enzyme values, there may be no detectable biochemical progression of liver disease over long periods of time. In patients with suspected liver involvement, the degree of dysfunction should be assessed at least annually using tests of synthetic function (albumin, prealbumin, prothrombin time [PT]/partial thromboplastin time [PTT]) and those that reflect liver cell damage (serum bilirubin, alanine aminotransferase, aspartate aminotransferase and alkaline phosphatase). Elevated GGT may reflect liver damage, even if other enzymes are normal.

Liver and spleen scans, computed tomography, and ultrasonography are useful in the diagnosis of hepatobiliary disease, but the findings do not always correlate with clinically apparent liver disease. The anatomy of the liver and spleen are well visualized by magnetic resonance imaging (MRI), and fatty infiltration is easily identified. Ultrasound can be helpful in identifying fatty infiltration, cirrhosis, portal vein dilatation, and ascites. Ultrasound can also demonstrate retrograde portal vein flow, which is indicative of portal hypertension. It is also excellent for evaluating the biliary tract. Endoscopic retrograde cholangiopancreatography (ERCP) can be used in patients with cholangitis-like illness to rule out intrahepatic cholelithiasis and bile duct stenosis. Hepatobiliary scintigraphy is the best functional test to image bile flow and can also provide information about hepatocyte function, liver size, and gallbladder filling. In a study of 50 CF patients with hepatomegaly or abnormal liver function test results, or both, hepatobiliary scanning showed evidence of a stricture of the distal common bile duct in 96% of cases (Gaskin, 1988). However, this observation was not confirmed in two other large studies, in which the incidence of common bile duct stenosis was 1% and 13% (Nagel, 1989; O'Brien, 1992). Liver biopsy is the definitive procedure to document cirrhosis, but its routine use is not indicated.

Patients with liver disease should have close monitoring of their nutritional status to optimize caloric intake and correct or prevent deficiencies of vitamins, minerals, carnitine, and essential fatty acids. Vitamin K supplementation should be given and the patient's clotting status followed closely. Aspirin-containing medications should be avoided and nonsteroidal antiinflammatory agents used with caution. Control of variceal bleeding can be achieved with sclerotherapy or endoscopic esophageal variceal ligation. Intravenous infusion of drugs such as vasopressin and somatostatin, which cause vasoconstriction and decreased splanchnic and hepatic blood flow, may result in at least initial control of variceal bleeding. Prophylactic sclerotherapy is not indicated. The transjugular intrahepatic portocaval shunt (TIPS) procedure can be used for short-term decompression in patients awaiting liver transplantation. Surgical decompression of the portal venous system by portosystemic shunting (e.g., distal splenorenal shunt) should be considered for long-term management of patients who continue to bleed following endoscopic procedures and who are not candidates for liver transplantation. Patients who have recurrent episodes of variceal bleeding or hepatocellular failure in the presence of good pulmonary status are candidates for liver transplantation. The results are similar to those obtained in non-CF patients.

The hydrophilic bile acid, ursodeoxycholate (UDCA), which has potent choleretic properties, is used in CF patients with liver disease and has a beneficial effect on liver function profiles, nutritional status, lipid profiles, and retinol status. However, there has not been a beneficial effect on fat absorption. After administration of UDCA for 2 months to 1 year, there is enrichment of the bile acid pool in UDCA and a reduction in chenodeoxycholic acid; UDCA becomes the predominant fecal bile acid excreted. Treatment over 1 to 2 years with UDCA at 10 to 15 mg/kg of body weight per day can normalize liver function tests and may improve liver morphology (less inflammation and bile duct proliferation) in CF patients with liver disease. However, improvement in long-term prognosis has not yet been demonstrated.

Gallbladder

Anatomic abnormalities of the gallbladder are present in approximately one-third of patients with CF. The gallbladder is often hypoplastic (microgallbladder) and filled with thick, colorless bile. There may be atresia and stricture of the cystic duct. Histologically, there are numerous multiloculated mucus-containing cysts in and beneath the mucosa.

A variety of gallbladder abnormalities occur in patients with CF. These include nonvisualization of the gallbladder on oral (31% to 33%) or IV cholecystography (12% to 23%), cholecystitis (5% to 10%), radiolucent gallstones (12% to 33%), and biliary sludge (6%). The incidence of these abnormalities increases with patient age. There are rare instances of atonic gallbladder, sclerosing cholangitis, and cholangiocarcinoma of the gallbladder. The high incidence of gallstones has been related to biliary stasis, increased bile viscosity secondary to the underlying defect in fluid and electrolyte transport, the presence of mucin glycoproteins which act as a so-called nucleating factor, and abnormalities of bile salt metabolism. In CF, there is interruption of enterohepatic circulation of bile leading to a reduction in the size of the bile salt pool and to an increased proportion of glycine conjugates (lithogenic bile). Early reports of an increase in the cholesterol saturation of bile have not been confirmed. The gallstones are composed of calcium bilirubinate, protein, and other unidentified materials.

Most CF patients with gallbladder abnormalities are asymptomatic, but recurrent episodes of abdominal pain (especially localized to the right upper quadrant) may occur secondary to bile duct obstruction from gallstones, sludge, stricture, or possibly an associated infection. In the largest reported series, only 24 (3.6%) of 670 patients developed symptomatic disease. All but one of these patients had exocrine pancreatic deficiency, and all but one were older than age 12 years. In patients with typical biliary colic, cholecystectomy leads to total cessation of symptoms. In patients who present with atypical symptoms, the results of cholecystectomy are often equivocal. Laparoscopic cholecystectomy under continuous epidural anesthesia is the preferred surgical option, especially in patients with severe pulmonary disease. Because the majority of gallstones in patients with CF contain little cholesterol, a litholytic agent such as UDCA would not be expected to be effective in dissolving these stones.

GASTROINTESTINAL COMPLICATIONS

Gastroesophageal Reflux

Although the exact prevalence of gastroesophageal reflux (GER) in patients with CF is not known, it appears to occur with considerable frequency. Heartburn and regurgitation are reported by more than 20% of all CF patients and by 80% of adult patients. GER has been documented in approximately 80% of unselected CF patients younger than 5 years of age, 75% of symptomatic patients older than 4 years of age, and 20% of infants younger than 6 months.

The mechanism leading to GER in patients with CF is not well understood. It is postulated that recurrent and chronic cough, chest hyperinflation, and an increased transdiaphragmatic pressure gradient may be contributory factors. GER has also been documented during chest physiotherapy, especially in head-down positions, and many experts now recommend avoiding these positions during chest PT in infants. The frequency and severity of GER has been correlated with the severity of the underlying pulmonary disease. It is known from esophageal manometry studies in patients with CF that resting lower esophageal sphincter pressure is normal. However, there may be transient, inappropriate episodes of lower esophageal sphincter (LES) relaxation, along with abnormal distal esophageal motility. It is likely that in some patients, underlying pulmonary disease facilitates GER, which, in turn, may contribute to the progression of pulmonary disease. However, there is evidence that in young infants with CF, GER may precede significant pulmonary disease. A relationship between GER and the use of methylxanthines has not been documented in patients with CF, but these agents and β agonists have been shown to decrease LES pressure.

Patients with GER may present with upper abdominal pain, epigastric or substernal burning (especially when supine), vomiting, hematemesis, dysphagia, failure to thrive, or pulmonary disease that does not respond to usual therapy. Esophageal strictures may develop secondary to chronic esophagitis. Infants with reflux esophagitis may manifest vomiting, regurgitation, irritability, poor oral intake, and growth failure. There have been patients in whom GER has dominated the clinical picture and has been the presenting manifestation of CF. The diagnosis is suspected on the basis of symptoms and then confirmed by prolonged intraesophageal pH monitoring, upper gastrointestinal endoscopy, and esophageal biopsy. Blind esophageal suction biopsies provide excellent histologic material from infants, obviate the need for anesthesia or prolonged monitoring, and are available in a few centers. An upper gastrointestinal series should be performed to exclude an anatomic lesion.

Treatment needs to be tailored to the individual patient but may include frequent small meals, avoidance of caffeine and theophylline, prone positioning—especially for sleep, antacids, H_2 blockers, and avoidance of head-down tilting during chest physiotherapy. Because of underlying pulmonary disease, the use of bethanechol is not generally recommended. The prokinetic agent cisapride has been shown to be effective in young CF patients with GER. In older patients, no therapy has been shown to be very effective. Reflux esophagitis often follows a relapsing course and may require repeated or chronic courses of therapy. In those instances in which medical management does not improve the patient's condition, a fundoplication may be indicated.

Peptic Ulcer Disease

Patients with CF would appear to be at increased risk for the development of peptic ulcer disease (PUD). They show hypersecretion of gastric acid in response to pentagastrin stimulation, and bicarbonate secretion from the pancreas is greatly reduced. The result is a duodenal content pH range of 5.5 to 6.5 compared with a normal pH of about 7.0. Also, a marked increase in the incidence of PUD has been reported in adults with chronic obstructive pulmonary disease and in patients with chronic pancreatitis and pancreatic insufficiency. However, an increased antemortem incidence of PUD has not been documented in patients with CF, with the exception of an unexplained cluster of cases in black adolescents (Rosenstein, et al., 1986). In a review of the pathologic findings in 146 autopsies of patients with CF, there were 12 instances (8%) of peptic ulcerations involving the stomach and duodenum (Oppenheimer, 1975). However, these may have represented an agonal feature of CF and its complications.

In the patient with symptoms suggestive of PUD, endoscopy is the diagnostic procedure of choice. Contrast radiography is not useful because of the underlying radiographic abnormalities of the duodenum that are seen in almost all CF patients.

Duodenal Abnormalities

Radiographically demonstrable abnormalities of the duodenum are present in approximately 85% of CF patients at all ages. These abnormalities consist of thickened and coarse mucosal folds, nodular indentations along the duodenal wall, smudging or poor definition of the normal mucosal pattern, and a redundant and distorted duodenal contour (Fig. 5–9). These findings are most prevalent in the first and second portions of the duodenum. There is no apparent relationship between the radiographic findings and the patient's symptoms. However, they can be confused with other diagnoses and this may interfere with the usefulness of radiographic studies in the diagnosis of PUD. The etiology of these abnormalities is unknown. It has been postulated that Brunner's gland hyperplasia, goblet cell

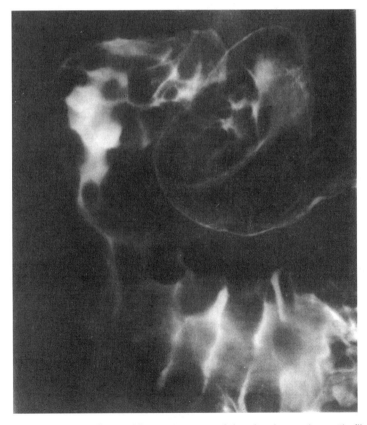

FIG. 5–9. Typical radiographic appearance of the duodenum in cystic fibrosis. Contrast material outlines thickened mucosal folds and nodular indentations along the duodenal wall (Courtesy John Dorst, M.D.).

hypertrophy, adherent mucus, and contraction of the underlying circular muscle may play a role.

Pancreatitis

Recurrent episodes of acute pancreatitis have been reported in 15% of pancreatic-sufficient CF patients. Most cases occur in older patients, but pancreatitis has been reported as early as 1 year of age. In some patients, pancreatitis is the initial or only feature suggesting the diagnosis of CF. Detection of CF mutations may be diagnostically helpful in such cases. Presumably, hyperconcentration of pancreatic secretions leads to obstruction of the pancreatic ducts, which provokes autodigestion of the pancreas by activated pancreatic proteolytic enzymes. Patients manifest severe abdominal pain, usually with vomiting, midepigastric tenderness, and elevated levels of serum and urinary amylase and serum lipase. Ultrasonography may demonstrate increased echogenicity of the pancreas. Serum amylase values may remain elevated for 4 to 6 months after resolution of symptoms. Attacks may be precipitated by ingestion of a fatty meal, alcohol, or tetracycline. Patients with pancreatitis may develop abdominal pain and hyperamylasemia in response to the intravenous administration of secretin and pancreozymin. Treatment consists of IV fluids, analgesics, antacids, H_2 blockers, and parenteral nutrition. There is some evidence that administration of pancreatic enzymes may inhibit pancreatic exocrine function, thus decreasing pancreatic autodigestion and pain. Pancreatic-sufficient patients who develop pancreatitis should be closely monitored for progression to pancreatic insufficiency.

Distal Intestinal Obstruction Syndrome

Distal intestinal obstruction syndrome (DIOS), previously referred to as MI equivalent, is a frequent cause of partial small bowel obstruction in patients with CF. It is caused by the impaction of mucofeculent material in the distal ileum, cecum, and proximal colon, and with rare exception, is seen only in those patients with pancreatic exocrine insufficiency. Contributing factors include abnormal intestinal mucins, undigested food residues, prolonged intestinal transit time, low dietary fiber content, bowel dilatation, and abnormal intestinal electrolyte and water transport. There may be a higher incidence in patients who had MI in the newborn period. There is often no identifiable precipitating event, but relative dehydration, inadequate enzyme supplementation, and change in diet have been implicated. The exact incidence is unknown, but DIOS has been reported in 9% to 40% of patients. It has been described in patients of all ages but is probably more common in adolescents and adults.

Clinical manifestations include crampy lower abdominal pain, distention, vomiting, anorexia, abdominal tenderness, and a palpable mass in the right lower quadrant. Episodes may occur within a normal stooling pattern, even during symptomatic periods, although the typical picture includes decreased stooling. There may be progression to complete obstruction, volvulus, or intussusception. Patients may have isolated episodes with long symptom-free periods or chronic symptoms with intermittent exacerbations.

In evaluating a CF patient who has abdominal pain, one needs to consider a wide range of possibilities, including DIOS, intussusception, volvulus, appendiceal disease, esophagitis, peptic ulcer disease, gallbladder disease, fibrosing colonopathy, pancreatitis, adhesions from prior surgery, and other conditions that may be unrelated to CF. In most cases, the diagnosis of DIOS is suspected on the basis of the history and physical findings. Abdominal radiographs show a bubbly granular appearance in the area of the ileum and cecum consistent with retained stool; there may be air-fluid levels (Fig. 5–10). An enema using an isoosmolar water-soluble contrast material may be both diagnostic and therapeutic. Hyperosmolar contrast agents are irritating to the colon and may cause large fluid and electrolyte shifts. Careful monitoring is essential if they are employed. The most specific radiologic finding is the presence of inspissated material demonstrated on reflux of contrast into the terminal ileum.

In the absence of complete obstruction, the treatment of choice is the administration of a balanced intestinal lavage solution (GoLYTELY and others) orally or by nasogastric tube at a dose of 20 to 40 mL/kg of body weight per hour, with a maximum of 1,200 mL/hour. Effective therapy may take 4 to 6 hours. The end point of therapy is determined by passage of stool, resolution of symptoms, and disappearance of a previously palpated right lower quadrant

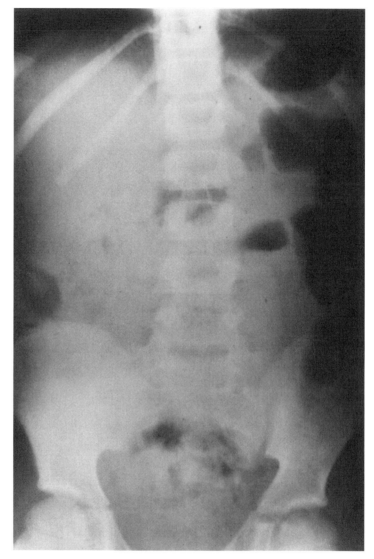

FIG. 5–10. Abdominal radiograph in a patient with distal intestinal obstruction syndrome. There is a diffuse granular appearance consistent with retained stool, along with scattered air-fluid levels.

mass. Clear effluent by itself is not an adequate end point. Follow-up abdominal radiographs can be helpful in documenting the resolution of DIOS. Balanced electrolyte solutions have largely replaced the use of *N*-acetylcysteine enemas and other previously reported methods. Early intervention with lactulose (starting dose of 1 tablespoon three times a day, and increasing until soft stools are produced) or an adult Fleet's enema in a child with decreased stooling may obviate the need for intestinal lavage.

In the absence of peritoneal irritation, nonoperative therapy is almost always successful, although full resolution of symptoms may take several days. If there is complete obstruction or signs of peritoneal irritation, surgical intervention is indicated. On occasion, a patient may develop chronic or recurrent abdominal symptoms in association with a persistent right lower quadrant mass representing a cecal mucocele. Contrast enema shows a smooth filling defect in the area of the cecum. Medical therapy is usually unsuccessful, and a partial colectomy is necessary.

Following an acute episode of DIOS, a variety of preventive measures can be instituted, including increased fluid intake, optimization of pancreatic enzyme supplementation, increased dietary fiber, lactulose, and laxatives.

Intussusception

Secondary to the accumulation of inspissated putty-like material in the cecum, terminal ileum, and ascending colon, CF patients with pancreatic insufficiency are at increased risk for the development of intussusception. Episodes tend to occur in older patients (4 to 16 years of age), may be recurrent, and occasionally precede the diagnosis of CF. It is probably part of the spectrum of DIOS. Patients usually present with the acute onset of intermittent crampy abdominal pain often accompanied by vomiting. Other manifestations include a palpable abdominal mass, rectal bleeding, and decreased or absent bowel movements. Twenty-five percent of patients with intussusception present with atypical or chronic symptoms. Most episodes are ileocolic, but ileoileal, ileocecal, colocolic, and even appendiceal locations have been reported.

Intussusception may be difficult to distinguish from uncomplicated DIOS. It should be suspected in the patient with a presumptive diagnosis of DIOS who does not respond to usual therapy. Plain radiographs of the abdomen and abdominal ultrasound may not be helpful in identifying the patient with an intussusception. The diagnosis is usually confirmed by contrast enema—which may also be therapeutic—but in some cases, the diagnosis is made only at laparotomy. Hydrostatic reduction with contrast enema may be successful, but most cases require surgery.

Appendiceal Disease

In patients with CF, there are typical histologic findings in the appendix. There is an increase in the number of goblet cells, and they are often markedly distended with mucous secretions. The crypts are dilated and appear wider, and at times deeper, owing to distention of the lumen by accumulated secretions. Eosinophilic casts of the crypts may extrude into the lumen of the appendix (Fig. 5–11). Inspissated secretions may extrude through the orifice of the appendix to form a local cecal mass. There is little or no cellular infiltration, and the muscularis layer is not affected. There also is an increased incidence of appendiceal diverticuli. In some patients, the diagnosis of CF has been suggested by the histologic appearance of an appendix removed from a patient with acute, or recurrent or chronic abdominal pain. An asymptomatic right lower quadrant mass secondary to mucoid impaction of the appendix also may be a presenting manifestation of CF.

The reported incidence of acute appendicitis in patients with CF is only 1% to 2%, compared with a rate of 7% in the general population. This incidence may be accounted for by the long-term use of antibiotics in many CF patients. Patients with CF who have acute appendicitis may present with classic symptoms, but the diagnosis is often delayed because of an atypical or subacute presentation and confusion with DIOS. At laparotomy, a high percentage of patients show appendiceal perforation and periappendiceal abscess formation.

Clinically, CF patients with acute appendicitis present with right lower quadrant pain, nausea, and anorexia. Fever and change in stool

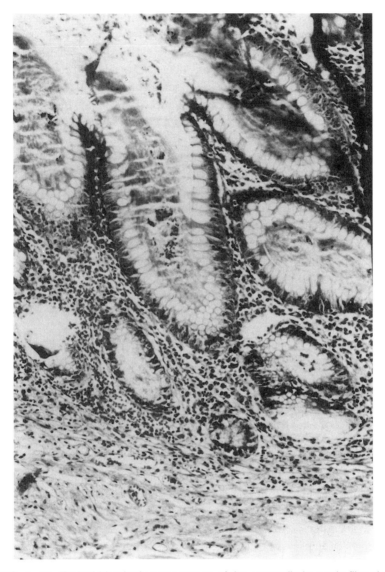

FIG. 5–11. Typical histologic appearance of the appendix in cystic fibrosis. There is an increased number of goblet cells that are distended with mucus, and eosinophilic casts of the crypts extrude into the lumen.

frequency may or may not be present. The initial diagnosis is usually DIOS. Abdominal ultrasound, computed tomography, and gallium scans generally have not been helpful in establishing a diagnosis. A contrast enema may be helpful if it shows extrinsic cecal compression or appendiceal filling. Filling the appendix implies the absence of appendicitis. However, failure to visualize (fill) the appendix before or after evacuation of contrast material cannot be used as a sign of appendicitis in patients with CF. Failure of visualization is most often related to mucus plugging of the appendiceal lumen.

The possibility of an appendiceal abscess needs to be considered when a patient with CF presents with pain, a mass, or drainage from the right flank; prolonged fever; a limp; or failure of suspected DIOS to respond to appropriate therapy. In patients with DIOS, abdominal radiographs usually show extensive stool accumulation and the white blood cell count is normal or only mildly elevated. Abdominal computed tomography may be a useful diagnostic tool. Treatment consists of surgical drainage and IV antibiotics, followed by an elective appendectomy.

Rectal Prolapse

Rectal prolapse occurs in approximately 20% of patients with CF, usually between 6 months and 3 years of age and often preceding the diagnosis of CF. Onset after age 5 years is thought to be unusual, but this occurrence may be underreported. The incidence is very low (2%) in patients diagnosed and treated before 3 months of age. In the United States, severe constipation is the most frequent cause of rectal prolapse but a sweat test is probably indicated in every child who presents with this complication. In patients with CF, episodes of prolapse are often recurrent and may range from a simple mucosal prolapse to prolapse of all layers of the anorectum (procidentia). There may be associated bleeding and pain. The occurrence of prolapse is probably related to malnutrition, poor muscle tone, and the passage of voluminous stools. Episodes may be precipitated by paroxysmal cough.

Following the initiation of pancreatic enzyme therapy, there is a marked reduction in the frequency of prolapse. Recurrences may indicate a need for increased pancreatic enzyme dosage. The prolapse can almost always be easily reduced manually by a parent. Older patients learn to prevent or reduce prolapses by voluntary muscle action. In those rare instances in which there are recurrent episodes of prolapse accompanied by pain, bleeding, or incontinence, submucosal injection of a sclerosing agent such as 30% saline, 70% ethyl alcohol, or D50W is usually curative. On rare occasions, a surgical procedure may be indicated.

MECONIUM ABNORMALITIES

In newborns with CF, there is a decrease in the mineral and water content of meconium; an increase in undigested serum proteins, especially albumin; and an increase in the disaccharidases, lactase, and β-*D*-fucosidase. Increased albumin concentration, abnormal salt and water transport, and excessive mucus production by intestinal goblet cells are thought to be responsible for inspissation of meconium and several clinical complications, including delayed passage of meconium, MI, and meconium plug syndrome (MPS).

Meconium Ileus

MI, in which there is intraluminal intestinal obstruction secondary to inspissation of tenacious meconium in the terminal ileum, occurs in 10% to 20% of newborns with CF. With rare exception, almost all full-term infants with MI eventually have a confirmed diagnosis of CF. There is a strong familial trend for the occurrence of MI, with a recurrence rate of 29% to 39% in subsequent CF-affected siblings. There is evidence that MI is, in part, genetically determined. There is a decreased risk in patients who carry R117H/A455E or other "mild" mutations that confer pancreatic sufficiency, and an increased risk in patients who carry certain "severe" mutations (e.g., 621+1G→T). With rare exception, MI is seen only in those patients who are later shown to have pancreatic insufficiency.

Affected infants present within the first 48 hours of life with abdominal distention, bilious vomiting, and failure to pass meconium. There may be a maternal history of polyhydramnios. As many as 50%

of cases are complicated by volvulus, atresia, perforation, ischemic necrosis, meconium peritonitis, or pseudocyst formation. The diagnosis of MI is supported by abdominal radiography (Fig. 5–12), which shows distended loops of bowel, usually without air-fluid levels, and a granular ground-glass appearance in the area of the terminal ileum, indicating the mixture of air bubbles with meconium (so-called soap-bubble sign). Contrast enema shows an unused microcolon. If there is associated meconium peritonitis, there may be flecks of intraperitoneal calcium throughout the abdomen. Intramural jejunal calcification has been reported in a newborn with CF who had MI complicated by jejunal atresia, and male infants with *in utero* meconium peritonitis may present with scrotal calcification. The presence of abdominal calcification, however, is usually associated with non-CF causes of meconium peritonitis; conversely, the absence of calcification favors CF as the etiology of meconium peritonitis. Isolated meconium peritonitis, in the absence of MI, or jejunal or ileal atresia or perforation, is not usually associated with CF. The diagnosis of MI is sometimes suggested by the prenatal ultrasound finding of a hyperechoic bowel

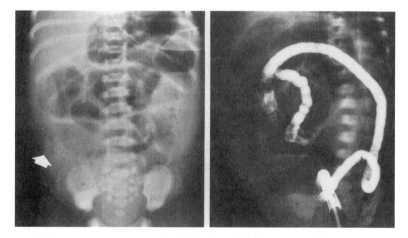

FIG. 5–12. Radiographic findings in a newborn infant with meconium ileus. There is a granular ground-glass appearance in the area of the terminal ileum (*arrow*), and a contrast enema shows an unused microcolon.

pattern that persists throughout pregnancy. The diagnosis of CF is confirmed, either prenatally or postnatally, in approximately 10% of such cases. In several cases, the obstruction has been relieved by intrauterine amniography with Urografin.

In the absence of complications, up to 50% of cases can be treated successfully by the administration of hyperosmolar (e.g., Gastrografin) or isoosmolar contrast enemas under fluoroscopic control. With this therapy, the patient's fluid and electrolyte status needs to be monitored closely to prevent hypovolemia. Repeated attempts to evacuate meconium may be required. If the patient's condition remains stable without change in abdominal findings, therapeutic enemas can be repeated over several days. However, the procedure may be complicated by intestinal perforation in up to 15% of cases. Patients who present with complications of MI or who do not respond to nonoperative therapy require surgical intervention. In some instances, the inspissated meconium can be cleared by intraoperative irrigation with acetylcysteine, hyperosmolar contrast, or saline. If irrigation is unsuccessful or if there are complications, patients are managed by resection of the involved bowel followed by primary anastomosis or a temporary double-barrel (side-by-side) enterostomy. The appendix should be removed to prevent later appendicitis. After surgery, most patients require a period of total parenteral nutrition followed by intensive enteral nutritional support.

Among patients with a history of MI, there is earlier acquisition of *Pseudomonas aeruginosa* in the respiratory tract, but at ages 8 and 13 years, pulmonary function is similar in patients with and without MI. There may be an increased incidence of later intestinal complications such as fibrosing colonopathy and DIOS. Long-term survival among males and females with MI is similar to that of females without MI but is significantly shorter than that of males without MI.

Meconium Plug Syndrome

MPS is a well-recognized cause of low intestinal obstruction in newborn infants secondary to inspissated meconium. It is manifest by progressive abdominal distention; vomiting, which is often bilious; and failure to pass meconium. There may be visible and palpable loops of tense bowel. Rectal examination may be normal, or the leading edge of the meconium may be felt. With a contrast enema, contrast material may mix with large pieces of meconium to produce radiolucent filling defects or may outline a long continuous meconium cast filling the colon (Fig. 5–13). The caliber of the colon is normal.

Meconium plug syndrome occurs in association with prematurity, hypotonia, and hypermagnesemia, and is the earliest manifestation of Hirschsprung's disease. It is well recognized that MPS may also occur as the presenting manifestation of CF. In one series (Rosenstein and Langbaum, 1980), MPS occurred in 12 of 87 newborns with CF in the absence of MI, and in another series (Olsen, et al., 1982), 6 of 25

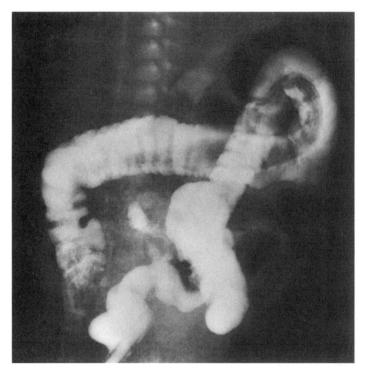

FIG. 5–13. Contrast enema in a newborn infant with signs of intestinal obstruction. The contrast material outlines a radiolucent meconium plug in the transverse colon and splenic flexure.

newborns who presented with MPS eventually had a diagnosis of CF. It is likely that MPS and MI represent gradations of the same underlying abnormality, differing only in degree of severity, and site of obstruction. In general, MPS is a benign condition that is usually relieved following anal stimulation, administration of enemas, or a diagnostic contrast enema. The success of nonoperative treatment is probably due to the lower site and significantly easier removal of the obstructing meconium in infants with MPS as compared with those with MI.

MISCELLANEOUS AND ASSOCIATED INTESTINAL ABNORMALITIES

Cancer

A large retrospective cohort study of US, Canadian, and European patients found that the overall cancer risk in CF patients was similar to that of the general population, but found a marked elevation in the risk ratio for digestive tract tumors (esophagus, small and large intestine, and pancreas) for the 20- to 29-year-old age group (Neglia et al., 1995). A case-control study did not identify any characteristics associated with an increased risk. The increased risk of digestive tract cancers may be related to differential localization and expression of the CFTR gene; persistent pathologic alterations in digestive tract organs, leading to increased cell turnover; and antioxidant deficiency.

Celiac Disease

In several patients, celiac disease (or a celiac-like syndrome) manifested by persistence of bulky stools, irritability, and growth failure, and documented by intestinal biopsy findings and response to a gluten-free diet has been reported to coexist with CF. This clinical picture may represent a chance association of these two conditions. Alternatively, increased intestinal permeability and impaired protein digestion secondary to lack of proteases could lead to a high antigen load to the small intestinal mucosa.

Clostridium difficile Colonization

Clostridium difficile colonization has been reported in up to 50% of CF patients. Many colonized patients also have cytotoxin recovered from their stools, even in the absence of symptoms. This may be attributable to the observation that CFTR mutations confer varying degrees of resistance to various bacterial toxins. However, *C. difficile*–associated disease has been reported in patients with CF, including cases of severe colitis and toxic megacolon. The diagnosis needs to be considered in the patient who develops crampy abdominal pain, fever, diarrhea, and abdominal tenderness following a course of antibiotics. Associated laboratory findings include leukocytes, blood, and mucus in the stool, and peripheral leukocytosis with a left shift. Colonic thickening can be demonstrated by ultrasound or computed tomography. The diagnosis is confirmed by the findings of pseudomembranous colitis on sigmoidoscopy and *C. difficile* toxin A in the stool. Vancomycin and metronidazole are the treatments of choice.

Colonic Wall Abnormalities

The most significant abnormality of the colonic wall in patients with CF is fibrosing colonopathy, a complication seen in young children in association with high-dose pancreatic enzyme replacement (see earlier discussion). Although there is no documented increase in the prevalence of colonic diverticuli in patients with CF, partial obstruction of the ascending colon secondary to diverticulitis may occur. The radiographic picture could be confused with that of a colonic stricture secondary to fibrosing colonopathy.

Even in the absence of obstruction, fibrosing colonopathy, or inflammatory bowel disease, computed tomography scans in patients with abdominal pain show characteristic findings of colonic wall thickening (mean 6.4 mm, range 4–10 mm, compared with the normal colonic wall thickness of 0.4–0.8 mm), mural striation, pericolonic mesenteric and soft tissue fatty infiltration. The cecum and ascending colon are most frequently involved, followed by the transverse and descending colon. The etiology of these findings remains speculative.

Crohn's Disease

Based on a number of case reports, it has recently been recognized that there is more than a coincidental association between CF and Crohn's disease. Such patients usually manifest significant weight loss, intestinal fistula formation, and perianal disease. There is evidence that CF patients operated on for MI may be at increased risk for the development of inflammatory bowel disease.

Giardiasis

Patients with CF have a significantly higher risk of giardiasis than expected, possibly related to abnormal bile composition.

Intestinal Permeability, Transit Time, and Absorption

In patients with CF, there is evidence of increased small intestinal permeability, which is probably related to the leakage of large molecules (disaccharides) through paracellular pathways. This increased intestinal permeability is probably related to underlying pancreatic dysfunction. The passive transcellular uptake of small molecules is preserved. Orocecal transit time has been shown to be prolonged both in children and adults with CF.

In general, small intestine biopsies from patients with CF show normal histology; however, there may be a thick mucus cover over the brush border membrane. Enhanced intestinal active transport of glucose has been demonstrated, possibly related to a decreased intestinal diffusion barrier. Enzyme-depleted small intestinal villi are present in some patients. It is postulated that this condition may be due to impaired maturation secondary to nutritional deficiencies, or failure of enterocytes to increase their brush border enzymes secondary to impaired absorption of nutrients.

Pneumatosis Intestinalis

Pneumatosis intestinalis is characterized by the presence of gaseous cysts in the wall of the bowel. It is associated with mechan-

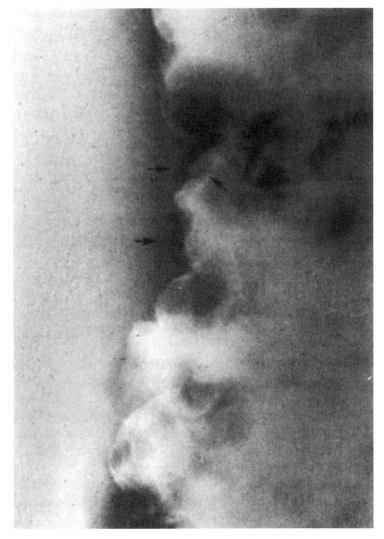

FIG. 5–14. Contrast enema in a patient with pneumatosis coli showing collections of air (arrows) within the wall of the colon. (From Wood RE, et al. Pneumatosis coli in cystic fibrosis. *Am J Dis Child* 1975;129:246.)

ical intestinal obstruction, immunosuppression (acquired immuno-deficiency syndrome [AIDS] and after transplantation), and chronic obstructive lung disease, and is often an incidental finding at laparo-tomy or autopsy. It has been found in as many as 5% of autopsies of patients with CF, and in all cases, it has been confined to the colon. Patients are usually asymptomatic, but there may be abdominal dis-tention and palpable crepitant abdominal masses. Cystic collections of air within the bowel wall can be seen on abdominal radiography, contrast enema studies (Fig. 5–14), MRIs, computed tomography scans, and ultrasound. Complications such as intestinal obstruction, volvulus, perforation, pneumoperitoneum, rectal prolapse, and intus-susception may occur. On pathologic examination, the intestinal mucosa appears to be stretched over a solid matting of air-filled blebs in the mucosa and submucosa surrounded by dense fibrous connective tissue. In patients with CF, pneumatosis probably occurs secondary to alveolar rupture, dissection of air interstitially along the bronchopulmonary bundles to the mediastinum and then retroperi-toneally along the vascular supply of the mucosa. It is usually seen in patients with advanced pulmonary disease, often in association with ectopic (both pulmonary and extrapulmonary) air. The natural history is variable, but in patients with CF, air collections tend to per-sist. In the absence of complications, treatment is not indicated.

REFERENCES

Pancreatic Exocrine Insufficiency

Beverley DW, Kelleher J, Macdonald A, et al. Comparison of four pancreatic extracts in cystic fibrosis. *Arch Dis Child* 1987;62:564–568.

Borowitz DS, Grand RJ, Durie PR, and the Consensus Committee: Use of pancre-atic enzyme supplements for patients with cystic fibrosis in the context of fibros-ing colonopathy. *J Pediatr* 1995;127:681–684.

Dominguez-Munoz JE, Hieronymus C, Sauerbruch T, Malfertheiner P. Fecal elas-tase test: Evaluation of a new noninvasive pancreatic function test. *Am J Gastro-enterol* 1995;90:1834–1837.

Durie PR, Fostner GG, Gaskin KJ, et al. Age-related alterations of immunoreactive pancreatic cationic trypsinogen in sera from cystic fibrosis patients with and without pancreatic insufficiency. *Pediatr Res* 1986;20:209–213.

FitzSimmons SC, Burkhart GA, Borowitz D, et al. High-dose pancreatic enzyme supplements and fibrosing colonopathy in children with cystic fibrosis. *N Engl J Med* 1997;336:1283–1289.

Heijerman HG, Lamers CB, Baker W. Omeprazole enhances the efficacy of pancreatin (pancrease) in cystic fibrosis. *Ann Intern Med* 1991;114:200–201.

Kristidis P, Bozon D, Corey M, et al. The relation between genotype and phenotype in cystic fibrosis—analysis of the most common mutation (ΔF508). *Am J Hum Genet* 1992;50:1178–1184.

Robinson PJ, Smith AL, Sly PD. Duodenal pH in cystic fibrosis and its relationship to fat malabsorption. *Dig Dis Sci* 1990;35:1299–1304.

Shepard RW, Cleghorn GJ. The pancreas: Clinical aspects and investigation of pancreatic function. In Shepherd RW, Cleghom GJ (eds), *Cystic fibrosis: nutritional and intestinal disorders.* Boca Raton, Florida: CRC Press 1989:87–90.

Shwachman H, Lebenthal E, Khaw K. Recurrent acute pancreatitis in patients with cystic fibrosis with normal pancreatic enzymes. *Pediatrics* 1975;55:86–95.

Smyth RL, Van Velzen D, Smyth AR, et al. Strictures of the ascending colon in cystic fibrosis and high-strength pancreatic enzymes. *Lancet* 1994;343:85–86.

Waters DL, Dorney SFA, Gaskin KJ, et al. Pancreatic function in infants identified as having cystic fibrosis in a neonatal screening program. *N Engl J Med* 1990; 322:303–308.

Electrolyte Abnormalities

Beckerman RC, Taussig LM. Hypoelectrolytemia and metabolic alkalosis in infants with cystic fibrosis. *Pediatrics* 1979;63:580–583.

di Sant'Agnese PA, Darlimg RC, Perera GA, Shea E. Abnormal electrolyte composition of sweat in cystic fibrosis of the pancreas. *Pediatrics* 1953;12:549–562.

Kessler WR, Andersen DH. Heat prostration in fibrocystic disease of the pancreas and other conditions. *Pediatrics* 1951;8:648–655.

Nussbaum E, Boat TF, Wood RE, Doershuk CF. Cystic fibrosis with acute hypoelectrolytemia and metabolic alkalosis in infancy. *Am J Dis Child* 1979;133:965–966.

Ruddy R, Anolik R, Scanlin TF. Hypoelectrolytemia as a presentation and complication of cystic fibrosis. *Clin Pediatr* 1982;21:367–369.

Nutrition and Nutrition Management

Cornelissen EAM, van Lieburg AF, Motohara K, van Oostrom CG. Vitamin K status in cystic fibrosis. *Acta Paediatr* 1992;81:658–661.

Durie PR, Pencharz PB. A rational approach to the nutritional care of patients with cystic fibrosis. *J R Soc Med* 1989;82:11–20.

Farrell PM, Bieri JG, Frantantoni JF, et al. The occurrence and effects of human vitamin E deficiency. *J Clin Invest* 1997;60:233–241.

Gunn T, Belmonte MM, Colle E, Dupont C. Edema as the presenting symptom of cystic fibrosis: Difficulties in diagnosis. *Am J Dis Child* 1978;132:317–318.

Henderson RC, Madsen CD. Bone density in children and adolescents with cystic fibrosis. *J Pediatr* 1996;128:28–34.

Kawchak DA, Zhao H, Scanlin TF, et al. Longitudinal prospective analysis of dietary intake in children with cystic fibrosis. *J Pediatr* 1996;129:119–129.

Steinkamp G, von der Hardt H. Improvement of nutritional status and lung function after long-term nocturnal gastrostomy feedings in cystic fibrosis. *J Pediatr* 1994; 124:244–249.

Pancreatic Endocrine Deficiency

Moran A. Diabetes and glucose intolerance in cystic fibrosis. *New Insights into Cystic Fibrosis* 1997;5:1–6.

Moran A, Diem P, Klein DJ, et al. Pancreatic endocrine function in cystic fibrosis. *J Pediatr* 1991;118:15–23.

Lanng S, Thorsteinsson B, Lund-Andersen C, et al. Diabetes mellitus in Danish cystic fibrosis patients: prevalence and late diabetic complications. *Acta Paediatr Scand* 1994;83:72–77.

Lanng S, Thorsteinsson B, Nerup J, Koch C. Influence of the development of diabetes mellitus on clinical status in patients with cystic fibrosis. *Eur J Pediatr* 1992;151:684–687.

Hepatobiliary Disease

Angelico M, Gandin C, Canuzzi P, et al. Gallstones in cystic fibrosis: A critical reappraisal. *Hepatology* 1991;14:768–1475.

Bern EM, Grand RJ. Management of therapy for hepatobiliary disease in cystic fibrosis. *New Insights into Cystic Fibrosis* 1996;4:4–8.

Colombo C, Apostolo MG, Ferrari M, et al. Analysis of risk factors for the development of liver disease associated with cystic fibrosis. *J Pediatr* 1994;124: 393–399.

Colombo C, Setchell KDR, Podda M, et al. Effects of ursodeoxycholic acid therapy for liver disease associated with cystic fibrosis. *J Pediatr* 1990;117:482–489.

Gaskin KJ, Waters DLM, Howman-Giles R, et al. Liver disease and common-bile-duct stenosis in cystic fibrosis. *N Engl J Med* 1988;318:340–346.

Mieles LA, Orenstein D, Teperman L, et al. Liver transplantation in cystic fibrosis. *Lancet* 1989;1:1073.

Nagel RA, Javaid A, Meire HB, et al. Liver disease and bile duct abnormalities in adults with cystic fibrosis. *Lancet* 1989;2:1422–1425.

O'Brien S, Keogan M, Casey M, et al. Biliary complications of cystic fibrosis. *Gut* 1992;33:387–391.

Scott-Jupp R, Lama M, Tanner MS. Prevalence of liver disease in cystic fibrosis. *Arch Dis Child* 1991;66:698–701.

Stern R, Rothstein FC, Doershuk CF. Treatment and prognosis of symptomatic gallbladder disease in patients with cystic fibrosis. *J Pediatr Gastroenterol Nutr* 1986;5:35–40.

Treem WR, Stanley CA. Massive hepatomegaly, steatosis, and secondary plasma carnitine deficiency in an infant with cystic fibrosis. *Pediatrics* 1989;83:993–997.

Wilroy RS, Crawford SE, Johnson WW. Cystic fibrosis with extensive fat replacement of the liver. *J Pediatr* 1966;68:67–73.

Gastrointestinal Complications

Allen ED, Pfaff JK, Taussig LM, McCoy KS. The clinical spectrum of chronic appendiceal abscess in cystic fibrosis. *Am J Dis Child* 1992;146:1190–1193.

Coughlin JP, Gauderer MWL, Stern RC, et al. The spectrum of appendiceal disease in cystic fibrosis. *J Pediatr Surg* 1990;25:834–839.

Gustafsson PM, Gransson S-G, Kjellman N-IM, Tibbling L. Gastro-oesophageal reflux and severity of pulmonary disease in cystic fibrosis. *Scand J Gastroenterol* 1991;26:449–456.

Holmes M, Murphy V, Taylor M, Denham B. Intussusception in cystic fibrosis. *Arch Dis Child* 1991;66:726–727.

Koletzko S, Corey M, Ellis L, et al. Effects of cisapride in patients with cystic fibrosis and distal intestinal obstruction syndrome. *J Pediatr* 1990;117:815–822.

Koletzko S, Stringer DA, Cleghorn GJ, Durie PR. Lavage treatment of distal intestinal obstruction syndrome in children with cystic fibrosis. *Pediatrics* 1989;83:727–733.

Malfroot A, Dab I. New insights on gastro-oesophageal reflux in cystic fibrosis by longitudinal follow up. *Arch Dis Child* 1991;66:1139–1145.

Neglia JP, FitzSimmons SC, Maisonneuve P, et al., and the Cystic Fibrosis and Cancer Study Group. The risk of cancer among patients with cystic fibrosis. *N Engl J Med* 1995;332:494–499.

Oppenheimer EH, Esterly J. Pathology of cystic fibrosis: review of the literature and comparison with 146 autopsied cases. *Perspectives in Pediatric Pathology, Volume 2.* Chicago: Year Book Publishers 1975:242–278.

Rosenstein BJ, Perman JA, Kramer SS. Peptic ulcer disease in cystic fibrosis: an unusual occurrence in black adolescents. *Am J Dis Child* 1986;140:966–968.

Rubenstein S, Moss R, Lewiston N. Constipation and meconium ileus equivalent in patients with cystic fibrosis. *Pediatrics* 1986;78:473–479.

Shields MD, Levison H, Reisman JJ, Durie PR, Canny GJ. Appendicitis in cystic fibrosis. *Arch Dis Child* 1991;65:307–310.

Stern RC, Izant RJ, Boat TF, et al. Treatment and prognosis of rectal prolapse in cystic fibrosis. *Gastroenterology* 1982;82:707–710.

Meconium Abnormalities

Foster MA, Nyberg DA, Mahony BS, et al. Meconium peritonitis: Prenatal sonographic findings and their clinical significance. *Radiology* 1987;165:661–665.

Kerem E, Corey M, Kerem B, et al. Clinical and genetic comparisons of patients with cystic fibrosis, with or without meconium ileus. *J Pediatr* 1989;114:767–773.

Olsen MM, Luck SR, Lloyd-Still J, Raffensperger JG. The spectrum of meconium disease in infancy. *J Ped Surg* 1982;17:479–481.

Rescorla FJ, Grosfeld JL, West KJ, Vane DW. Changing patterns of treatment and survival in neonates with meconium ileus. *Arch Surg* 1989;142:837–846.

Rosenstein BJ, Langbaum TS. Incidence of meconium abnormalities in newborn infants with cystic fibrosis. *Am J Dis Child* 1980;134:72–73.

6

Other Organ Systems

CARDIOVASCULAR COMPLICATIONS

Cor pulmonale (enlargement of the right ventricle) secondary to chronic hypoxemia is a frequent complication in patients with cystic fibrosis (CF) with advanced pulmonary disease. Cor pulmonale can be present for years as a successful compensation for increased pulmonary artery pressure. The more ominous finding of overt heart failure is a significant cause of morbidity and mortality. In addition, a number of other cardiovascular complications have been documented.

Evaluation of Cardiac Status

Physical Examination. The early clinical recognition of cor pulmonale may be difficult in patients with CF. Tachypnea, tachycardia, and hepatomegaly occur commonly secondary to underlying pulmonary disease. However, an enlarged tender liver is often an early clue to right ventricular failure. An accentuated second heart sound in the pulmonic area may be a helpful sign but is often blunted by an anterior chest wall deformity and air-trapping. Patients may develop a tricuspid insufficiency murmur, either simultaneously with or shortly after the onset of cardiac enlargement. Peripheral edema is not a common finding and usually appears late in the clinical course. In patients with heart failure, weight loss is as common as weight gain.

Laboratory Findings. There is a close correlation between the degree of hypoxemia and pulmonary artery pressure. A PaO_2 of less than 50 mm Hg (Fig. 6–1) and a PCO_2 of greater than 45 mm Hg are consistently associated with severe cor pulmonale. Hypoalbumine-

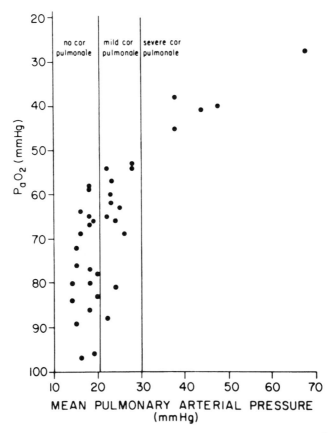

FIG. 6–1. Relationship between pulmonary artery pressure and PaO₂ in 34 patients with cystic fibrosis. All patients with pulmonary artery pressures greater than 30 mm Hg had PaO₂ values less than 50 mm Hg. (From Siassi B, et al. *J Pediatr* 1971;78:794.)

mia secondary to expansion of plasma volume may be a helpful early clue to right ventricular failure but may also reflect poor nutrition.

Chest Radiograph. Because of severe air-trapping in patients with CF, it is often difficult to assess heart size; in general, there is poor correlation between echocardiographic findings and cardiothoracic ratio. Cardiomegaly may be obvious only in patients with overt right heart failure. However, an increase in heart size by 1 cm or more can point to cardiac enlargement, even if the cardiac silhouette does not seem especially large. There may be enlargement of the main pulmonary arteries, but this finding is often obscured by striking hilar adenopathy and parenchymal disease.

Electrocardiogram. The electrocardiogram (ECG) is not generally helpful in the diagnosis of cor pulmonale in patients with CF. The majority of patients with confirmed right ventricular hypertrophy have a normal ECG. In some patients, however, especially those with heart failure, the ECG may show evidence of right ventricular hypertrophy, right atrial hypertrophy, left ventricular hypertrophy, ST- and T-wave abnormalities and low voltage.

Echocardiogram. Although the quality of echo images may be poor, especially in patients with severe pulmonary disease, echo is the most useful noninvasive clinical tool for the early diagnosis and longitudinal assessment of cor pulmonale in patients with CF. Even in patients with clinically mild disease, there is thickening of the anterior wall of the right ventricle, which progresses to enlargement (dilation) of the right ventricular cavity and right ventricular outflow tract, along with abnormal right ventricular systolic time intervals. Patients with advanced disease may show left ventricular wall hypertrophy, a decrease in the size of the left ventricular cavity, and abnormal septal motion (flattened or reversed). Echocardiographic changes correlate with clinical CF (e.g., Shwachman-Kulczycki) score, chest radiograph score, pulmonary function, and postmortem cardiac findings. A composite echo scoring system has been proposed and has been shown to correlate with clinical score, chest radiograph score, pulmonary function, and prognosis.

Radionuclide Scans. Quantitative radionuclide angiography is a reproducible technique used to assess biventricular function. Using this technique to measure ejection fractions, right ventricular dysfunction at rest has been demonstrated in 41% to 72% of patients and a significant percentage of patients exhibit an abnormal right ventricular response to exercise. Abnormal left ventricular function at rest is present in up to 25% of patients, with a variable response to exercise. Radionuclide perfusion studies suggest that in CF, abnormal right ventricular function may occur before clinically significant cardiac disease is present and that the stress of exercise may uncover right ventricular and left ventricular dysfunction. Thallium myocardial perfusion scans can be used to assess right ventricular hypertrophy, but in patients with CF, this technique offers no advantage over echo.

Cardiac Catheterization. Right-sided heart catheterization with direct measurement of pulmonary artery pressure remains the gold standard for evaluation of pulmonary hypertension. Although this procedure is too invasive for the routine assessment of cor pulmonale, it can be used to monitor the response to various therapeutic interventions and to assess patients before lung transplantation.

Cor Pulmonale

Secondary to alveolar hypoventilation, chronic hypoxemia, and pulmonary vasoconstriction, up to 70% of patients eventually develop pulmonary hypertension and hypertrophy of the right ventricle (cor pulmonale). A clear relationship has been demonstrated between the degree of hypoxemia and pulmonary artery pressure (Fig. 6–1). Airflow obstruction and wide ranges in intrathoracic pressure may augment venous return to the right side of the heart, with resultant increase in pulmonary artery flow and aggravation of an already increased right ventricle afterload. In patients with CF, there is probably slowly progressive hypertrophy and dilation of the right ventricle over a period of years. At one extreme, there may be only mild pulmonary hypertension with minimal right ventricular hypertrophy, whereas at the other extreme, there may be severe right ventricular overload with overt right-sided heart failure.

In the absence of obvious heart failure, the diagnosis of cor pulmonale by clinical findings may be difficult. Pulmonary hypertension is often severe and most likely irreversible by the time clinical parameters such as arterial desaturation, right ventricular hypertrophy, x-ray evidence of pulmonary artery enlargement, and clinical signs of congestive heart failure are present. Echocardiography is the most sensitive noninvasive technique for the early recognition and monitoring of cor pulmonale. For practical purposes, cor pulmonale is assumed to be present when one or more of the following is present: right ventricular hypertrophy by ECG; PaO_2 less than 50 mm Hg; signs of heart failure; and radiographic evidence of enlarged pulmonary arteries.

Approximately one-third of patients with CF have right-sided failure during the terminal phase of their illness. Clinical features include enlargement and tenderness of the liver (90%), peripheral edema (64%), and weight gain (37%). Such patients usually have markedly abnormal pulmonary function, severe hypoxemia, ECG changes of right ventricular hypertrophy, and abnormal echo. At catheterization, pulmonary artery pressure is elevated but the range of values is considerable.

Treatment of heart failure consists of oxygen, lowered salt intake, diuretics, and aggressive treatment of underlying pulmonary obstruction and infection, but the response is often unsatisfactory. There is no demonstrated benefit to the use of digitalis. Tolazoline transiently reduces pulmonary artery pressure but has not been shown to be of long-term benefit. Other pulmonary vasodilators, including phentolamine, hydralazine, and nifedipine, have not reduced pulmonary artery pressure in patients with CF and prior episodes of right-sided heart failure. After the onset of right-sided heart failure, most patients are significantly disabled, and mean survival is 8 months (range 1 to 63 months). Although there are data to support a role for chronic oxygen therapy in reducing pulmonary hypertension in adults with chronic obstructive pulmonary disease (COPD), this therapy has not been adequately studied in patients with CF. However, supplemental oxygen has been shown to minimize oxyhemoglobin desaturation in CF patients who desaturate during exercise in room air and to improve exercise tolerance. Acute administration of aminophylline and digoxin has not been shown to improve cardiac function in CF patients, either at rest or during exercise, and heart failure increases the risk for aminophylline toxicity.

Myocardial Lesions

There have been several reports of focal areas of myocardial necrosis and fibrosis in patients with CF who were younger than age 3 years. Lesions involve mainly the left ventricle and spare the endocardium, pericardium, atria, and coronary vessels. Microscopically, the lesions consist of connective tissue or fibrosis in the absence of any inflammatory reaction. Patients may present with the sudden onset of congestive heart failure or asystole preceded by episodes of dyspnea, pallor, and tachycardia. Radiographs may be normal or show cardiomegaly. Metabolic and nutritional factors have been postulated, but the etiology of these lesions remains unknown.

Arrhythmias

Recurrent episodes of supraventricular tachycardia (SVT) have been observed in a small number of patients with CF. Patients have baseline tachycardia, but there is no correlation between severity of pulmonary disease and frequency of SVT. The etiology of the arrhythmia is unclear, but possible causes include myocardial fibrosis and necrosis, stimulation of pressure receptors in a distended right atrium, intracardiac autonomic imbalance, and reaction to combination bronchodilator therapy. Acute management consists of vagal maneuvers or intravenous verapamil. Long-term management consists of digoxin or verapamil, or both. Bronchodilator therapy should be reduced as clinically indicated.

There is a single report of an adolescent with CF who showed first-degree atrioventricular (A-V) block, ventricular trigeminy, and multiple premature ventricular contractions. Echocardiogram and thallium scan were suggestive of an infiltrative process in the anteroseptal region.

ENDOCRINE-METABOLIC

Parathyroid Gland

In some patients with CF, there is evidence of secondary hyperparathyroidism, as evidenced by elevated levels of immunoreactive parathyroid hormone. There are conflicting results as to whether the elevated levels correlate with low serum concentrations of 25-hydroxyvitamin D and the degree of bone demineralization. The absence of secondary hyperparathyroidism in the majority of patients, in the presence of subnormal 25-hydroxyvitamin D concentrations, is probably explained by normal serum concentrations of 1, 25-dihydroxyvitamin D_3. Gastrointestinal absorption of calcium is normal, and there is normal end-organ responsiveness to parathyroid extract.

Pituitary Gland

In patients with CF, there is retardation of physical growth in all age groups and an average delay of 2 years in pubertal development. Skeletal maturation is delayed in approximately 40% of patients. There is a significant correlation among growth retardation, severity of pulmonary disease and survival. The hypothalamic-pituitary-gonadal axis is intact, but there is a substantial delay in the normal pubertal rise of gonadotropins and testicular androgens. Plasma growth hormone and somatomedin C levels are normal. Short-course testosterone therapy has been shown to be a safe and effective means of improving the growth rate in male adolescents with CF and pubertal delay. Isolated growth hormone deficiency has been reported in several patients with CF, probably as a chance coincidence of the two disorders. Among nine prepubertal endocrinologically normal CF patients, a 12-month trial of biosynthetic recombinant human growth hormone resulted in a significant anabolic effect, as shown by increased growth velocity, somatomedin C values, and protein stores. However, a long-term benefit from such therapy has not been demonstrated.

Thyroid Gland

At autopsy, the thyroid gland of older CF patients contains excessive quantities of lipofuscin (ceroid) pigment in follicular epithelial cells, possibly related to the autooxidation of cellular lipids secondary to chronic vitamin E deficiency. The development of a goiter with or without hypothyroidism has been well documented in patients with CF following chronic administration of iodide. In several patients treated with iodide, hypothyroidism has occurred in the absence of a goiter. Studies of thyroid metabolism in patients with CF have failed to explain the apparently enhanced sensitivity of the thyroid gland to the inhibitory action of iodides on hormone synthesis. Although serum thyroxine (T_4) concentrations are within the normal range, there may be significantly low triiodothyroxine (T_3) concentrations, suggesting a defect in the peripheral deiodination of T_4 to T_3. No defects in thyroidal iodide organification have been seen with iodide-perchlorate discharge tests. Thyroid-stimulating hormone (TSH) reserve was normal, and there was a normal response to endogenous TSH stimulation. Dysgenetic congenital hypothyroidism has been recognized in association with CF. Gastrointestinal absorption of L-thyroxine may be reduced in such a patient.

Adrenal Gland

Cortex. It has been demonstrated in autopsy material that there is hyperplasia of the zona glomerulosa (the site of aldosterone production) in the adrenal cortex of children with CF. The other zones are normal, and there are no other characteristic histologic changes in the adrenal gland. Older nonstressed patients show normal to slightly elevated urinary aldosterone excretion, plasma aldosterone levels, and aldosterone secretion rates. These results are consistent with a state of secondary hyperaldosteronism, probably related to excessive loss of sodium in sweat. Young CF patients who present with dehydration, hypoelectrolytemia, and metabolic alkalosis have elevated plasma renin activity, hyperaldosteronemia, and hyperaldosteronuria secondary to sodium depletion and intravascular volume contraction; plasma and urinary levels of mineralocorticoids are elevated. All values return to normal on restoration of fluid and electrolyte balance and maintenance on a high sodium diet. CF patients show normal aldosterone responses to exercise and heat stress.

Medulla. There is histologic evidence of adrenal medullary hyperplasia. Studies of circulating plasma catecholamines, their precursors, metabolites, and major urinary products have yielded somewhat conflicting results. Plasma norepinephrine levels have been reported to be normal or slightly elevated. Free plasma dopamine levels have been reported to be significantly elevated, but in this group of patients, there was no concomitant increase in urinary levels of dopamine or homovanillic acid, the final breakdown product of dopamine. The significance of these findings and their relationship to autonomic dysfunction and clinical outcomes in patients with CF are not clear.

RENAL ABNORMALITIES

Although renal involvement is not a major clinical concern in CF, a number of conditions are present, including immune-complex deposition, heavy exposure to aminoglycosides and other nephrotoxic antibiotics, diabetes mellitus, steatorrhea, and cor pulmonale, which place patients at increased risk of renal injury. Hypoxemia and the use of diuretics may increase the nephrotoxic potential of these risk factors. Histologic abnormalities, described largely in autopsy material, include glomerular alterations, glomerulomegaly, amyloid deposition, glomerulosclerosis, mesangial proliferation, mesangial deposits of IgM and C3 (suggestive of immune-complex mediated injuries); tubulointerstitial lesions, tubular lysosomal proliferation, lymphoplasmocytic infiltration, fibrosis, and tubular atrophy (suggestive of chronic aminoglycoside injury); and microscopic nephrocalcinosis. Changes consistent with diabetic nephropathy have also been described.

Patients may manifest proteinuria, nephrotic syndrome, renal colic and hematuria, severe nephropathy with progressive renal insufficiency, or end-stage renal disease. These conditions may be related to renal amyloidosis, IgA nephropathy, aminoglycoside or ibuprofen nephrotoxicity, nephrocalcinosis, diabetic nephropathy or nephrolithiasis. Patients are also at high risk of developing calcium oxalate renal stones. This possibility needs to be considered in patients who present with abdominal or flank pain, or hematuria. Stone formation is probably related to enteric hyperoxaluria secondary to pancreatic exocrine deficiency in association with a reduction in the anaerobic degradation of intestinal oxalate due to an absence or reduction of the intestinal bacterium *Oxalobacter formigenes*. Patients with secondary amyloidosis may present with proteinuria, which progresses rapidly to nephrotic syndrome and then end-stage renal disease. Proteinuria greater than 1 g/24 hours is uncommon in patients with CF and warrants further investigation. Nephrotic syndrome may occur coincidentally with CF, unrelated to amyloidosis. In such patients, unlike those with amyloidosis, response to glucocorticoid therapy has been good.

Renal physiology studies in patients with CF reveal that the glomerular filtration rate is slightly decreased, normal, or slightly increased, probably depending on experimental conditions of salt and water balance. Effective renal plasma flow is normal. Patients are capable of lowering urinary excretion of sodium when placed on a moderately reduced sodium intake, or when they lose excessive salt through the sweat, as with exercise and heat stress, and renal tubular anion–secreting mechanisms are intact. There is evidence, however, of decreased free water clearance and impaired ability to excrete sodium in response to an oral or intravenous sodium load. These findings are consistent with increased sodium reabsorption in the renal proximal tubule and decreased delivery of sodium to more distal segments of the nephron. CF patients are at increased risk of magnesium loss. The finding of microscopic nephrocalcinosis in a high percentage of patients, including those younger than 1 year of age, suggests that a primary renal defect may be present in CF.

FEMALE REPRODUCTIVE TRACT

Genital Abnormalities

An excess of cytoplasmic and extracellular cervical mucus is present in patients with CF in the absence of inflammation or other obvious contributory factors. This is a consistent finding in newborns, and although it decreases in frequency, it remains a common finding throughout infancy and childhood (Fig. 6–2). The submucosal glands, uterine cavity, and cervical os may also be filled with mucin-rich material. In one-third of adult patients, multicystic ovaries and reduced uterine size are demonstrated on ultrasonography, especially in patients with amenorrhea or irregular menstrual cycles. The histologic appearance of the endometrium, fallopian tubes, and ovaries is otherwise normal.

Cervical mucus is scanty and dehydrated, usually containing less than 80% water. This is below the minimum critical water level of 93% to 95% believed to be essential for sperm migration. Moreover, the typical midcycle increase in water content and the accompanying thinning of cervical mucus that occurs in normal subjects are not seen in patients with CF. This may result in the formation of a tenacious mucus plug in the os that impedes sperm penetration. The electrolyte pattern of the cervical mucus is noncyclic; the average

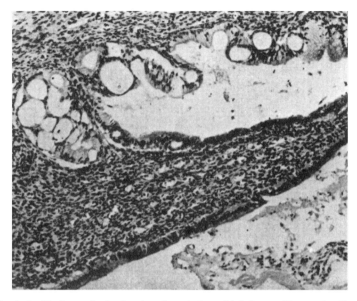

FIG. 6–2. Endocervical glands of a 4-day-old infant with cystic fibrosis showing so-called balloon cells with excessive intracellular mucus. Mucoid exudate is present in the cervical cells. (From Oppenheimer EH, Esterly JR. Observations on cystic fibrosis of the pancreas. VI. The uterine cervix. *J Pediatr* 1970;77:991.)

sodium concentration in the dry residue is only one-tenth of normal during the critical midcycle period.

Pubertal Delay

In girls with CF, there is an average delay of 2 years in age at menarche (14.5 to 14.9 years). Delay in pubertal increases of serum gonadotropin and sex steroid levels suggests late maturation of the reproductive endocrine system. Generally, appropriate levels of these hormones are finally attained in most patients by the late teenage years. There is evidence that the neuroendocrine mechanism controlling onset of puberty can be modified by various factors, including inadequate fat reserve. In patients with CF, pubertal development may be related to the severity of disease and nutritional status, but pubertal delay also occurs in patients who have good clinical and nutritional status. In these patients, genotype, maternal menarchal age, and abnormal glucose tolerance may influence timing of puberty.

Menstrual Abnormalities

Among adolescent and adult patients with CF, primary and secondary amenorrhea and irregular cycles (missed periods, prolonged cycle lengths) are common.

Fertility

Despite reduced fertility in patients with CF, the potential for pregnancy exists and is likely to increase in association with improved survival. Patients wishing to avoid pregnancy need to employ adequate methods of contraception. Barrier methods are safe and highly effective in the well-motivated patient but are associated with unacceptably high failure rates in adolescents. The use of oral contraceptives has been somewhat controversial because of potential CF-related side effects such as diabetes, cholelithiasis, hepatic dysfunction, and bronchial mucous obstruction. There is one report of atypical polypoid endocervical hyperplasia in CF patients using combination birth control pills. However, use of a combination contraceptive pill has not been associated with cervical changes or decline in pulmonary function, even in women with moderate-to-severe pulmonary disease.

Pregnancy

In recent years, there has been a dramatic increase in the number of reported pregnancies among women with CF. In 1996, 145 pregnancies were reported to the Cystic Fibrosis Foundation Patient Registry, compared with 52 pregnancies in 1986. Normal physiologic adaptations seen during pregnancy, such as an increase in minute ventilation, alterations in gas exchange, a decrease in residual volume and functional residual capacity, and an increase in blood volume and cardiac output, place the patient with CF at risk for respiratory failure and right ventricular decompensation. Closure of the small airways at the lung bases may accentuate ventilation-perfusion mismatch and hypoxemia. In addition, the increased nutritional demands during pregnancy may be unattainable.

Early reports of pregnancy outcomes among patients with CF suggested a significant risk, both for the mother and fetus, including decline in pulmonary status and increased rates of stillbirth and prematurity. It is not clear, however, whether pregnancy per se was responsible for the clinical decline or whether this was the natural history of CF in patients of this age and severity. More recently, it has been shown that pregnancy in patients with mild disease is well tolerated with little decline in pulmonary and nutritional status 1 year after pregnancy. Prepregnancy pulmonary function is the best predictor of outcome. A prepregnancy FEV_1 of more than 60% generally predicts a good outcome, and a significant decline in FEV_1 during pregnancy is associated with significant postpregnancy mortality. Approximately one-quarter of CF pregnancies result in preterm labor and delivery. The duration of pregnancy and birth weight correlate most closely with prepregnancy pulmonary function. Women with CF are at high risk of developing gestational diabetes; this complication may be associated with unusually rapid deterioration of pulmonary function in the years following pregnancy.

Patients contemplating pregnancy require counseling regarding the advisability of and potential risks associated with pregnancy. Patients who become pregnant require close supervision by an obstetrician skilled in high-risk obstetrics, a pulmonologist, dietitian, and respiratory therapist. Pulmonary exacerbations require aggressive management including intravenous antipseudomonal penicillins and cephalosporins. The use of intravenous aminoglycosides is generally discouraged because of concerns of fetal ototoxicity. In patients with severe exacerbations, however, the benefit of their use may outweigh the potential risk. Tetracyclines, fluoroquinolones, and trimethoprim-sulfamethoxazole should be avoided. The safety of dornase alfa (Pulmozyme) during pregnancy has not been established. The decision to terminate a pregnancy should be weighed in favor of protecting the immediate health of the mother. Indications for pregnancy termination include marked and sustained decline in pulmonary function, development of right-sided heart failure, refractory hypoxemia, and progressive hypercapnia and respiratory acidosis.

Genetic counseling and mutation screening of the prospective father should be offered to all couples contemplating a pregnancy. All offspring will be obligate carriers of a CF mutation. For a woman with CF whose partner does not carry a common CF mutation, the risk of an affected infant is 1:160. Couples also need to be counseled as to nonmedical issues including the additional demands of child-rearing, financial aspects of parenting, and the potential premature loss of a parent.

Breast Feeding

Mothers with CF can successfully breast feed, but they and their infants need careful nutrition monitoring. Studies of CF breast milk composition indicate a normal electrolyte composition, increased protein content, and a slight decrease in lipid levels. The lipid pattern of CF breast milk (decreased content of linoleic and arachidonic acid) reflects the blood lipid pattern of CF patients.

MALE REPRODUCTIVE TRACT

Genital Abnormalities

The external genitalia are normal. The testes are usually normal in size and contour but may be reduced in size in the presence of advanced disease or malnutrition. There are, however, abnormalities of wolffian duct–derived structures. The epididymis is either not palpable or reduced in size, soft, and poorly formed. In almost all patients, there is bilateral absence or atresia of the vas deferens. Pathologic studies reveal absence of epididymal ducts and vas deferens, and atrophy and fibrosis of the body and tail of the epididymis. The presence of normal ureters and kidneys (metanephroi) indicates that the wolffian duct was present in early embryonic life but disappeared during development. However, the presence of normal vas deferens in CF-affected fetuses and in some prepubertal boys suggests that the observed genital tract abnormalities may be secondary to intraluminal obstruction by abnormally viscous secretions and subsequent atrophy. There is an increased incidence of abnormalities associated with testicular descent including inguinal hernia, hydrocele, and undescended testicle. Testicular function and male sexual activity are otherwise normal, but testosterone levels are low in approximately 20% of men.

Pubertal Delay

Linear growth and onset of puberty are frequently retarded in men with CF. There is an intact hypothalamic-pituitary-gonadal axis, but the normal pubertal rise of gonadotropins and testicular androgens is substantially delayed. Generally, this is accompanied by retardation of skeletal maturation reflected in delayed bone age and short stature. Maximal growth velocity is shifted from age 13 years in normal subjects to age 15 years in patients with CF. Short-term treatment with testosterone enanthate, 200 mg IM every 3 weeks for a total of four injections, has been associated with significantly increased growth velocity, along with objective and subjective improvement in self-image.

Azoospermia

Almost all postpubescent boys and men with CF demonstrate obstructive azoospermia. Characteristically, the ejaculate is of low volume (0.5 to 1.0 mL) and acidic (pH less than 7.2) compared with that of controls (volume 3.0 to 5.0 mL; pH 7.2 to 8.0). The concentration of fructose, which is of seminal vesicle origin, is diminished (less than 1 g/L), whereas the concentration of citric acid and the activity of acid phosphatase, both of which are of prostatic origin, are increased. Microscopic examination of the testes shows active meiosis and spermatogenesis, but there is a reduction in the number of mature spermatozoa produced, with up to 50% abnormal forms. In men who present with azoospermia and chronic sinopulmonary infection, the differential diagnosis includes CF, Young's syndrome, and ciliary dyskinesia (immotile cilia syndrome). Testicular biopsy, electron microscopy of bronchial mucosal biopsy specimens, sweat testing, measurement of transepithelial potential differences, and genotype analysis can be helpful in arriving at a conclusive diagnosis.

Of particular interest are otherwise healthy men who present with obstructive azoospermia secondary to bilateral absence or atresia of the vas deferens. Most have no pulmonary or gastrointestinal manifestations. Among such cases, 50% to 65% have one detectable CF mutation or an incompletely penetrant mutation (5T) on a noncoding region of the CF transmembrane conductance regulator (CFTR) gene and 10% to 15% are compound heterozygotes. Sweat electrolyte levels are usually normal but may be intermediate or elevated. A diagnosis of CF in patients with obstructive azoospermia can be made only by mutation analysis or by demonstration of an abnormality of CFTR function by sweat test or nasal potential difference measurement. The prognosis for such individuals appears to be excellent, but they should be monitored for the development of CF-related complications, and genetic counseling should be offered to their relatives.

Fertility

Although the overwhelming majority of men with CF are infertile secondary to obstructive azoospermia, fertility has been documented in 2% to 3% of men, usually those with mild pulmonary disease or specific mutations, such as 3849+10 kb C→T. For purposes of reproductive counseling, semen analysis should be offered to all postpubescent boys. The finding on testicular biopsy of active spermatogenesis in patients with CF has raised the possibility of microscopic sperm aspiration from the epididymal remnant combined with in vitro fertilization and tubal embryo transfer. In such cases, including men with the syndrome of congenital bilateral absence or atresia of the vas deferens, it is important to test the partner for CF mutations in order to predict the risk of CF in their offspring.

HEMATOLOGIC ABNORMALITIES

In patients with CF, there is an inverse relationship between PaO_2 levels and hemoglobin and hematocrit, but the degree of compensatory polycythemia is less than expected. Although there is a blunted compensatory increase in erythropoietin relative to the degree of underlying anemia and hypoxemia, red blood cell (RBC) mass in hypoxemic CF patients increases similarly to that of healthy individuals living at high altitude. The lack of polycythemia is related more to a disproportionate rise in plasma volume relative to RBC mass.

Iron deficiency anemia is present in 33% to 66% of patients with CF. The etiology involves several factors, including inadequate dietary iron intake, blood loss, iron malabsorption, and chronic infection. *In vitro* and *in vivo* studies suggest that iron absorption is increased with exocrine pancreatic insufficiency and that the administration of pancreatic enzymes may impair oral iron absorption. The mechanism by which pancreatic enzymes impair iron absorption is not clear. The iron status of patients should be routinely monitored. A low serum ferritin level is a useful measure of decreased total body iron stores; however, an elevated level may not be a reliable indicator of adequate iron stores, because ferritin is an acute-phase reactant that is often elevated in CF patients secondary to lung infection and inflammation. If supplemental iron is given, it should not be in close proximity to the administration of pancreatic enzyme supplements.

An early report of hemosiderosis in patients with CF is probably explained by the persistence of fetal iron in the livers of young infants. Beyond infancy, there is no evidence of increased hepatic iron stores in patients with CF.

A moderate degree of thrombocytosis is a common finding, probably secondary to chronic infection and inflammation. Thrombocytopenia in patients with CF is almost always related to hypersplenism secondary to cirrhosis and portal hypertension.

CENTRAL NERVOUS SYSTEM COMPLICATIONS

Brain Abscess

Brain abscess has been reported in a small number of adolescents and adults with CF, usually in association with advanced pulmonary disease. In most cases, there have been multiple abscesses remote from the paranasal sinuses. The responsible organisms are aerobic and anaerobic mouth bacteria of low virulence, suggesting hematogenous spread from a site other than the lungs. The possibility of a brain abscess should be pursued vigorously in patients with CF who have a compatible clinical history.

Increased Intracranial Pressure

Transient increased intracranial pressure (pseudotumor cerebri), manifested by a bulging fontanel, irritability, and rapid head growth may occur in malnourished infants with CF shortly after initiation of nutritional therapy. There are usually no associated neurologic abnormalities. On lumbar puncture, cerebrospinal fluid (CSF) pressure may be increased; computed tomography (CT) is usually normal. The fontanel returns to normal over a period of several days to several months. In the patient who develops a cranial nerve palsy or who does not improve over 1 to 2 weeks, a magnetic resonance imaging (MRI) or CT study should be performed to rule out an underlying anatomic abnormality. The etiology of the increased intracranial pressure is unclear. Postulated mechanisms include vitamin A deficiency, intrathoracic obstruction to venous return, or shifts in fluid compartments of the brain. The rapidity of onset and resolution suggests a mechanism other than catch-up brain growth.

There are several reports of CF patients who developed convulsions following treatment with intranasal desmopressin. The probable mechanism was water intoxication. It is probably prudent to avoid the use of this drug in patients with CF.

Neurologic Dysfunction Related to Vitamin E Deficiency

Neuropathologic changes and a spinocerebellar syndrome have been described in patients with CF in association with vitamin E deficiency. Patients with liver disease and decreased intraluminal bile salt concentrations may be at particular risk. Neuropathologic studies have demonstrated a high incidence of axonal degeneration in the rostral parts of the posterior columns in the spinal cord of patients with CF, a lesion characteristic of vitamin E deficiency. The incidence of this finding increases with age in untreated patients. Among 89 patients who died after the age of 5 years, 17 (19%) had evidence at autopsy of posterior column degeneration. Most often, there was bilateral degeneration limited to the fasciculus gracilis extending from thoracic through cervical segments. The lesions involve both axons and myelin, and the site of degeneration is marked by cellular and fibrillary astrogliosis.

Patients may manifest ophthalmoplegia, peripheral and truncal ataxia, peripheral neuropathy, proximal muscle weakness, areflexia, and decreased vibratory and proprioceptive sensation. In vitamin E–deficient patients, sural nerve conduction latency is increased and action potential amplitude is decreased. Somatosensory and visual evoked potentials are abnormal. Although the relationship between vitamin E deficiency and neurologic dysfunction is not clear-cut, significant clinical improvement or stabilization of neurologic status has been documented following vitamin E supplementation.

OCULAR COMPLICATIONS

Ocular abnormalities in CF include visual field defects, venous engorgement, tortuosity, hyperemia and blurring of the optic nerve head, abnormal pupillary responses, and decreased contrast sensitivity. Examination of the ocular surface shows an increase in fluorescein staining and clinical blepharitis, as well as decreased tearing (by Schirmer testing) and tear lysozyme. Conjunctival epithelial cell morphology is normal. Adolescents and young adults who are vitamin A deficient may manifest night blindness and subnormal dark adaptation. In patients with CF-related diabetes mellitus (CFRDM), there is evidence of breakdown of the blood–retinal barrier; this is considered to represent a functional abnormality that is a precursor to diabetic microangiopathy. Proliferative diabetic retinopathy with blurred vision, neovascularization, vitreous hemorrhages, and cataract formation occurs in CF patients with long-standing diabetes. Patients with CFRDM should have an annual ophthalmologic evaluation. Acute hemorrhagic retinopathy may occur at high altitudes. Optic atrophy and neuropathy with decreased contrast sensitivity and visual acuity have been observed in patients treated with chloramphenicol.

SALIVARY GLANDS

In patients with CF, there are characteristic histologic abnormalities of the salivary glands. In the submaxillary glands, there are dilated mucous acini and ductules filled with inspissated mucous secretions. In the labial (mucus) glands, there are dilated ducts with inspissated mucus, atrophy and cystlike dilation of acini, and metaplasia of the ductule epithelium. Enlargement of the submaxillary glands has been observed in 90% of patients of all ages (Fig. 6–3). Parotid gland enlargement is rare, and there is no evidence of sialoangiectasis.

Studies of flow rates and constituent composition of the various salivary glands have yielded somewhat conflicting data, probably

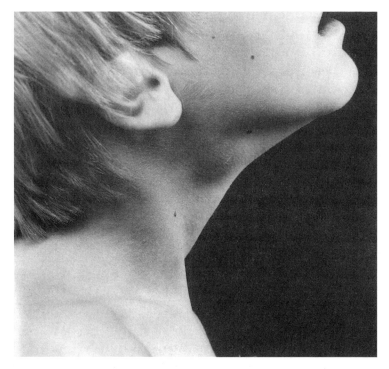

FIG. 6–3. Enlarged submaxillary gland in a patient with cystic fibrosis.

related to differences in methods of salivary gland stimulation and saliva collection. In the parotid gland (serous), there is an increased flow rate and increases in the concentrations of urea nitrogen and uric acid. Amylase activity and sodium concentration are normal. In the submaxillary gland (seromucoid), the flow rate is normal to slightly decreased and concentrations of calcium, amylase, total protein, acid and alkaline ribonuclease, lysozyme, and immunoglobulin A are increased. Sodium and chloride concentrations are normal. There is increased turbidity of submaxillary gland saliva, probably accounted for by the formation of high-molecular-weight calcium and glycoprotein precipitates. In the small salivary glands (mixed type), there is a moderately decreased flow rate and a markedly increased sodium concentration. This is the only exocrine gland (apart from the eccrine sweat glands) that consistently exhibits the sodium abnormality characteristic of CF. The increased sodium concentration observed in mixed mouth saliva is probably due to the sodium contribution by the small salivary glands.

SKIN MANIFESTATIONS

Skin manifestations occur in patients with CF secondary to nutritional deficiencies and vasculitis. Patients with vasculitis may develop sudden onset of raised, palpable, petechial lesions over the lower extremities. The rash is frequently associated with pruritus, a burning sensation, slight edema of the feet, and concomitant arthritis. It fades spontaneously in 3 to 7 days but is followed by multiple recurrences and eventually a diffuse purple-brown pigmentation of the affected areas. Skin biopsy shows vasculitis and perivascular infiltrates. Most of these patients have evidence of advanced pulmonary disease, elevated serum immunoglobulin G levels, and circulating immune complexes. There is usually no response to anti-inflammatory agents.

Infants with CF may present with a periorificial dermatitis that closely resembles acrodermatitis enteropathica (Fig. 6–4). The rash consists of extensive dry, scaling, fissured, erythematous plaques, and papules involving the diaper region, extremities, shoulders, and perioral area. It may be pruritic, with extensive excoriation. Mucous

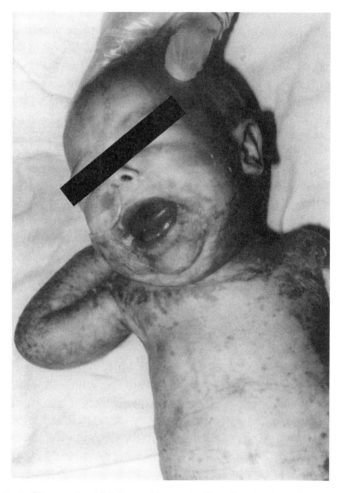

FIG. 6–4. Six-month-old infant with cystic fibrosis who initially presented with extensive dry, scaling, fissured erythematous plaques, and papules involving the diaper region, extremities, shoulders, and perioral area. Clinically, it closely resembled acrodermatitis enteropathica.

membranes and nails are not affected. There may be mild diffuse alopecia. The rash is usually seen in association with failure to thrive, hypoalbuminemia, anemia, and hepatomegaly. Although the pathogenesis of the rash is not entirely clear, it is probably related to deficiencies of zinc, protein, and essential fatty acids, along with altered prostaglandin metabolism. It responds rapidly to nutritional therapy, including protein, essential fatty acids, zinc, and pancreatic enzyme supplementation.

MUSCULOSKELETAL ABNORMALITIES

Digital Clubbing

Digital clubbing is an almost universal finding in patients with CF. In most instances, both the fingers and toes are involved. The diagnosis is based on finding bulbous enlargement of the distal segment of the digit, a change in the angle between the nail and the proximal skin to greater than 180 degrees, sponginess of the nail bed when pressure is applied, and increased nail curvature (Fig. 6–5). When the dorsal surfaces of the terminal phalanges of both long fingers are placed together, there is a prominent distal angle between the ends of

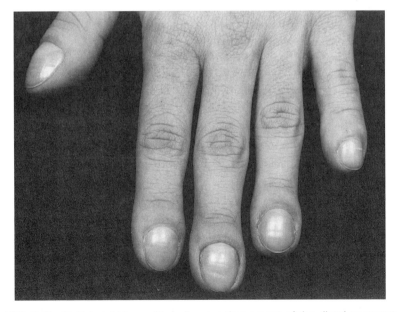

FIG. 6–5. Digital clubbing, with bulbous enlargement of the distal segment of the digit and increased nail curvature.

the nails and loss of the normal diamond-shaped window at the base of the nail beds. The degree of clubbing is related to the severity of the patient's pulmonary disease, but the correlation is often poor; the relative importance of hypoxemia and lung suppuration has not been determined. It has been hypothesized that the increased digital blood flow observed in clubbed digits may be caused by increased plasma levels of prostaglandin E or other vasoactive substances.

Pulmonary Hypertrophic Osteoarthropathy

Pulmonary hypertrophic osteoarthropathy (PHOA) occurs in 5% to 15% of patients with CF, usually in those older than 12 years of age and with advanced suppurative lung disease. It manifests as bilateral painful swelling of the distal third of affected bones (Fig. 6–6). Most commonly involved are the femur, tibia, fibula, radius, ulna, and humerus. Metacarpals and metatarsals are less commonly involved. There may be arthralgia, stiffness, joint swelling, and effusion. Radiographic findings are diagnostic and include periostitis and subperiosteal new bone formation. Periarticular manifestations may precede radiographic findings by months. The arthropathy is usually chronic, with intermittent exacerbations at times of pulmonary exacerbations. Pathologically, there is edematous thickening of the periosteum, inflammatory periostitis, and subperiosteal new bone formation. On synovial biopsy, there is cellular infiltration, hyperplasia of synovial cells, and fibrosis. The pathogenesis of PHOA is obscure. Treatment with nonsteroidal antiinflammatory agents usually produces symptomatic improvement, and symptoms usually remit when lung disease is better controlled.

Episodic Arthritis

Transient episodic seronegative arthritis has been described in 1.5% to 5% of patients with CF and in up to 8.5% of adult patients. The most commonly affected joints in decreasing order of frequency are the knees, ankles, wrists, proximal interphalangeal joints of the hands, shoulders, elbows, and hips. The pattern may be monarticular, pauciarticular, or polyarticular. Episodes last from 1 to 10 days

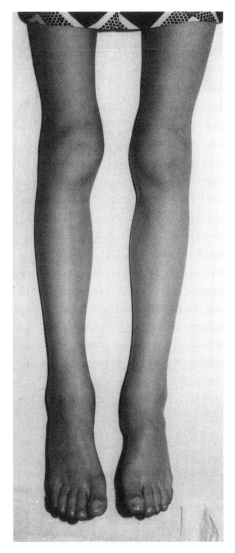

FIG. 6–6. Adolescent with cystic fibrosis and hypertrophic pulmonary osteoarthropathy, manifested as painful swelling of the distal ends of the long bones.

and recur at intervals ranging from several weeks to several months. Marked joint stiffness and deformity are rare. Episodes may be accompanied by low-grade fever, generalized or localized erythematous maculopapular rash, painful erythematous nodules over the anterior tibia (erythema nodosum), or vascular purpura over the lower extremities. In general, there is no relationship between the episodes of arthritis and the severity of the underlying pulmonary disease. There are reports, however, in which episodes of arthritis occurred in association with infectious respiratory exacerbations and improved with antibiotic therapy for the lung infection.

Positive laboratory findings include a moderately elevated sedimentation rate, detectable circulating immune complexes, and elevated immunoglobulin G (IgG) levels. These latter findings suggest an immune-mediated basis for the arthritis. Rheumatoid factor and antinuclear antibodies are not present. Radiographic studies are normal except for joint effusions and soft tissue swelling. Synovial biopsy shows nonspecific subacute synovitis; on immunofluorescent staining, there may be deposits of IgM, IgG, and complement components. Episodes usually respond to nonsteroidal antiinflammatory agents, although in some cases, a short course of glucocorticoids may be required.

Seropositive Rheumatoid Arthritis

Seropositive rheumatoid arthritis has been reported in several patients with CF, probably as a coincidental finding. The arthritis is progressive, sustained, and unassociated with rash.

Back Pain and Spinal Deformity

Recurring back pain is eventually present in most patients with CF and relates to the severity of the underlying pulmonary disease. Pain varies in intensity from mild to severe, and it affects both the mid and lower back. Episodes often occur in association with paroxysms of cough, position, and respiratory infection. Associated findings include decreased range of motion and muscle strength. Patients with CF often assume a kyphotic, hunched-over posture secondary to abdominal flexion, shoulder protraction, and increased anteroposterior chest diameter. Among patients older than 15 years of age, kyphosis is present in three-fourths of women and one-third of men. Radiographs of the spine may show apical vertebral wedging, probably related to underlying osteopenia. Postural abnormalities may be improved by appropriate exercises and postural counseling.

Osteopenia and Fractures

Osteopenia is well documented in CF patients. It may occur as early as the third decade and accelerates during adolescence and young adulthood. Men and women are affected equally. Dual energy x-ray absorptiometry (DEXA) scans show decreased lumbar spine, femoral neck, and whole-body mineralization consistent with a reduction in both cortical and trabecular bone mineral.

The pathogenesis of osteopenia in CF patients is not entirely clear, but it is likely that there is increased bone resorption and decreased bone formation. Potential contributory factors are reduced intestinal absorption of calcium and vitamin D, delayed and reduced production of sex steroids, use of glucocorticoids, reduced physical activity, advanced pulmonary disease, and increased concentrations of circulating osteoclast-activating factors. The relative importance of these factors probably varies from patient to patient. Low 25-hydroxy-vitamin D levels, delayed puberty, low testosterone levels in men and an increased incidence of primary and secondary amenorrhea are seen with increased frequency in patients with advanced osteopenia, but there are conflicting data regarding the correlation with disease severity and glucocorticoid use.

Clinically, there is an increased incidence of traumatic fractures among adult male and female CF patients and 6- to 16-year-old girls. There is also a high incidence of unrecognized vertebral compression and rib fractures and kyphosis in adult patients. Vertebral wedging and kyphosis contribute to diminished stature in adults with CF and probably account for the increased frequency of back pain. The fracture rate increases and kyphosis occurs at least three decades before it would normally be expected.

Preventive measures include maintaining good nutrition, minimizing long-term glucocorticoid use, encouraging physical activity and regular exercise, and maintaining normal serum levels of vitamin D. Higher than recommended daily allowances of vitamin D may be required. The efficacy of antiresorptive agents such as calcitonin or biphosphonates has not been assessed in CF patients. Testosterone has been shown to enhance bone mineral status in men with idiopathic hypogonadism, but its long-term efficacy in CF patients has not been determined.

REFERENCES

Cardiovascular Complications

Stern RC, Borkat G, Hirschfeld SS, et al. Heart failure in cystic fibrosis. *Am J Dis Child* 1980;134:267–272.

Endocrine-Metabolic

Beckerman RC, Taussig LM. Hypoelectrolytemia and metabolic alkalosis in infants with cystic fibrosis. *Pediatrics* 1979;63:580–583.
Huseman CA, Colombo JL, Brooks MA, et al. Anabolic effect of biosynthetic growth hormone in cystic fibrosis patients. *Pediatr Pulmonol* 1996;22:90–95.
Ruddy R, Anolik R, Scanlin TF. Hypoelectrolytemia as a presentation and complication of cystic fibrosis. *Clin Pediatr* 1982;21:367–369.

Renal Abnormalities

Abramowsky CR, Swinehart GL. The nephropathy of cystic fibrosis: A human model of chronic nephrotoxicity. *Hum Pathol* 1982;13:934–939.
Strandvik B, Hjeltel L. Nephrolithiasis in cystic fibrosis. *Acta Paediatr* 1993;82:306–307.

Female Reproductive Tract

Edenborough FP, Stableforth DE, Webb AK, et al. Outcome of pregnancy in women with cystic fibrosis. *Thorax* 1995;50:170–174.
Kotloff RM, FitzSimmons SC, Fiel SB. Fertility and pregnancy in patients with cystic fibrosis. *Clin Chest Med* 1992;13:623–635.

Stead RJ, Hodson ME, Batten JC, et al. Amenorrhoea in cystic fibrosis. *Clin Endocrinol* 1987;26:187–195.

Male Reproductive Tract

Anguiano A, Oates RD, Amos JA, et al. Congenital bilateral absence of the vas deferens. *JAMA* 1992;267:1794–1797.

Chillon M, Casals T, Mercier B, et al. Mutations in the cystic fibrosis gene in patients with congenital absence of the vas deferens. *N Engl J Med* 1995;332: 1475–1480.

Colin AA, Sawyer SM, Mickle JE, et al. Pulmonary function and clinical observations in men with congenital bilateral absence of the vas deferens. *Chest* 1996; 110:440–445.

Oates RD, Honig S, Berger MJ, Harris D. Microscopic epididymal sperm aspiration (MESA): A new option for treatment of the obstructive azoospermia associated with cystic fibrosis. *J Assist Reprod Genet* 1992;9:36–40.

Central Nervous System Complications

Roach ES, Sinal SH. Initial treatment of cystic-fibrosis: Frequency of transient bulging fontanel. *Clin Pediatr* 1989;28:371–373.

Ocular Complications

Spaide RF, Diamond G, D'Amico RA, et al. Ocular findings in cystic fibrosis. *Am J Opthalmol* 1987;103:204–210.

Musculoskeletal Abnormalities

Cohen AM, Yulish BS, Wasser KB, et al. Evaluation of pulmonary hypertrophic osteoarthropathy in cystic fibrosis. *Am J Dis Child* 1986;140:74–77.

Pertuiset E, Menkes CJ, Lenoir G, et al. Cystic fibrosis arthritis. A report of five cases. *Br J Rheumatol* 1992;31:535–538.

Rose J, Gamble J, Schultz A, Lewiston N. Back pain and spinal deformity in cystic fibrosis. *Am J Dis Child* 1987;141:1313–1316.

7

Exercise

The ability to perform muscular work—to exercise—is one of the key elements that contribute to one's quality of life. And impairment of stamina and strength is one important factor that diminishes quality of life as lung disease progresses in CF patients. Exercise can serve as an important diagnostic, prognostic, and therapeutic tool in CF patients, as well as being the medium for play, recreation, and employment for patients of all ages.

In this chapter, we review the response of CF patients to single bouts of exercise, their response to exercise in the heat, and their response to exercise programs. We then discuss exercise testing, exercise as therapy, and the relationship between exercise tolerance and prognosis.

EXERCISE TOLERANCE—RESPONSE TO SINGLE BOUTS OF EXERCISE

Cardiopulmonary Fitness

Patients with CF have a wide range of physical fitness as measured on exercise testing (Fig. 7–1). This should come as no surprise to anyone familiar with a cross-section of the CF population, because some patients are nearly bedridden and some are extremely athletic (CF patients have completed marathons and so-called Ironman-distance triathlons [2.4-mile swim, 112-mile bike race, 26.2-mile run]). As an entire population, CF patients have lower than normal fitness, measured as Physical Working Capacity or maximum oxygen consumption—$\dot{V}O_{2MAX}$—on a progressively increasing exercise test to exhaustion. For the whole population, fitness varies with resting pulmonary function, but there is tremendous interindividual variation, with a

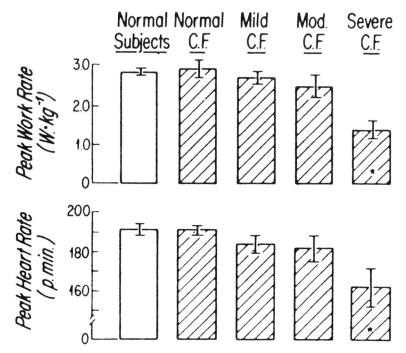

FIG. 7–1. Fitness of a group of CF patients with normal resting pulmonary function ("normal CF"), mildly, moderately, and severely compromised pulmonary function ("mild CF," "mod. CF," and "severe CF," respectively), compared with a group of normal resting children. Note the normal peak rate for the CF patients with normal resting pulmonary function, nearly normal work rate for those with mild pulmonary dysfunction, and progressively worse work rate for the more severely affected patients. Note too the normal heart rate for those with normal work tolerance, and the lower-than-normal peak heart rate in those who exercise a shorter time, before they have pushed their heart rates to the normal range. (From Cropp GJ, Pullano TP, Cerny FJ, Nathanion IT. Exercise tolerance and cardiorespiratory adjustments at peak work capacity in cystic fibrosis. *Am Rev Respir Dis* 1982;126:211–216, with permission.)

wide range of fitness levels for any given pulmonary function level. Once again, this finding corresponds to the everyday observation that some patients with fairly good pulmonary function seem unable to do very much, whereas others with poor pulmonary function carry a full load of school courses, captain the cheering squad, and dance into the wee hours.

Cardiovascular Responses

Patients with CF have normal cardiovascular responses to exercise, with appropriate increases in heart rate and appropriate blood pressure control during progressively more difficult workloads (Fig. 7–2).

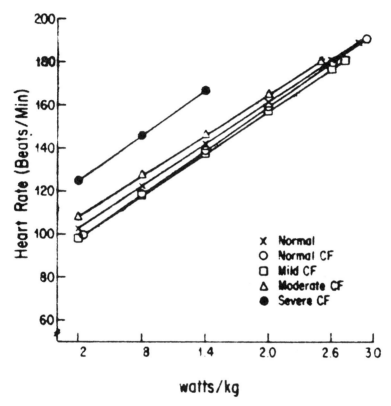

FIG. 7–2. Cardiovascular responses to progressively more difficult exercise (expressed as workload in watts per kg of body weight) among a group of CF patients with normal resting pulmonary function ("normal CF"), mildly, moderately, and severely compromised pulmonary function ("mild CF," "mod. CF," and "severe CF," respectively), compared with a group of normal, healthy children. Normal increase in heart rate with increasing workload in all groups. Patients with severe pulmonary dysfunction at rest have higher baseline heart rate, and lower peak workload, but a normal heart rate response. (From Cerney FJ, Pullano TP, Cropp GJA. Cardiorespiratory adaptations to exercise in cystic fibrosis. *Am Rev Respir Dis* 1982;126: 217–220, with permission.)

Patients with normal or near-normal pulmonary function have normal maximum heart rates for age. Patients with compromised lung function have lower than normal maximal heart rates, not because of a chronotropic abnormality, but because exercise is limited by pulmonary factors before the heart rate reaches normal maximum rates.

Ventilatory Responses

Minute ventilation increases with workload, as in normal, healthy subjects. However, patients with CF tend to use a higher minute ventilation for a given workload, presumably because of having greater than normal dead space—areas through which air moves but does not participate in gas exchange. This greater than normal ventilatory demand serves as the limiting factor for most patients with CF engag-

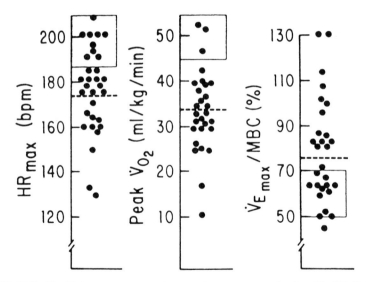

FIG. 7–3. Ventilatory responses to exercise among patients with CF. Data from maximal exercise testing in 31 patients with CF (normal ranges are delineated within the black borders). Minute ventilation ($\dot{V}_E$ max) at maximum exercise in many of these patients exceeded the normal 50–70% of resting maximum breathing capacity (MBC)(currently more often referred to as maximum voluntary ventilation, or MVV). Although a few patients had peak oxygen consumption ($\dot{V}_{O2}$) in the normal range, most were below normal, and most patients were limited in their exercise before they had pushed their heart rates into the normal maximum range.

ing in progressively more difficult exercise. At maximum exercise, most healthy subjects employ a minute ventilation ($\dot{V}_E$) somewhere between 50% and 70% of their resting maximum voluntary ventilation (MVV). In contrast, patients with CF may employ a $\dot{V}_E$ of 80% to 110% of MVV (Fig. 7–3). Patients cannot be expected to breathe more than their maximum capacity, so it is no wonder that when ventilation reaches these extremes, patients stop exercising, even if this occurs with a relatively low heart rate. Accordingly, the $\dot{V}_E$/MVV ratio is useful in evaluating an exercise test in CF patients, with values greater than 80% to 90% indicating a ventilatory limitation.

Gas Exchange

Oxygen. Most patients with CF, even those with severe pulmonary disease, can exercise without significantly affecting gas exchange. Oxygen levels usually do not decrease significantly. Some patients whose resting FEV_1 is below 50% of predicted values will desaturate with exercise (Fig. 7–4). Note in the figure that even among those patients with resting FEV_1 below 50% of predicted values, most do not desaturate. Note also that virtually no patient with an FEV_1 greater than 50% predicted desaturates. Therefore, it makes sense for patients with a resting FEV_1 below 50% of predicted values to have an exercise test before engaging in strenuous exercise in order to identify those patients who do desaturate and at what intensity of exercise (e.g., at what heart rate) the desaturation occurs. These patients can then be counseled to exercise at a lower intensity than the one at which desaturation occurred, or to use supplemental oxygen when they exercise.

Carbon Dioxide. In normal, healthy subjects, arterial and end-tidal carbon dioxide levels remain fairly constant until close-to-maximal exercise, at which point they may decrease slightly. Most CF patients follow this same pattern, with the exception of those who experience oxyhemoglobin desaturation with exercise; these patients almost invariably have slightly elevated carbon dioxide levels. Thus, even though their minute ventilation is relatively high for a given workload, they are hypoventilating.

Supplemental Oxygen for Exercise. Patients who desaturate while breathing room air during exercise can accomplish the same exercise without desaturation, if they exercise with supplemental oxygen. Dur-

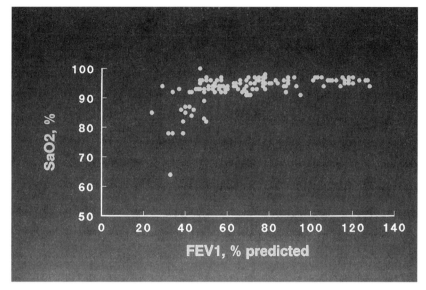

FIG. 7–4. Oxygenation at peak exercise in patients with CF. No patients with resting FEV$_1$ > 50% predicted had oxyhemoglobin saturation below 90% at peak exercise. Even most patients with resting FEV$_1$ < 50% predicted maintain oxygenation at peak exercise, but some of these patients do desaturate during exercise.

ing exercise with supplemental oxygen, they require lower minute ventilation and lower heart rate for each workload. The extra oxygen may or may not enable them to reach a higher maximal workload on a progressive exercise challenge to exhaustion, but it makes less-than-maximal exercise easier and safer. And, although the progressive exercise test to exhaustion has become the gold standard for assessing cardiopulmonary fitness, it does not represent the type of exercise most people engage in, so the results with submaximal workloads are much more relevant to everyday life.

EXERCISE IN THE HEAT

Single Session of Exercise and Heat Stress

It has been recognized for more than 50 years that patients with CF can have difficulty in the heat. It was the recognition that many babies with CF suffered heat exhaustion during the heat wave of 1948 that led to the discovery of the CF sweat defect. A number of studies have confirmed that CF patients are at greater risk for heat illness because of greater than normal salt loss. Patients have normal cardiovascular and hormonal responses to exercise in the heat, and have normal core body temperatures and heart rates, but they continue to lose sweat that is high in sodium and chloride, leading to hypochloremia (if they drink water during these stresses). They have normal renal salt preservation, but it is not adequate to make up for the excessive sweat electrolyte losses. CF patients also underestimate their fluid needs during exercise in the heat and, given a choice of how much to drink, will drink less than they need. This underestimation ("voluntary hypohydration") is probably explained as follows: one of the main thirst stimuli in normal, healthy subjects is a relative hemoconcentration that comes about with loss of hypotonic sweat. CF patients lose a much more concentrated sweat, and therefore, their intravascular volume is close to isotonic, thus robbing them of an important hypothalamic stimulus to drinking. Despite their poor sense of fluid and salt losses during exercise in the heat, CF patients have superb regulatory sense between such bouts and choose intake exactly appropriate to replace fluid and electrolytes. So patients with CF should be encouraged to drink more fluid than they think they need during prolonged exercise in the heat, ideally with an electrolyte-rich sport drink such as Gatorade, AllSport, or PowerAde, and they should not be restricted from taking as much salt as they want at other times (the rare exceptions being those in frank heart or liver failure with ascites). Salt tablets are neither effective nor needed.

Heat Acclimatization

With repeated bouts of exercise in the heat, over 7 to 14 days, normal, healthy subjects develop certain adjustments in their response to exercise and heat stress: They have a lower heart rate and lower core body temperature for an equal challenge, they have earlier onset of sweating, and their sweat is more dilute. CF patients can also adjust to repeated bouts of exercise in the heat. They, too, have lower heart rate and lower core body temperature during peak exercise, but they do not alter their sweat composition. They still lose significantly more sodium and chloride in their sweat than their non-CF peers. It is not known if they have earlier onset of sweating with acclimatization.

EXERCISE TESTING

Among diagnostic modalities, exercise testing is probably one of the most underused (see also Appendix B, Laboratory Testing). Formal exercise testing may give the best measure of overall health (see below, Exercise Tolerance and Prognosis), incorporating at least pulmonary, cardiac, and musculoskeletal function, and depending additionally on nutritional and even motivational factors, all of which must be important for length and quality of life. Additionally, exercise testing is particularly important for patients with more severe pulmonary dysfunction before they embark on an exercise program. This test can identify which patients desaturate during exercise and can identify the level of intensity of exercise (heart rate) at which the oxygen level drops. A repeat test can document progress from the program. An exercise test can help determine factors that may or may not contribute to exercise intolerance or exercise-related symptoms, including fatigue, shortness of breath, cough, and chest pain. In different patients, these factors can include deconditioning, exercise-induced asthma, ventilatory limitations of CF lung disease, and cardiac dysfunction. On occasion, an exercise test might show changes in exercise tolerance, even in the absence of pulmonary function changes.

EXERCISE PROGRAMS

Numerous studies since the early 1980's have tested the effects of various kinds of exercise programs for patients with CF, including upper body exercise (canoeing, swimming) and sustained isocapnic hyperventilation, jogging, swimming, combined aerobic exercises, and weight training. Various benefits, including improved ventilatory muscle strength and endurance, improved work tolerance, improved cardiopulmonary fitness (measured as maximum oxygen consumption, $\dot{V}O_{2MAX}$), and decreased dyspnea, have been documented from aerobic exercise programs (rhythmic exercise that is sustained over 15 to 30 minutes or longer, and repeated several times per week, such as swimming, jogging, bicycling, and the like). A weight-training program has been shown to increase strength and weight. In no study has a detrimental effect been shown. However, in quite a few studies, unsupervised programs have had little or no effect, and like exercise programs in the general population or other disease populations, there are high drop-out rates.

Effect on Pulmonary Function

Most studies have shown no effect on resting pulmonary function, but several have shown improvements in expiratory flow rates during the program, with prompt return to the preprogram baseline after the program has ended. The weight-training program demonstrated a decrease in trapped gas. No program has resulted in worse pulmonary function.

EXERCISE AS THERAPY

The exact role of exercise in CF therapy is still unclear. It is clear that exercise can improve patients' exercise tolerance: Patients can usually do more after an exercise program than before. As noted earlier, pulmonary function may or may not improve during an exercise program. Skeletal muscle strength can improve, and the most important skeletal muscles, namely, the ventilatory muscles, can increase strength and endurance. The main question usually asked is whether exercise has a useful role in airway clearance, and here, the answer is controversial. Airway mucus clearance is greater with exercise than at rest but not as good as with traditional chest physical therapy (and presumably, therefore, not as good as with any of the newer airway clearance techniques such as Flutter, percussive vest, or PEP mask). Thus, the idea that exercise obviates the need for mucus clearance is false. However, teenagers who will not do any of the standard airway clearance techniques are better off if they exercise than if they do not, but they would be better off still with exercise and airway clearance.

RELATIONSHIP BETWEEN EXERCISE TOLERANCE AND PROGNOSIS

There is some suggestion that exercise tolerance improves the prognosis in patients with CF. Causality is difficult to establish, but there is a striking and statistically significant correlation between fitness measured on an exercise test and survival—a correlation that is stronger for exercise than for virtually any other parameter, including pulmonary function and nutrition. One hundred patients were divided in tertiles based on exercise test results, and they were followed for 8 years. Patients in the top tertile were more than three times likely to survive 8 years than those in the less fit groups. It is not clear what it is about fitness that confers this improved prognosis, and it is possible that it is not fitness itself but rather that fitness serves as a marker for overall integrated health, incorporating aspects of pulmonary, cardiac, musculoskeletal, nutritional, and even psychological health. Regardless of the explanation, the correlation between fitness and survival is striking.

DESIGNING AN EXERCISE PROGRAM

Whether an exercise program is intended to improve airway clearance, boost ventilatory muscle function, keep patients lively and active, or even improve prognosis, there are certain guidelines that can help establish a successful program (Table 7–1). For a program to be successful, it must be sustained and therefore should be enjoyable. The particular forms of exercise should be ones that the patient has access to and enjoys. A swimming program will not work if there is no ready access to a pool or lake during the whole year. Running can be excellent, but arrangements must be made to ensure the patient's safety if the running is to done before or after school, when it might be dark, and footing is uneven, especially if there is ice. Roads need to have generous shoulders or sidewalks, and joggers need to wear bright, reflective clothing. These considerations also apply to a biking pro-

TABLE 7–1. *Designing an Exercise Program*

---

1. Preprogram exercise test (required for those with FEV_1 <50% predicted, unless supplemental oxygen is being prescribed empirically)
2. Select the exercise or exercises to be used.
3. "FIT" (frequency, intensity, time)
    Frequency:
        3–5 times per week
    Intensity
        'pleasantly tired' (see text)
        70%–85% of patient's own maximum heart rate
    Time
        1st week: 10 minutes
        2nd week: 12 minutes
        3rd week: 14 minutes
Safety:
    Follow the same safety guidelines as would apply to non-CF patients,
    plus always have a companion for anyone exercising with
    supplemental oxygen; be sensible about avoiding overexertion

---

gram, although a stationary bike can provide a safe substitute for road biking, and one that provides protection from extremes of weather. Exercise on pieces of apparatus such as stationary bikes, stair-steppers, rowing machines, or treadmills is excellent, safe, weather-irrelevant, and at least potentially boring. The boredom of these forms of exercise can be decreased considerably by placing the apparatus in front of the TV or VCR, or having the patient listen to music on headphones. Another way to fight boredom is to vary the form of exercise used; for example, jogging can be alternated with stair-stepping.

Children are more likely to sustain an exercise program if exercise is valued in the family. Having family members share exercise time can be beneficial on several levels, including the increased chance that the child will continue to exercise.

Pre-conditioning Exercise Test

Exercise testing should be done for any CF patient whose FEV_1 is less than 50% predicted, in order to identify the patient who desaturates with exercise, and the heart rate at which the desaturation occurs, to prescribe exercise intensity below that associated with desaturation, or to prescribe supplemental oxygen for use during the training sessions. Alternatively, any patient with marginal pulmonary function (especially those with resting hypoxemia) can be given oxygen for exercise, even without pretesting. The preconditioning exercise test can also be used as a baseline against which to compare values periodically during the ensuing months and years, to document improved—and then sustained—fitness.

The exercise sessions should be carried out at least three times a week. More is better, but seven times a week is too much. It is important for injury prevention to take at least 1 day off each week for recovery. Some people—especially adults—will find that they do better if they take a day off after each day that they exercise.

Some experts recommend beginning each session with gentle warm up and stretching for a few minutes. The main portion of the exercise session should then begin at a comfortable intensity. Walking or jogging very easily is a good way to start each running session, before increasing the intensity to that which will be sustained for the bulk of the exercise time. That intensity can be prescribed with a heart rate range (typically 70% to 85% of the patient's maximum heart rate, as measured in the preconditioning maximal exercise test, not a predicted maximum heart rate based on normals). Many CF patients have maximum heart rates considerably below those predicted for healthy subjects their age, and their prescribed exercise intensity would be too great if based on normal predicted values. We have found that exercise intensity based on the subjective feeling of "pleasantly tired" works just as well. This indicator usually correlates with the heart rate range with this intensity. Patients are told to aim for that feeling; if they feel just pleasant, they need to work harder; if they feel just tired, they should reduce the intensity of the exercise. For a jogging program, this intensity is likely to correspond to starting out with jogging until they feel more tired than pleasant, then walking for a while to reestablish the pleasant and tired balance, then resuming jogging. As the patients become more fit, and particularly as younger children learn the concept of pacing themselves, they will be able to jog for the entire session.

The main part of the session should last about 30 minutes, but most people are not ready to start out at 30 minutes. Rather, 10 minutes is a good starting time, with gradual increases. For people who need explicit guidance, the main part of the session should increase by 2 minutes each week until reaching 30 minutes. For example, the patient will walk and jog for 10 minutes three or four times the first week, for 12 minutes the second week, 14 the third week, and so on.

REFERENCES

Asher MI, et al. The effects of inspiratory muscle training in patients with cystic fibrosis. *Am Rev Respir Dis* 1982;126:855–859.

Bar-Or O, et al. Voluntary dehydration and heat intolerance in cystic fibrosis. *Lancet* 1992:339:696–699.

Cerny FJ, Pullano TP, and Cropp GJ. Cardiorespiratory adaptations to exercise in cystic fibrosis. *Am Rev Respir Dis* 1982;126: 217–220.

Cropp GJ, et al. Exercise tolerance and cardiorespiratory adjustments at peak work capacity in cystic fibrosis. *Am Rev Respir Dis* 1986;126:211–216.

di Sant' Agnese PA, et al. Abnormal electrolyte composition of sweat in cystic fibrosis of the pancreas. *Pediatrics* 1953;12:549–563.

Edlund LD, et al. Effects of a swimming program on children with cystic fibrosis. *Am J Dis Child* 1986;140:80–83.

Heijerman HGM, et al. Oxygen-assisted exercise training in adult cystic fibrosis patients with pulmonary limitation to exercise. *Int J Rehabil Res* 1991;14: 101–115.

Henke KG, Orenstein DM. Oxygen saturation during exercise in cystic fibrosis. *Am Rev Respir Dis* 1984;129:708–711.

Keens TG, et al. Ventilatory muscle endurance training in normal subjects and patients with cystic fibrosis. *Am Rev Respir Dis* 1977;116:853–860.

Nixon PA, et al. The prognostic value of exercise testing in patients with cystic fibrosis. *N Engl J Med* 1992;327:1785–1788.

Nixon PA, et al. Oxygen supplementation during exercise in cystic fibrosis. *Am Rev Respir Dis* 1990;142:807–811.

Orenstein DM. *Cystic fibrosis: a guide for patient and family,* 2nd ed. Philadelphia: Lippincott-Raven, 1997.

Orenstein DM. Exercise tolerance and exercise conditioning in children with chronic lung disease. *J Pediatr* 1988;112:1043–1047.

Orenstein DM, Henke KG, Green CG. Heat acclimation in cystic fibrosis. *J Appl Physiol* 1984;57:408–412.

Orenstein DM, Nixon PA. Exercise performance and breathing patterns in cystic fibrosis: male-female differences and influence of resting pulmonary function. *Pediatr Pulmonol* 1991;10:101–105.

Orenstein DM, et al. Exercise conditioning and cardiopulmonary fitness in cystic fibrosis. The effects of a three-month supervised running program. *Chest* 1981; 80:392–398.

Orenstein DM, et al. Exercise and heat stress in cystic fibrosis patients. *Pediatr Res* 1983;17:267–269.

Salh W, et al. Effect of exercise and physiotherapy in aiding sputum expectoration in adults with cystic fibrosis. *Thorax* 1989;44:1006–1008.

Sawyer EH, Clanton TL. Improved pulmonary function and exercise tolerance with inspiratory muscle conditioning in children with cystic fibrosis. *Chest* 1993;104: 1490–1497.

Zach M, Oberwaldner B, and Hausler F. Cystic fibrosis: physical exercise versus chest physiotherapy. *Arch J Dis Child* 1982;57:587–589.

Zach MS, Purrer B, and Oberwaldner B. Effect of swimming on forced expiration and sputum clearance in cystic fibrosis. *Lancet* 1981;ii:1201–1203.

Zach MS, Oberwaldner B. Influence of a swimming program on the lung function status of children with cystic fibrosis [Letter]. *Am J Dis Child* 1986;140:9.

8
Hospitalization

INDICATIONS

Philosophy

Hospital admission is indicated if the short-term and long-term health and economic advantages outweigh the immediate inconvenience, risks, and expense. Severity of illness is a factor but may not be decisive: A very ill, perhaps terminal, patient may be appropriately managed at home, whereas an energetic, virtually asymptomatic newly diagnosed 3-year-old child (and his or her family) may greatly benefit from hospitalization to initiate a comprehensive treatment program. Patients with theoretically identical medical situations may differ considerably in their need for hospitalization: The 23-year-old patient with moderate lung disease and many prior episodes of hemoptysis may deserve hospitalization if he or she lives alone and far from family; the same patient with a strong family support system may be able to be followed at home.

Types of Admission

Categories of admission criteria are shown in Table 8–1. It is not possible to list every possible admission criterion and its modifiers. For some, the need for hospitalization is obvious and absolute (e.g., those with massive hemoptysis). For others, there will be variations among centers, as well as among patients and physicians (e.g., initiation and regulation of home oxygen) even within the same center. Unfortunately, an algorithm that accurately identifies all CF patients

TABLE 8–1. *Categories of Admission Criteria (With Examples)*

1. Failure of outpatient treatment to bring
   a. Resolution of pulmonary symptoms
   b. Improvement in pulmonary function test results
2. Possibility of rapid progression or development or recurrence of a dangerous complication
   A. Pneumothorax
   B. Intussusception
   C. Hyponatremic dehydration
3. Need for close observation (e.g., hemoptysis)
4. Use of a dangerous drug or treatment (e.g., intravenous colistin)
5. Surgery and/or pre- and postperative stabilization for surgery management
6. Terminal care (often best done in hospital)
7. Rapid deterioration (multiorgan failure)
8. Observation of an (e.g., puzzling abdominal pain) unusual complaint
9. Serious concurrent illness (e.g., influenza or diabetes)
10. Low-level danger (e.g., adult who lives alone) but high-risk patient

who should (and should not) be admitted would be extremely difficult to create.

Insurance Considerations

The primary goal of medical care should be to optimize short-term and long-term survival, comfort, and function by using the safest, cheapest, easiest, and least invasive methods. As medical costs rise, however, third-party payors increasingly search for short-term economy with minimal legal risk.

For example, a newly diagnosed infant may have treatment initiated as an outpatient, even if the physician suspects that the parents do not fully grasp the implications of the diagnosis. Even though they may obediently return for the outpatient instruction sessions, they will be too insecure and overwhelmed to provide optimal care. Short-term savings have been achieved at a high long-term price.

This example illustrates the long-term destructive effect of short-term economy when a patient with cystic fibrosis who has much to gain by preservation of good health is denied hospitalization.

Another example is the noncompliant patient who needs intravenous (IV) antibiotics but is not admitted (or is discharged early), thus risking both an unsatisfactory immediate outcome and the emergence of resistant organisms.

Although the infrastructure on which home treatment rests has improved, the concepts underlying the admission decision should remain unchanged. The newly diagnosed infant may not be admitted for economic reasons, but that should not change how physicians think; the physician should not conclude from the denial by the insurance company that, ". . . well, all things considered, maybe the patient really is better off at home." In the absence of new treatment (which makes home treatment better or safer) or new knowledge (e.g., the risk of a complication is less than previously thought), the real indications for admission do not change. Both psychosocial and medical issues (as well as economics) must be weighed in the decision.

GENERAL CARE

Physician Continuity

Patient satisfaction is enhanced and medical care is almost always better if the patient's usual outpatient physician is also his or her inpatient attending physician as well. Outpatients often choose their regular physicians, whereas inpatients may be assigned to a team. Arguments to the contrary, for example, "It often works to the patient's advantage if another physician (or group of physicians) thinks about your case as well" or "The inpatient physicians are not subject to distraction from outpatients" may have some validity, but few would honestly argue that discontinuity is intrinsically better. Much of the enormous amount that the physician knows about each of his or her patients is never recorded. If the center's operation precludes physician continuity, the patient should be assured that steps have been taken to ensure that all important information has been transferred to the attending physician and that the initial inpatient care has been determined, in large part, by the admitting (outpatient) physician.

The Need for Instruction on How To Be a Successful Hospital Patient

Patients and their families who are not familiar with hospital routine benefit from a comprehensive course that is taught by the physician or nurse coordinator, covering basic facts, helpful hints, patient rights, and patient resources. For elective admissions, this process can occasionally be done several days in advance; usually, however, the need for admission is relatively sudden, and this course should be completed simultaneously with the institution of hospital care or on the next day. If a critical pathway (care map) is in place, this can be a useful tool to review hospital procedures and expectations. Some topics to be covered in the course are shown in Table 8–2.

Psychosocial Issues

Common Psychosocial Concerns. Although many patients and families do not initiate discussion about psychosocial matters, some are nearly universal. These problems can be of equal immediate importance to the patient as the medical complication that has resulted in admission. A family may feel isolated because they do not consider the possibility that the medical team can help with their psychosocial concerns.

The medical team should explore the impact of the admission on the patient's nonmedical life, for example, school or work issues, social responsibilities, guilt about inconveniencing family members, and loss of privacy about the diagnosis. At the least, the team can be sympathetic. In many cases, the patient can benefit from a discussion of how other families have addressed the problem, and on occasion, the problem can be solved completely (and simply) by a letter from the center physician or other administrative action.

Other common psychosocial problems are hospital or illness-based, for example, concerns about the prognostic meaning of the need for hospitalization or rehospitalization, precipitation (or reactivation) of fears about death and dying (perhaps following a death, whether of a CF patient or not, on the ward), concerns about being labeled as a carrier of a dangerous pathogen, perhaps resulting in iso-

TABLE 8–2. *How To Be a Well-Adjusted and Successful Hospital Patient*

Topic	Examples of material to be covered
Personnel	Who's who in the hospital. Categories of personnel (e.g., those involved with direct and essential patient care) versus those who are more peripheral, including those who are doing research or who are involved with administrative issues, such as insurance status. Role of the Attending physician as opposed to Consultants. Role of housestaff and fellows.
Physician's orders	How treatments and drugs get from the doctor's mind to the patient's body, and examples of how errors can be made, and how they are minimized.
Other hospital routines	Appropriate use or collection of vital signs, weights, calorie counts, intake and output, routine blood tests, etc.
Painful procedures	IVs; ABGs; etc. What degree of analgesia should the patient expect? Should the patient watch the procedure or look away? Who performs procedures, and how many attempts are reasonable?
Risks of hospitalization	Medical risks: Treatment/medication errors; contagion; sleep deprivation. Psychosocial risks: Bad habits (e.g., contact with noncompliant patients); exposure to death and awareness of dying patients; falling behind in school-work or job, kidnapping or random violence; theft.
Nonmedical benefits	Learning to cope with disease and learning to interact with medical personnel. For children, learning to survive without a parent present. Learning about how hospitals work. Exposure to people at work—possibly influencing choice of career.
Intravenous lines and treatment	1. Why IVs are needed; 2. Risks of having an IV line; 3. Nonrisks of having an IV line (e.g., unlikeliness of dying of a "bubble of air"; if a gravity-driven IV runs dry, air will not rush into the vein, and neither will large quantities of blood back up and fill the IV bottle; 4. Why people "run out of veins"—advantages and disadvantages of central venous lines; 5. Variability of vein quality between patients is not correlated to cystic fibrosis health status; 6. Variability of insertion skill is not directly correlated to other aspects of physician skill or knowledge.
Insurance issues	Who is responsible for what? Hospital or center personnel are available to help family.
Maintaining school or career	Not only does this ease the transition back to "real life," but it conveys an important message: the medical establishment believes that the patient is going to improve and resume normal activities.

lation measures. These issues are more obvious to medical personnel who may even be able to anticipate them and intercede proactively.

The Patient and Family Attempts To Prolong Hospitalization. The possibility of Munchausen's syndrome (or Munchausen's syndrome by proxy) should be considered for any patient whose course takes unexpected turns (with many new complications and complaints), all of which delay discharge. However, the absence of serious psychopathology does not exclude the possibility of a psychosocial obstacle to successful medical care (or hospital discharge). For example, the child whose hospital life is better than his or her chaotic home social situation may be making a perfectly sane decision to prolong the hospital stay. School phobia may present with puzzling medical complaints that lead to hospitalization.

Some patients who have supplemental hospitalization insurance that pays (the patient) by the day may attempt to prolong their stay as well. This may be inappropriate and dishonest, but it is not overt psychopathology.

Drug Abuse. CF patients are by no means immune to recreational drug use and overt addiction. In fact, they may be at increased risk for these problems. In addition to the possibility of social use of alcohol, marijuana, and cocaine, they have access to medical equipment, are often not reticent about performing procedures on themselves, and may have substantial medical or social problems from which they would like to escape.

Unexpected requests for narcotics (especially for specific drugs), the sudden onset of a new problem (e.g., renal colic) on the first day of hospitalization, and resistance to the discontinuation of opiates several days after surgery warrant sympathetic, but probing, investigation. IV drug abuse should be considered in patients who have IV access devices and who repeatedly request oral antiemetics and antihistamines but who never swallow the capsules in the presence of the nurse.

For relatively well patients, opiate addiction is a serious impediment to health and is well worth confronting and treating. These patients can devote almost all their mental energy to the combined goals of concealing their addiction and maintaining their drug supply. On the other hand, opiate addiction is unavoidable in a small number of CF patients, including those with recurrent severe pancreatitis or those who are discovered to be addicted but are believed to be too sick to withstand the rigors of withdrawal.

Group Meetings. Support group meetings with patients and their families and facilitators are widely advocated and often attempted. Unfortunately, the benefit of such meetings is infrequent at best and is extremely unlikely, unless (a) the leader or facilitator is experienced and a regular member of the CF team (as opposed to a psychology, social work, or postgraduate nursing student who is rotating through the service); (b) patient and family attendance (and continued attendance) is optional, and no one is coaxed to attend; and (c) the meetings occur at off hours so that interruption for procedures or rounds is minimized.

Establishing Rapport. Rapport and trust are the factors that physicians depend on to elicit accurate historical information and achieve optimal compliance. Unfortunately, no one can earn the patient's trust without some personal investment of time and effort. Child life personnel have no trouble building trust by providing companionship and play, but the doctor does not derive much from that relationship. Hospital services (e.g., daily newspaper, computer hook-ups) help hospital public relations, but again, they do not do much for the physician/patient relationship.

Competence, empathy, and honesty are critical to building patient/physician trust, but spending time (and especially leisure time) with the patient is best. However, not much time is needed. Minimal play with a young child, a joke, or magic trick for an older child or teenager, and sports talk for just about anyone can be as important to medical care as up-to-date medical knowledge.

Depression. In view of ample reasons to be depressed, for example, failing health or disability and the likelihood of death at an early age, deteriorating physical appearance, economic worries, and new complications (such as diabetes), it is amazing that clinically important depression (and even suicide) is not more common in patients with CF. Although it is easy to diagnose depression when the patient complains of being depressed, sad, or suicidal, it is important to consider the diagnosis for less subtle but equally common manifestations, such as insomnia, inability to concentrate, and anorexia. Psychotherapeutic intervention may be helpful, but pharmacologic treatment is often extremely effective and can be used safely if it is properly monitored. All hospitalized children should be encouraged to dress in their everyday street clothes, but depressed patients may also benefit from therapeutic leaves of absence (with reasons clearly documented in the chart).

Medical Issues

Contagion. There are now incontrovertible epidemiologic data indicating that the acquisition of *Burkholderia cepacia* is a risk factor for mortality and morbidity, and there is equally solid evidence that noncolonized CF patients can acquire the pathogen from infected CF patients. Although the exact mechanism of transmission remains unknown, there are also good data supporting the effectiveness of physical separation of these patients in the hospital. Ideally, this goal is achieved by having them on separate wards (although still using [if appropriate and at different times] certain common facilities, such as the elevators, cafeteria, pulmonary function laboratory, and radiology). If this is not possible, the patient with *B. cepacia* should be isolated in a single room, and the use of a contact precaution (gown-and-glove technique) by medical personnel should be mandatory.

Similar data do not exist, at least as of now, for other multiply resistant gram-negative pathogens (e.g., *Stenotrophomonas maltophilia, Alcaligenes xylosoxidans*) or for nontuberculous mycobacteria. However, some centers use some isolation measures to protect patients with relatively susceptible *Pseudomonas aeruginosa* from those whose organisms are multiply resistant. Patients who do not harbor any gram-negative pathogens (including pseudomonas) should be protected, to the greatest extent possible, from other CF patients.

Some centers have adopted universal contagion control practices for all CF patients to avoid stigmatizing those known to be infected with certain "bad" organisms and to avoid exposing patients to organisms not yet isolated from other patients' previous cultures. These practices typically include rules against CF patients rooming together and require them to wear masks and use handwashing when they visit each other or go to a community area together (teen lounge, playroom, cafeteria).

Management of patients with methicillin-resistant *Staphylococcus aureus* (MRSA) and vancomycin-resistant enterococci should follow Centers for Disease Control and Prevention (CDC) and local hospital guidelines. These organisms usually do not pose a major health threat to CF patients, but MRSA lung infections can be difficult to treat.

Maintenance of Immunization Schedules. In general, subspecialists and their clinics try not to intrude on routine well-child care. However, the large number of immunizations now required by normal children almost necessitates that the schedule be maintained if an infant with CF is hospitalized for more than a few days. Prolonged interruption may result in having to restart a series, and equally important, many of the diseases these immunizations prevent (e.g., pertussis, rubeola, haemophilus influenzae B (HiB)) are pulmonary diseases that could be harmful to a CF patient, especially one who is already sick enough to require hospitalization during infancy.

Non-CF Medical Issues. Just because a problem is not related to CF does not mean that it will not drain mental and physical energy and therefore impede recovery. Any substantive complaint, that is, one that causes pain, loss of function, and substantial anxiety should be investigated and treated as definitively as possible. A relatively trivial problem (e.g., worsening acne in a teenager), if not appropriately addressed, may prompt the patient to request discharge before the indication for his or her CF admission has been adequately treated.

Fever. Transient fever should be assessed and treated as it would be in a patient without CF. Persistent fever (lasting over several days) without an obvious localizing symptom or sign (other than the patient's usual pulmonary symptoms) merits additional investigation. Some CF-related causes are shown in Table 8–3. Epstein-Barr virus (EBV) infection (mononucleosis) is a common cause of fever, and its course is often somewhat atypical (e.g., lacking pharyngitis or splenomegaly, or both).

Effective Patient and Family Communication About Medical Issues. Without effective communication, even the best therapeutic plan is likely to fail. Some common pitfalls and suggested solutions are listed in Table 8–4.

TABLE 8–3. *Causes of Fever in Cystic Fibrosis Patients**

1. Related to Cystic Fibrosis Pulmonary Disease
   A. Fever due to otherwise uncomplicated, but severe, cystic fibrosis (CF) pulmonary infection (e.g., with *Pseudomonas aeruginosa* and/or *Staphylococcus aureus*). This problem is not common but does occur occasionally.
   B. New onset *Burkholderia cepacia* (and, less commonly, *Stenotrophomonas maltophilia*) infection. Should be evident from culture results.
   C. Infection with atypical mycobacteria. Colonization with these organisms is common; infection is uncommon. Most patients with convincing evidence for infection have a positive AFB smear as well as a positive culture.
   D. Pulmonary fungal infections. More likely in patients on systemic corticosteroids and with central venous access devices, but can occur in other patients. This problem is not a common cause of fever in cystic fibrosis.
2. Unrelated to Cystic Fibrosis Pulmonary Disease
   A. Infection of central venous access device (e.g., Mediport). Usually very high daily fever. Blood cultures usually yield *Staphylococcus epidermidis* and/or yeast within a couple of days of incubation. However, culture may not reveal bacteria because of antibiotic treatment.
   B. Brain abscess. Rare in CF but more common than in general population. Usually due to streptococci. Headache is almost always present; localizing neurologic findings may not be present.
   C. Chronic partially treated abscess. Chronic appendicitis and periappendiceal abscess are common in CF, and presentations are atypical (vomiting, constipation, history of periumbilical pain, etc., may all be absent, and the patient may not be discernibly anorectic).
   D. Vasculitis and collagen disease appear to have an increased incidence in CF patients. Workup and management is similar to that for non-CF patients except that some routine laboratory tests (e.g., erythrocyte sedimentation rate [1] (ESR)) may not be as helpful in CF.
   E. Drug fever, usually from a drug begun after admission.

*The items in this table relate directly or indirectly to CF. Obviously, the patient can have any non-CF cause of fever, and the usual age-appropriate differential diagnosis of fever of uncertain origin should be considered in the workup.

Recruitment for Research Projects and Protection From Research Abuses. Important pathophysiologic and therapeutic studies are being proposed with increasing frequency since the discovery of the CFTR gene. It is clearly in everyone's best interest for the CF center director and the patient's CF physician to select the best subjects for

TABLE 8–4. *Pitfalls in Patient and Family Communication*

Pitfall or Error	Preventive Action
1. Attempting communication of complex information while standing. The patient and family concludes (often correctly) that the informant is in a hurry and will not be patient if they do not understand the material immediately.	1. Sit down. 2. Use diagrams (see below).
2. Attempting communication of complex information to parents in the presence of the young child or infant patient. This may occasionally be unavoidable but is always suboptimal. If the patient is "sick," such a meeting is almost totally worthless.	1. Get help from a child life worker, nurse or another family member.
3. Failure to draw and use diagrams. Visual aids are essential. Preprinted diagrams are often less effective (and much less personal) than a diagram drawn for or in the presence of the patient or family. Extraneous information can be omitted, and the patient and family has something to take home and look at later.	1. Draw diagrams that family or patient can take home.
4. Using medical terms without definition and/or using medical terms incorrectly and/or inappropriate ambiguous (or undefined) layman's language. Once the educator has said "alveolus" or "gas exchange" without explanation, she or he has lost the battle. Once the educator calls an acute gastrointestinal illness the flu, it will be understandably difficult to convince that patient to get influenza vaccine the next year (since it obviously failed this year). Once one person calls "intensive IV antibiotic treatment" (the correct and unambiguous term), a "clean-out," the same term cannot be used by another medical person to indicate bronchoscopy and lavage.	1. Use correct medical terms. 2. Be sure the listener understands your meaning.
5. Failure to explain normal (physiology) before abnormal (pathophysiology). Surprisingly few people, even high school (and college) graduates, know very much about the inside of the body!	1. Give the 1-minute course in normal physiology before launching into the explanation of the abnormal.
6. Failure to cover the usual patient and family concerns or failure to allow time for questions. "What do I have, and how was the diagnosis made?" "What is the prognosis with and without treatment?" "What is your medical recommendation?" "How (genetics/infection/accident) and why (is it my or someone else's fault) did I get it?" "How much will treatment cost, and does the treatment hurt?"	1. Answer the "universal questions."
7. Different information from different members of the team. Difficult to prevent but very disconcerting to patients and families.	1. Coordinate your communication efforts. 2. Limit the number of persons who can give information.
8. Failure to seize on the optimal moment for communication. For example, discussion of an acutely worse prognosis (e.g., after a pneumothorax or after the onset of hypercapnia) is best delayed until the patient is getting better (even if improvement is expected to be temporary). Or failure to discuss death (whether it be imminent or remote in time) when the patient brings up the subject. Although presentation of medical information to outpatients is often appropriate, there is obviously less leeway with regard to timing in the outpatient setting.	1. The "right" moment for the patient is not always the best time for the doctor, but it is wise to make every effort to use it.

approved protocols and to participate in their recruitment. Also, it is important that the CF patient volunteers for important studies, particularly if he or she is one of a very limited pool who meet the criteria for entry.

On the other hand, it is also important that the patient feels confident that he or she will not be deceived into participating in so-called fluff experiments with questionable science or unimportant goals. Some fluff experiments may be important for education or other purposes, but patients who are recruited for them should be told that the likelihood of the project directly benefitting them or helping in the elucidation of pathophysiology is minimal. Patients should be recruited only for studies that have been approved by an institutional review board.

VENIPUNCTURE, VENOUS ACCESS, AND ARTERIAL BLOOD SAMPLING

Maintaining Venipuncture Sites

Chemical analysis of blood samples is by far the most common source of laboratory data in medicine. However, considering the dominant role of blood tests in both diagnosis and treatment, surprisingly little attention is given to maintaining easily accessible venipuncture sites in patients with a chronic illness. All medical personnel who are responsible for obtaining blood samples readily understand the problems faced by patients with poor peripheral veins.

CF centers should have specific policies directed at maintaining these veins. Antecubital veins should never be used for infusion or IV injections unless failure to do so would create (or fail to treat) an emergent problem and substantial threat to life or would involve a substantial risk of irreversible loss of function. Patients whose antecubital veins have already been destroyed should have other veins designated for venipuncture, and these veins should not be used for any other purpose. Because home care companies often deliver IV treatment (and do so with many different providers), the only person who can really enforce this policy is the informed patient and family. "Just say no" is a perfectly appropriate approach, and families and patients should be instructed (and feel empowered) to use it. Routine tests (those that do not affect day-to-day treatment or a decision to discharge) should be grouped on 1 or 2 days a week.

Gaining and Preserving Venous Access

For many patients and their families, the ease of IV insertion and infusions is a major determinant of satisfaction with medical care and their acceptance of a subsequent recommendation to treat a pulmonary exacerbation with IV antibiotics (or to enter the hospital for any reason). This is an area where a little common sense can go a long way.

CF centers should develop general policies concerning IV insertion and maintenance. These policies should address

1. Who should be allowed to insert IV lines (this can sometimes vary depending on the quality of the individual patient's veins). Patients and families often have favorite infusion nurses, and to the greatest extent possible, family requests should be honored.
2. Which veins should be used (e.g., use of the upper arm for any IV access other than percutaneously inserted central catheter (PICCs) is probably unwise).
3. Criteria for arbitrary removal of a functioning IV line (rarely necessary in CF patients).
4. Allowable activity (generally almost anything). Patients should have a cavalier attitude about their veins and should not be encouraged to guard the IV against every possible threat.
5. Early insertion of PICC lines in patients who are going to receive very corrosive antibiotics (or other IV drugs), such as imipenem, some penicillins, and vancomycin, rather than destroying several peripheral veins and then having to resort to central venous access anyway.
6. When peripheral access becomes more difficult, and the need to employ a logical sequence that ends with placement of a semi-permanent central venous access device (e.g., Mediport).
7. Development of a relationship with a small number of surgeons who then become very familiar with the problems of placing

semipermanent lines in CF patients (e.g., increased risk of pneumothorax) and who are willing to modify their techniques accordingly (e.g., have the catheter enter the venous system via the external jugular vein, rather than the subclavian).

8. Ensure that only experienced personnel are authorized to maintain PICC or semipermanent venous access devices when they are not being used for treatment.

Obtaining Arterial Blood Samples

Except in the most urgent situation, an Allen test should be performed before arterial puncture at the wrist to help ensure that the palmar arterial arches are intact so that vascular spasm or injury does not cause necrosis of distal structures. If the Allen test is unilaterally abnormal, the other side should be used (or at least used for the initial attempt) for arterial sampling. If the test is abnormal at the only available arterial puncture site or sites, the test indications should be reviewed; perhaps slightly less definitive (but still clinically useful) information can be derived from other sources (e.g., using serum chemistries to detect indirect evidence of CO_2 retention [high bicarbonate] or using a venous sample or mixed venous sample, or end-tidal expired air to assess hypercapnia—a normal or near-normal P_{CO_2} from any venous source excludes arterial hypercapnia, and a normal expired P_{CO_2} makes it unlikely).

The pain of arterial puncture can be minimized and the chance for success maximized by using some or all of the following methods:

1. The patient's wrist should be hyperextended over the corner of a table or bedside stand. Either the patient or an assistant can hold the hand down so it does not curl up when the operator inserts the needle.
2. The smallest possible needle (26 gauge) and a thin blood gas syringe (total syringe volume 1 mL) that allows blood to enter to a preset volume should be used.
3. The operator should feel for the artery, not the pulse. Although they seem to be the same, they are not. For consistent success, the operator should have the shape of the artery in his mind's eye when inserting the needle.

4. The needle should be inserted at no more than a 20- to 25-degree angle to the forearm. There is no reason for a perpendicular insertion with the intent to impale the artery against the radius. The needle need not be inserted very far; in most people, the artery is very superficial at the wrist. Initial misses require complete or nearly complete withdrawal of the needle before readvancing it.

5. Obtain enough of a sample to allow for some laboratory error. This is usually not the time to worry about conserving the patient's blood volume. There are few patients who will be endangered by removing an extra 0.2 to 0.3 mL.

6. Be very careful about labeling the sample. Some laboratories discard incorrectly labeled samples.

7. Resampling the same artery is often easier if the needle is reinserted in precisely the same location as a previous success.

8. Be sure that the sample arrives at the laboratory in the time window allowed by the hospital; most laboratories discard samples if they do not arrive within an arbitrary time window from the time they were drawn (these time limits are often unnecessarily short, but the lab will enforce them anyway). The operator should keep track of the specimen until it leaves the hospital ward or clinic.

Use of Local Anesthesia

There is legitimate difference of opinion concerning the use of local anesthesia (by either subcutaneous injection or by topical application) for venipuncture, insertion of IV lines, and arterial puncture. The operator must weigh the following factors.

Venipuncture for Blood Sampling or Simple Intravenous Injection (e.g., for an Imaging Procedure). Subcutaneous injection of a local anesthetic is almost always as painful as the venipuncture itself. The topical anesthetic cream, euecic mixture of lidocaine anoprilocaine (EMLA), can be effective and has the following advantages: (a) the procedure can be done with less pain; (b) the patient and family may have better acceptance of future venipunctures; (c) the use of EMLA shows that the operator is sympathetic with the patient's and family's anxiety about pain. However, EMLA also has formidable disadvantages: (a) its use implies that the pain of venipuncture is so great that no one can be expected to stand it, and therefore, if venipuncture is ever needed in less than the 45 to 60 minutes required for EMLA's action, the patient will be frantic; (b) it causes local vasoconstriction and therefore increases the likelihood of failure; (c) it creates problems for the patient when venipuncture is to be performed by physicians or other medical personnel who do not use it. Overall, EMLA for simple venipuncture is probably not a good idea for most patients.

Intravenous Insertion. EMLA or subcutaneous injection can be considered: EMLA has the advantage of easy (nonpainful) application, but the disadvantages of requiring a postponement of the procedure by 45 to 60 minutes for the anesthetic to act. Also, the local blanching and vasoconstriction caused by the drug increase the chance of failure. In addition, its effect is less predictable than that of subcutaneous injection.

Subcutaneous injection has the advantages of immediate onset of action and the guarantee that the patient will experience the same level of pain regardless of whether the venipuncture is a success or a failure. Many patients gladly accept the pain (burning) of the local injection in return for uniformity of pain from one IV attempt to the next. A local anaesthetic has the potential disadvantage of interfering with the operator's ability to feel the vein, but this can usually be circumvented by massaging the location of the injection so the vein is not lost in the anaesthetic bleb.

Arterial Puncture. Subcutaneous injection of a local anesthetic (at the wrist) may not be less painful than the arterial puncture itself. Furthermore, it is very difficult to anesthetize the arterial wall. Finally, the additional fluid of the anesthetic may greatly interfere with the operator's ability to feel the artery. EMLA may have some use in anesthetizing the skin of the wrist, but it may also cause arterial spasm. For experienced operators, the use of local anesthesia for this procedure is unnecessary.

9
Surgery

Surgery may be required for patients with cystic fibrosis (CF) for many different indications (Table 9–1). In this chapter, we concentrate on the conditions for which surgery is indicated, or for which surgery should be considered that are specifically related to CF, which may be more common in patients with CF, or which raise special considerations when they occur in people with CF. This chapter is organized by organ system, beginning at the head and working south.

HEAD, EYES, EARS, NOSE, AND THROAT

Head and Brain

There have been several cases of brain abscess reported in patients with CF. Surgery is indicated for these rare cases in order to drain the abscesses, relieve pressure, and obtain cultures. The surgical approach is no different in CF patients from that in other patients with brain abscess.

Nose and Sinuses

Approximately 20% of patients with CF develop nasal polyps, and each year, about 3% of CF patients undergo surgical removal of polyps. Broadly speaking, there are two surgical approaches to removing polyps, namely, simple polypectomy and polypectomy combined with functional endoscopic sinus surgery (FESS). The

TABLE 9–1. *Indications for Surgery in Cystic Fibrosis*

System/ location	Indication/ procedure	Frequency*	Urgency
HEENT	Brain abscess	Rare	Urgent
	Nasal polyps	3%/year†	Elective
	Symptomatic sinusitis	<3%/year	Elective
	Sinus mucocele	Rare	Urgent‡
Chest/ respiratory	Pneumothorax: chest tube	1%†	Urgent
	Pneumothorax: pleurodesis	1%†	Semi-urgent
	Empyema drainage	Very rare	Semi-elective
	Lobectomy for isolated bronchiectasis	Rare	Elective
	Lobectomy for isolated hemoptysis	Rare	Semi-elective
Abdomen/GI	Gastroesophageal reflux/fundoplication	Common†	Elective
	Gastrostomy/jejunostomy	7%	Elective
	Meconium ileus	5–10%§	Urgent
	Distal intestinal obstruction syndrome	3%†	
	Intussusception	Rare	Urgent or semi-urgent‖
	Appendiceal abscess/ phlegmon	Uncommon	Semi-elective
	Fibrosing colonopathy	Rare	Urgent
	Recurrent rectal prolapse	Up to 20%†	Elective
	Gallstones	Uncommon	Semi-elective
	Portal hypertension/ portosystemic shunting	3–5%†	Elective/semi- elective or urgent
GU	Male infertility/obstructive azoospermia: MESA	98%†	Elective
Vascular	Vascular access	Common	Usually elective/ semi-elective

*Frequency estimates from various sources, including CF Data Registry

†The condition is common, but the procedure is required/or has been reported much less commonly. The incidence cited is for the condition itself, not the intervention.

‡If erosion of sinus wall or impingement on orbit or brain.

§Based on 10% to 20% incidence of meconium ileus and roughly 50% of babies with meconium ileus requiring surgery

‖Intussusception may present as an acute surgical abdomen or much more benignly, with recurrent episodes of abdominal pain. The urgency of a surgical approach varies accordingly.

GI, gastrointestinal; GU, genitourinary; HEENT, head, ears, eyes, nose, and throat; MESA, microsurgical epididymal sperm aspiration.

more extensive procedure usually also includes creating maxillary drainage windows, opening the ethmoid cells, opening the frontal sinuses (if they are present), removing impacted mucus, and sometimes, placing catheters through the nose into the maxillary sinuses on each side. These catheters are used to instill tobramycin into the sinuses twice daily for 1 to 4 weeks.

Opacification of the sinuses is a nearly universal roentgenographic finding among patients with CF. A relatively small but important minority of CF patients develop symptomatic sinusitis, with obstruction of nasal airflow, purulent nasal discharge, postnasal drip, headache, facial pain, sore throat, or a combination of these features. Some physicians and families believe that uncontrolled sinus infection may seed the lower airway and worsen CF lung disease. It is widely believed that this route of infection may complicate the course of CF patients after lung transplantation. If medical treatment with oral antibiotics, saline irrigations, topical decongestants, topical corticosteroids, or a combination of these agents is unsuccessful, surgery may be indicated. The results of this surgery are difficult to assess, largely owing to the lack of controlled studies. One study (Moss and King, 1995) claims that the surgery greatly reduces the need for repeat sinus surgery, whereas another study (Cuyler, 1992) reports subjective improvement in spite of objective evidence of persistent sinus disease (based on otolaryngologic exam and computed tomographic studies). Some centers believe that sinus surgery may improve pulmonary function in selected patients, whereas one retrospective study failed to show such improvement (Madonna, et al., 1997). Extensive sinus surgery is employed frequently—even routinely—before or soon after lung transplantation in some lung transplant centers in an attempt to diminish posttransplant lung infection. There are no controlled studies documenting the effectiveness of this approach.

Rarely, a mucopyocele—especially of the frontal sinus—may develop and may erode the sinus wall. Symptoms may include severe headache, double vision, proptosis, or a combination of these. In these rare cases, surgery is indicated urgently. Removal of the mucopyocele and obliteration of the frontal sinus with adipose tissue from the abdominal wall or buttock is often attempted.

CHEST AND RESPIRATORY SYSTEM

Symptomatic pneumothorax occurs in almost 1% of all CF patients each year. Surgical intervention is indicated in the majority of these cases.

Except in the cases of the tiniest rim of extrapulmonary air, some intervention is usually warranted in CF patients who have developed pneumothorax. Because the lung in patients with CF tends to be stiff, it may not collapse even when a fairly large collection of air presses on it. Therefore, describing a pneumothorax as 15% or 25% may not give useful information, because a small pneumothorax may be under tension and thereby be of physiologic import. Beyond the physiologic consequences of an episode of pneumothorax in CF is the fact that, without preventive measures, the recurrence rate for ipsilateral pneumothorax is at least 50%.

Therefore, the conservative approach to pneumothorax in patients with CF has been to use a single procedure to treat the current episode and prevent recurrences. This was accomplished most reliably with pleural ablation. Pleural ablation can be carried out through a chest tube with instillation of a sclerosing agent, such as atabrine (no longer available), tetracycline, or talc, or with an open thoracotomy, with identification, excision, and sewing of discrete blebs (usually apical), stripping the visceral pleura where possible, and manual abrasion of the remaining lung surface. These procedures help seal the current leak and, by assuring adherence of the surface of the lung to the inside of the chest wall, prevent recurrent leaks. The advent of lung transplantation has complicated this sit-

TABLE 9–2. *Surgical Approach to Pneumothorax in Patients with Cystic Fibrosis*

Step One
  Thoracostomy tube drainage
Step Two
  Identification and oversewing of leaks/blebectomy (via thoracotomy or
    thoracoscopy)
Step Three
  Pleurodesis
    via open thoracotomy or via thoracoscopy

uation, because the extensive adhesions created with mechanical or chemical pleurodesis make removal of the native lung a difficult and bloody undertaking. In some lung transplant centers, prior pleurabrasion is an absolute contraindication to transplant (in others, it is a relative contraindication). Because of the difficulty pleural adhesions present for transplantation, we recommend the following approach to treatment of pneumothorax in patients with CF (Table 9–2).

A chest tube should be inserted and attached to continuous suction through a water-seal system, with 15 to 30 cm H_2O pressure as soon as the pneumothorax is diagnosed. A small bore pigtail catheter may be used in this first step because it is less painful than a larger tube and therefore interferes less with deep breathing, coughing, and airway clearance. Care must be taken in placing the tube to use the smallest skin incision possible. An oversized skin and muscle incision readily allows air to enter the pleural space from outside the body. The tube should remain in place until the leak seals (the bubbling in the water in the drainage tube under the water seal stops). The lung should become fully inflated because apposition of the visceral and parietal pleural surfaces helps seal any leaks. If the lung does not come into full apposition with the chest wall within a day or two, more suction should be used (as much as 40 cm H_2O pressure), additional or larger bore tube or tubes should be inserted, or a combination of these approaches may be chosen. If the lung does inflate fully and the leaking stops, the tube should be left in place under water seal, with no negative pressure applied for 4 to 24 hours. If the lung remains inflated, the tube should be withdrawn. If extrapleural air reaccumulates, another tube should be inserted and suction should be reapplied. If the leaking does not stop within 5 days, a more invasive approach should be undertaken. Although it may be tempting to avoid invasive procedures, in the case of a prolonged indwelling chest tube, the dictum *primum no nocere* calls for moving to the more invasive step, because there is substantial morbidity and mortality among CF patients with chest tubes in place for longer than 7 days. Chest tubes are painful and interfere with deep breathing, coughing, and airway clearance techniques. Adequate ongoing analgesia must be given, to allow for airway clearance, as well as for the obvious humane considerations.

Without prompt resolution of the air leak, the next step should probably be an attempt to identify and staple or oversew the leak or leaks (so-called blebectomy) through open thoracotomy or—preferably—thoracoscopy. Discrete leaks can be found in over 80% of cases of pneumothorax in CF patients. There is inadequate experience with this approach to know its likely success rate, but it has been successful in the treatment of idiopathic pneumothorax and avoids the extensive adhesions that result from pleurodesis (see later) and that make subsequent lung transplantation difficult.

If the air leak persists or pneumothorax recurs after blebectomy, a definitive approach is indicated. The definitive approach to pneumothorax involves creating extensive adhesions between the lung surface and the chest wall. These adhesions can be created by open thoracotomy with pleural stripping and manual abrasion of the remainder of the lung surface, or instillation of sclerosing chemicals (e.g., atabrine—no longer available, or tetracycline) through a chest tube. With the advent of video-assisted thoracoscopic surgery (VATS), the definitive procedure can be done less invasively, an apparent contradiction in terms that does not seem to compromise patient care. As with simple blebectomy, there have not yet been extensive published series to allow solid conclusions to be drawn about the efficacy of this approach, but it seems attractive: actively leaking areas and tenuous-seeming blebs can be identified, excised, and stapled. After the stapling, talc can be blown in through the thoracoscope, taking care to distribute the talc to all surfaces of the lung. Talc induces an avid inflammatory response, creating dense adhesions. Talc may injure the diaphragm, and therefore should be avoided in patients who might be candidates for lung transplantation.

Empyema is surprisingly uncommon in CF. It can occur, however, and requires a surgical approach, usually with tube drainage being adequate. In very rare circumstances, open thoracotomy, with creation of a pleural window or even decortication of underlying lung, may be indicated.

Lung resection for localized bronchiectasis is rarely indicated and should be approached with great caution. In the very unusual patient, severe disease may be localized to one lobe (most often the right upper), with relatively mild disease elsewhere. In such a patient, if there are serious problems referable to the diseased lobe, such as the frequent need for hospitalization, lobectomy may be useful. This is especially true if the patient's functional status improves substantially with control of the localized disease, as for example, after hospitalization and intravenous antibiotics, and yet recurs frequently. Because lobectomy almost always requires removing healthy tissue along with the unsalvageable tissue, the physician should be reluctant to advise this course in the absence of compelling evidence that it will help. In the few patients in whom it is indicated, lobectomy carries a relatively small short-term and intermediate-term morbidity. Most of the morbidity can be attributed to chest pain, both from the incision and the chest tube, which is left in place for several days after surgery. Pain control is essential so that deep breathing, coughing, and airway clearance can take place. Pain control can be accomplished pharmacologically, in some cases, with local nerve blocks, and with teaching patients techniques like squeezing a pillow to the chest during coughing.

Lung resection for intractable hemoptysis is likewise rarely indicated, but in these cases, can be lifesaving. Exquisite care must be taken to ascertain the source of bleeding (see Chapter 4), before the step of lobectomy, which should be used only in desperation. Probably more common than the lifesaving lobectomy for hemoptysis is the unsuccessful lobectomy for hemoptysis. Once the lobes are gone, they are gone forever, and most large CF centers have had to care for patients transferred from other locations with persistent bleeding after one or two lobes have been removed. The huge disadvantage for the CF patient forced to struggle through life with only three lobes is obvious.

ABDOMEN AND GASTROINTESTINAL SYSTEM

Gastroesophageal reflux (GER) occurs in 20% to 50% of patients with CF, and the condition is especially common among those with severe lung disease. GER may contribute to the severity of lung disease. Fundoplication may be indicated in those patients who have persistent disease, be it gastrointestinal (e.g., erosive esophagitis) or pulmonary (e.g., from aspiration or reflex bronchospasm), despite maximal medical therapy. The goal of fundoplication is to augment the antireflux function of the lower esophageal sphincter. This is accomplished by wrapping part of the stomach around the lower esophagus. The surgeon faces a difficult challenge in fashioning the perfect wrap because one that is too loose does not solve the initial problem and reflux continues, whereas too tight a wrap may prevent belching, and cause bloating and dysphagia. The most commonly used procedure is the Nissen fundoplication, which entails a 360-degree wrap of the gastric fundus around the lower esophagus. The Thal and Toupet procedures are partial wraps, either anterior (Thal) or posterior (Toupet), with the theoretic advantage of causing less bloating and dysphagia than the Nissen procedure. This advantage has not been demonstrated for the Toupet.

The decision to perform a fundoplication must consider not only the type of wrap to employ but also the operative approach, namely, the traditional open technique or laparoscopy. Laparoscopy is, in some sense, less invasive (it creates a smaller abdominal incision), but it has other problems (Table 9–3). The best approach varies from patient to patient and particularly from center to center, depending on the experience of the pediatric surgeon.

No matter which procedure is done by which approach, failure of wrap can occur, particularly with disruption of the wrap or prolapse of the wrap into the posterior mediastinum. Wrap failure is especially likely to occur in patients with chronic lung disease, probably because of increased intraabdominal pressure (coughing) and perhaps because of overfilling of the stomach with air, as is common with anyone who breathes hard.

TABLE 9–3. *Laparoscopic Versus Open Fundoplication*

	Laparoscopic	Open
Advantages	Smaller incision	Better ability to feel tightness of wrap
	Faster recovery from incision	More experience
Disadvantages	Abdomen filled with air, impeding diaphragm movement	Larger incision
	Fewer surgeons with experience	

Enteral feeds are given to 8% of CF patients. Most (86%) of these patients have feeds administered via gastrostomy tubes, and some (3%) are administered via jejunostomy tubes. Jejunostomy tubes have the advantage of not agravating gastroesophageal reflux (GER), but are more difficult to place initially and are usually more difficult to replace if they are dislodged. Placement of gastrostomy tubes can be done with an open procedure by a surgeon, with a percutaneous endoscopic procedure (PEG) by a gastroenterologist (sometimes with, sometimes without, the assistance of a surgeon), or by an interventional radiologist. Patients should be studied for GER before tube placement. In a patient with severe reflux before tube placement, the open approach, combined with fundoplication, may be indicated. In those with absent or mild reflux, the incidence of postprocedure GER is relatively low, but some experts prefer to use tube placement in the jejunum or a combined fundoplication-gastrostomy procedure in anyone with any degree of reflux. One approach may help solve these conflicts: placement of a gastrostomy, and feeding the distal end of the tube through the pylorus into the jejunum (often referred to, somewhat inaccurately, as a gastrojejunostomy). The immediate postoperative treatment of the stomas, the tubes, and patient as a whole is very important, and differs widely among physicians and centers. The conservative approach allows for only the smallest oral sips and uses continuous slow infusion of formula via the new tube for as long as 3 to 4 weeks after the procedure. Some surgeons allow oral and tube feedings to resume or commence within 24 hours after tube placement. The relatively long tube placed initially can be changed to a flat button device that fits flatly against the abdomen, and is nearly invisible under even fairly tight clothes. In the hands of conservative physicians, the change to the button occurs only after weeks to months, to allow the stomach to heal to the abdominal wall, so that button insertion does not disrupt that attachment. In others' hands, the button may be placed as the initial procedure and feedings withheld for a mere 24 hours. Whichever approach is taken, it is essential that the patient and family (and primary physician) be fully informed before agreeing to, and be fully prepared before undergoing, the procedure.

Meconium ileus occurs in 20% of newborns with CF. In 10% to 50% of these babies, the condition is complicated by perforation (meconium peritonitis), ileal atresia, or meconium cyst. In uncomplicated meconium ileus, which is diagnosed by contrast enema, usually using barium, nonoperative treatment should be attempted. Hyperosmolar contrast preparations are administered by rectum under fluoroscopic guidance. The first agent to be used for these procedures was diatrizoate meglumine (Gastrografin), and although other agents are now also used, the procedure is often referred to generically as a Gastrografin enema. Other contrast agents, including diatrizoate sodium (Hypaque) and iothalamate meglumine (Conray) have also been used. None of these agents should be used undiluted because of the greatly increased risk of complications (Gastrografin has an osmolality of 1900 mOsm/L). Different centers have developed their own favorite combinations for these therapeutic contrast enemas. Most use a 2:1 or 3:1 dilution of the contrast agent with water (i.e., two or three parts water to one part contrast). The mixture is infused gently per rectum until it refluxes into the terminal ileum. Over the ensuing 12 to 48 hours, most infants pass semiliquid meconium. Some centers use warm saline enemas with 1% acetylcysteine after the contrast enema, and many also administer 5% to 10% acetylcysteine by nasogastric tube (5 to 10 mL every 6 hours) to help liquefy obstructing mucus from above. The procedure may have to be repeated one or two times over the next day or two. Because the procedure works by pulling fluid into the bowel lumen, one of its main dangers is dehydration. Aggressive fluid replacement must begin even before the procedure and for approximately 24 hours afterward. One suggested regimen is 150 mL/kg/day, with careful monitoring of the patient's hydration status. The success rate of hyperosmolar enemas for meconium ileus should be at least 50%. In a minority of cases, operative intervention is necessary. There have been several different operative approaches described, but if the entire bowel is viable (as is usually the case in uncomplicated meconium ileus), the most commonly used approach is creation of a tube enterostomy (Fig. 9–1). A small enterotomy is formed, through which a tube is passed into the ileum. The tube is held in place with a purse-string suture. Saline (and sometimes acetylcysteine or Gastrografin) is used to irrigate the bowel, helping to liquefy the meconium, which can then be removed through the enterotomy or flushed distally through the bowel. This technique has the advantage of avoiding both bowel resection and the necessity of a

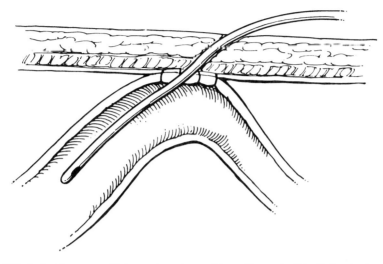

FIG. 9–1. Diagram of tube enterostomy. (From Rescorla FJ. Abdominal and general surgery. In: Orenstein DM, Stern RC, eds. *Treatment of the hospitalized cystic fibrosis patient*. New York: Marcel Dekker, Inc., l998:258. Vol. 109 of *Lung Biology in Health and Disease*, Lenfant C, ed.)

second operative procedure. Other operative approaches include resecting the dilated segment of bowel (proximal to the obstruction) and forming a double-barreled (Mikulicz) enterostomy, resecting the dilated segment with the formation of an enterostomy with the distal bowel and an end-to-side anastomosis (end of the proximal ileum anastomosed to the side of the distal ileum [Bishop-Coop procedure]), or resecting the dilated segment, with the formation of a proximal enterostomy and distal end-to-proximal side anastomosis (Santulli-Blanc procedure).

Complicated meconium ileus must always be treated surgically. In the case of volvulus or ileal atresia, the dilated segment is resected, usually with end-to-end anastomosis of the remaining bowel. If peritonitis is present, the extensive adhesions may make any procedure difficult and may threaten lengths of bowel such that short gut may result. In most cases of meconium peritonitis, the proximal bowel is used to form a temporary stoma, while the distal bowel is either brought to the abdominal wall as a mucous fistula or closed and left within the abdomen. After 4 to 6 weeks peritoneal inflammation is likely to have resolved and atonic bowel to have regained function, and the stomas can be closed, with reanastomosis of the bowel. During these weeks, some infants require parenteral nutrition, whereas others are be able to tolerate and absorb enteral feeds. Elemental formulas should be employed. Elemental formulas will obviate the need for pancreatic enzyme supplements, but these enzymes should probably be used if the fat source in the formula is long-chain fatty acids or even medium-chain triglycerides. Salt supplementation is required in infants with ileostomies, because ileal effluent contains as much as 100 mEq/L of sodium (compared with 20 mEq/L for infant stool).

Distal intestinal obstruction syndrome (DIOS; formerly referred to as meconium ileus equivalent) occurs in approximately 15% of patients with CF, mostly adolescents and adults. A fuller description of DIOS can be found in Chapter 5. The overwhelming majority of cases can be treated nonoperatively, with Gastrografin (or other contrast) enemas, intestinal lavage with GoLYTELY (or similar solution), or even standard (e.g., Fleet's) enemas or oral lactulose, if the obstruction is discovered early. There are a few patients, particularly those whose obstruction is associated with intraabdominal adhesions from previous surgery, who require abdominal exploration, freeing of adhesions, and perhaps opening the bowel to lavage the thick contents.

Intussusception occurs much more commonly (and at an older age) in patients with CF than in the general population and may be difficult to distinguish from DIOS. Its presentation may be acute with severe pain, bloody diarrhea, and shock, or much more insidious with recurrent low-level abdominal pain. The diagnosis is made by contrast enema, which may also reduce the intussusception. Operative intervention, perhaps including cecectomy, is sometimes required. Appendectomy should always be performed when intussusception is approached surgically, both to prevent the appendix from serving as a lead point for further episodes and to eliminate appendicitis from the differential diagnosis of future episodes of abdominal pain.

Appendicitis occurs in patients with CF in roughly the same frequency as in the general population. However, the signs of appendicitis may be obscured by antibiotic treatment, and a walled-off appendiceal abscess (phlegmon) may be present. In some CF patients, the appendix can become painfully distended with mucus, in the absence of inflammation. Appendectomy is required in these cases and may be accomplished laparoscopically. In some institutions, interventional radiologists may be able to provide percutaneous drainage of appendiceal abscesses.

Fibrosing colonopathy, first discovered in 1994, is a newly recognized and fortunately unusual complication of CF seen only in patients taking very high doses (greater than 5,000 units of lipase/kg body weight per meal) of pancreatic enzymes. This disorder presents with abdominal pain, diarrhea (perhaps bloody), or both. Even with early recognition of the problem, reduction of enzyme dosage seldom obviates the need for surgery. Some patients may require bowel rest, with parenteral nutrition. In most cases, the colonic strictures have developed by the time of diagnosis, and surgery is required, with resection of the involved bowel. Although most cases have been described in the ascending colon, any part of the large bowel may be involved, and there have even been some cases of pancolonic and rectal involvement. In these latter cases, an ostomy is required, but in other cases, children may be treated with resection of the involved segment and primary anastomosis.

Rectal prolapse is common, and usually responds to adjustment of pancreatic enzyme dosing. In a few patients, however, the problem continues to recur and requires further intervention. The least invasive of these further interventions is circumferential injections into the rectal submucosa with hypertonic (30%) saline, 5% phenol in almond oil, or 50% dextrose. If injection therapy is not successful, several operative options are available, none with perfect track records. Insertion of a Silastic ring has been helpful in some children, whereas some surgeons prefer to fix the rectum to the sacrum or to suspend the rectum and repair the levator ani muscle.

Gallstones are relatively uncommon in CF, but they are far from rare and may cause considerable morbidity. Symptomatic gallstones are a clear indication for a cholecystectomy, which can be carried out laparoscopically.

Portal hypertension occurs in 2% to 5% of patients with CF, with attendant complications, including formation of varices (especially esophageal) and hypersplenism. In years gone by, extensive surgical portosystemic shunting procedures were carried out to relieve the pressure. These procedures were reasonably successful but were exhausting for both the patient and surgeon alike, and created extensive intraabdominal adhesions that complicate or even prevent liver transplantation. In more recent years, the interventional radiologic procedure of transjugular intrahepatic portosystemic shunting (TIPS) has largely replaced the more extensive open surgical procedures and has been able to provide elective or urgent decompression of the portal venous system, relieving ascites and GI hemorrhage and allowing for future liver transplantation.

GENITOURINARY SYSTEM

Infertility on the basis of obstructive azoospermia occurs in 98% to 99% of men with CF, despite normal testicular sperm formation. In recent years, a very few men have had microsurgical epididymal sperm aspiration (MESA), with aspiration of sperm from the epididymis for direct injection into a readied egg for a variation on standard *in vitro* fertilization techniques. The direct injection is necessary because sperm aspirated from the epididymis are too immature to fertilize eggs on their own, as would be expected with standard *in vitro* fertilization. After fertilization, which occurs in as many as 50% of first attempts with this technique, gene analysis can be carried out before the fertilized egg is implanted into the mother's uterus. The technique is expensive and is not covered by most insurance policies.

VASCULAR ACCESS

Nearly 40% of all CF patients require one or more courses of intravenous antibiotics each year, so reliable hassle-free venous access is a common necessity. Peripheral intravenous lines sometimes suffice, but the availability of percutaneously insertable central lines has helped greatly, and these lines are much less likely to "go bad" than the peripheral IVs. Percutaneously inserted central catheters (PICC lines) can be placed by a surgeon, interventional radiologist, or the occasional generalist or CF specialist. These lines are usually inserted in the antecubital fossa or low upper arm, advanced into the basilic or cephalic vein and then into the superior vena cava or right atrium.

Some techniques require that the line be held in place with a single suture. PICC lines can also be placed directly into the subclavian, or internal or external jugular veins. With these routes, care must be taken not to puncture the apex of the almost-always overinflated CF lung. Although PICC lines have served many patients well, their useful lifetime is measured in days or weeks; whereas some patients require much longer treatment. In fact, some 12% of CF patients require three or more courses of intravenous antibiotics each year. For these patients, a permanent indwelling line can be very helpful, particularly one with a subcutaneous port for percutaneous access. Mediport and Portacath are two of the more popular options. The port can be placed on the anterior chest wall, the lower abdomen, or the upper inner thigh. The longevity of subcutaneous ports is measured in years.

ANESTHESIA

CF raises some special considerations regarding anesthesia (Table 9–4). Altered electrolytes from salt loss can complicate anesthetic management, as can decreased serum albumin (increased anesthetic drug potency). The coagulopathies of vitamin K deficiency or liver disease (with or without hypersplenism) can increase intraoperative and postoperative bleeding.

Nasal polyps can make passage of any nasal tube difficult or impossible; interfere with the ability to measure end-tidal gas concentrations in the non-intubated, spontaneously breathing patient; and even delay or prevent nasal delivery of inhalational anesthetic agents given by mask.

The lung disease that characterizes CF can also make anesthetic management more difficult: Copious secretions can block endotracheal tubes and interfere with the delivery of anesthetic gases. In this way, induction of anesthesia, as well as recovery from it, are often much delayed. Airway inflammation makes coughing a problem during many procedures for patients with CF and requires more local airway anesthesia and often deeper sedation than with patients with other conditions. Airway obstruction and lung overinflation increase the risk of further overdistention and bleb rupture with positive pressure ventilation.

TABLE 9–4. *Anesthesia and Cystic Fibrosis*

Cystic fibrosis feature or condition	Possible impact on anesthesia
Metabolic/nutritional/hematologic	
Decreased serum albumin	Increased drug potency
Electrolyte imbalance	Cardiovascular/drug effects
Decreased intravascular volume	Hypotension
Coagulopathy*	Increased blood loss
Upper airway	
Nasal polyps	Difficulty of passing nasal tubes; slower gas delivery to lungs; inaccurate nasal end-tidal gas measurement
Lower airways	
Copious secretions	Slow, uneven gas distribution: hypoxemia; delayed inhalant anesthesia induction and recovery; possible blockage of endotracheal tube
Air trapping	Danger of overdistention and rupture of blebs
Airway inflammation	Coughing

*Coagulopathy, such as from decreased vitamin K absorption, liver disease (increased prothrombin time) or hypersplenism (thrombocytopenia).

Special considerations concerning laparoscopic and thoracoscopic procedures: For both of these types of procedures, the surgeon gains visibility by collapsing structures through the instillation of sometimes large amounts of air. In thoracoscopic procedures, this process can impede lung filling on the side being examined. In laparoscopy, the abdomen is filled with air, impeding diaphragmatic excursion.

Specific drug considerations (Table 9–5): Ketamine can cause increased secretions and laryngospasm, and nitrous oxide can expand and thereby further increase pulmonary overdistention. On the other hand, halothane has bronchodilator properties, and anticholinergic agents (e.g., atropine or ipratropium bromide [Atrovent]) may provide weak bronchodilation and decrease secretions. Traditionally, physicians have avoided using atropine and atropine-like agents for fear of drying intrapulmonary secretions excessively. However, clinical practice indicates that this occurrence is unlikely,

TABLE 9–5. *Anesthetic Drugs and Cystic Fibrosis: Special Considerations*

Drugs to be avoided	Reason
Nitrous oxide	Possible expansion, with worsening lung distention
Ketamine	Possible increased secretions and laryngospasm
Useful drugs	Reason
Halothane	Bronchodilation
Anticholinergics	Decreased secretions*

*Atropine decreases the quantity of secretions without changing viscosity; the fear that atropine may excessively dry secretions is probably unfounded.

and some studies have shown that atropine diminishes the volume of secretions but does not change secretion viscosity.

It might be useful to schedule elective surgery for adolescent and adult patients who are in worse condition later in the day, in order that they have some hours after awakening on the day of surgery to work on airway clearance. Although the practice of starting an IV once a patient has been anesthetized with inhalational agent(s) is humane, it may be misguided in patients with CF, as the induction phase of anesthesia may be more difficult and delayed in CF, and intravenous access could be lifesaving. During and especially at the end of general endotracheal anesthesia, gentle suctioning of the thick tracheobronchial secretions can be helpful, but too vigorous suctioning may be counterproductive. Certainly, delaying a patient's extubation for continued suctioning is almost never justified, because the patient can do a better job by coughing. With any procedure involving endotracheal intubation, an excellent opportunity does exist for obtaining a specimen for culture, and the CF physician and anesthesiologist should always discuss whether such a culture should be obtained. During anesthesia, particularly in patients in worse condition, it is important to measure baseline blood gases and then monitor them throughout the procedure to ensure adequate, but not overzealous, ventilation and oxygenation. The chronic CO_2-retaining patient who is overventilated to a normal $PaCO_2$ may have dreadful acid–base imbalance as a result, with sudden respiratory alkalosis.

REFERENCES

General

Cystic Fibrosis Foundation. *Cystic Fibrosis Foundation patient registry annual data report 1997.* Bethesda, MD: Cystic Fibrosis Foundation, 1998.

Davis PB, Drumm M, Konstan MW. Cystic fibrosis. State of the art. *Am J Respir Crit Care Med* 1996;154:1229–1256.

Doershuk CF, et al. Anesthesia and surgery in cystic fibrosis. *Anesth Analg* 1972; 51:413–421.

Oppenheimer EH, Esterly JR. Pathology of cystic fibrosis review of the literature and comparison with 146 autopsied cases. *Persp Pediatr Pathol* 1975;2:241–278.

Rescorla FJ. Abdominal and general surgery. In: Orenstein DM, Stern RC, eds. *Treatment of the hospitalized cystic fibrosis patient.* New York: Marcel Dekker, Inc., 1998:249–281. Vol. 109 of *Lung Biology in Health and Disease.* Ed. Claude Lenfant.

Head, Eyes, Ears, Nose, and Throat

Batsakis, JG, El-Naggar AK. Cystic fibrosis and the sinonasal tract. *Ann Otol Rhinol Laryngol* 1996;105:329–330.

Brihaye P, Jorissen M, Clement PA. Chronic rhinosinusitis in cystic fibrosis (mucoviscidosis). *Acta Otorhinolaryngol Belg* 1997;51:323–337.

Cepero R, et al. Cystic fibrosis—an otolaryngologic perspective. *Otolaryngol Head Neck Surg* 1987;97:356–360.

Cipolli M, et al. Bronchial artery embolization in the management of hemoptysis in cystic fibrosis. *Pediatr Pulmonol* 1995;19:344–347.

Cooper DM, Russell LE, Henry RL. Cerebral abscess as a complication of cystic fibrosis. *Pediatr Pulmonol* 1994;17:390–392.

Cuyler JP. Follow-up of endoscopic sinus surgery on children with cystic fibrosis. *Arch Otolaryngol Head Neck Surg* 1992;118:505–506.

Davidson TM, et al. Management of chronic sinusitis in cystic fibrosis. *Laryngoscope* 1995;105(Pt 1):354–358.

Drake-Lee AB. Medical treatment of nasal polyps. *Rhinology* 1994;32:1–4.

Duplechain JK, White JA, Miller RH. Pediatric sinusitis. The role of endoscopic sinus surgery in cystic fibrosis and other forms of sinonasal disease. *Arch Otolaryngol Head Neck Surg* 1991;117:422–426.

Gentile VG, Isaacson G. Patterns of sinusitis in cystic fibrosis. *Laryngoscope* 1996;106:1005–1009.

Hebert RL 2nd, Bent JP 3rd. Meta-analysis of outcomes of pediatric functional endoscopic sinus surgery. *Laryngoscope* 1998;108:796–769.

Madonna D, Isaacson G, Rosenfeld RM, Pavitch H. Effect of sinus surgery on pulmonary function in patients with cystic fibrosis. *Laryngoscope* 1997;107: 328–331.

Moss RB, King VV. Management of sinusitis in cystic fibrosis by endoscopic surgery and serial antimicrobial lavage. Reduction in recurrence requiring surgery. *Arch Otolaryngol Head Neck Surg* 1995;121:566–572.

Nishioka GJ, et al. Symptom outcome after functional endoscopic sinus surgery in patients with cystic fibrosis: a prospective study [see comments]. *Otolaryngol Head Neck Surg* 1995;113:440–445.

Nishioka GJ, Cook PR. Paranasal sinus disease in patients with cystic fibrosis. *Otolaryngol Clin North Am* 1996;29:193–205.

Olsen MM, et al. Surgery in patients with cystic fibrosis. *J Pediatr Surg* 1987;22: 613–618.

Reilly JS, et al. Nasal surgery in children with cystic fibrosis: complications and risk management. *Laryngoscope* 1985;95:1491–1493.

Sharma GD, Doershuk CF, Stern RC. Erosion of the wall of the frontal sinus caused by mucopyocele in cystic fibrosis. *J Pediatr* 1994;124(Pt 1):745–747.

Stern RC, et al. Treatment and prognosis of nasal polyps in cystic fibrosis. *Am J Dis Child* 1982;136:1067–1070.

Walner DL, et al. The role of second-look nasal endoscopy after pediatric functional endoscopic sinus surgery. *Arch Otolaryngol Head Neck Surg* 1998;124:425–428.

Abdomen and Gastrointestinal System

Ade-Ajayi N, et al. Surgery for pancreatic cystosis with pancreatitis in cystic fibrosis. *Br J Surg* 1997;84:312.

Adinolfi A, Adinolfi M, Lessof. Alpha-feto-protein during development and in disease. *J Med Genet* 1975;12:138–151.

Amodio J, et al. Microcolon of prematurity: a form of functional obstruction. *AJR Am J Roentgenol* 1986;146:239–244.

Anagnostopoulos D, et al. Gallbladder disease in patients with cystic fibrosis. *Eur J Pediatr Surg* 1993;3:348–351.

Angelico M, et al. Gallstones in cystic fibrosis: a critical reappraisal. *Hepatology* 1991;14:768–775.

Bilton D, et al. Pathology of common bile duct stenosis in cystic fibrosis. *Gut* 1990; 31:236–238.

Boswell WC, Boyd CR, Lord SA. Percutaneous endoscopic gastrostomy with T-bar fixation in children. *Surg Laparosc Endosc* 1996;6:262–265.

Burton EM, et al. Neonatal jaundice: clinical and ultrasonographic findings. *South Afr Med J* 1990;83:294–302.

Chappell JS. Management of meconium ileus by resection and end-to-end anastomosis. *South Afr Med J* 1977;52:1093–1094.

Crisci KL, et al. Contrast enema findings of fibrosing colonopathy. *Pediatr Radiol* 1997;27:315–316.

Dogan AS, Conway JJ, Lloyd-Still JD. Hepatobiliary scintigraphy in children with cystic fibrosis and liver disease [see comments]. *J Nucl Med* 1994;35:432–435.

Donovan TJ, Ward M, Shepherd RW. Evaluation of endoscopic sclerotherapy of esophageal varices in children. *J Pediatr Gastroenterol Nutr* 1986;5:696–700.

Duchatel F, et al. Prenatal diagnosis of cystic fibrosis: ultrasonography of the gallbladder at 17–19 weeks of gestation. *Fetal Diagn Ther* 1993;8:28–36.

Edge WE, Nuss D, Loening WE. Late-onset intestinal obstruction in cystic fibrosis—meconium ileus equivalent. *South Afr Med J* 1977;52:271–274.

Feigelson J, et al. Late and unusual intestinal features in cystic fibrosis–pseudotumoral intestinal wall thickening. *Acta Universitatis Carolinae Medica* 1990;36: 144–147.

Fig LM, et al. Common bile duct obstruction in cystic fibrosis: utility of hepatobiliary scintigraphy. *American Journal of Physiologic Imaging* 1991;6:194–196.

FitzSimmons SC, et al. High-dose pancreatic-enzyme supplements and fibrosing colonopathy in children with cystic fibrosis. *N Engl J Med* 1997;336:1283–1289.

Fletcher BD, Abramowsky CR. Contrast enemas in cystic fibrosis: implications of appendiceal nonfilling. *AJR Am J Roentgenol* 1981;137:323–326.

Freiman JP, FitzSimmons SC. Colonic strictures in patients with cystic fibrosis: results of a survey of 114 cystic fibrosis care centers in the United States. *J Pediatr Gastroenterol Nutr* 1996;22:153–156.

Holmes M, et al. Intussusception in cystic fibrosis. *Arch Dis Child* 1991;66: 726–727.

King SJ, et al. Strictures of the colon in cystic fibrosis. *Clin Radiol* 1994;49: 476–477.

Kumari-Subaiya S, et al. Portal vein measurement by ultrasonography in patients with long-standing cystic fibrosis: preliminary observations. *J Pediatr Gastroenterol Nutr* 1987;6:71–78.

Lloyd-Still JD. Crohn's disease and cystic fibrosis. *Digest Dis Sci* 1994;39:880–885.

Lloyd-Still JD. Cystic fibrosis and colonic strictures. A new "iatrogenic" disease [Editorial]. *J Clin Gastroenterol* 1995;21:2–5.

Maurage C, et al. Meconium ileus and its equivalent as a risk factor for the development of cirrhosis: an autopsy study in cystic fibrosis. *J Pediatr Gastroenterol Nutr* 1989;9:17–20.

McCabe AJ, et al. The surgical aspects of gastrointestinal disease in cystic fibrosis. *New Insights Into Cystic Fibrosis* 1999;6:1–8.

Patrick MK, et al. Common bile duct obstruction causing right upper abdominal pain in cystic fibrosis. *J Pediatr* 1986;108:101–102.

Pawel BR, de Chadarevian JP, Franco ME. The pathology of fibrosing colonopathy of cystic fibrosis: a study of 12 cases and review of the literature. *Hum Pathol* 1997;28:395–399.

Reichard KW, et al. Fibrosing colonopathy in children with cystic fibrosis. *J Pediatr Surg* 1997;32:237–241; discussion 241–242.

Rescorla F, et al. Changing patterns of treatment and survival in neonates with meconium ileus. *Arch Surg* 1989;124:837–840.

Shields MD, et al. Appendicitis in cystic fibrosis. *Arch Dis Child* 1991;66:307–310.

Siegel MJ, Shackelford GD, McAlister WH. Neonatal meconium blockage in the ileum and proximal colon. *Radiology* 1979;132:79–82.

Smyth RL, et al. Fibrosing colonopathy in cystic fibrosis: results of a case-control study. *Lancet* 1995;346:1247–1251.

Smyth RL, et al. Strictures of ascending colon in cystic fibrosis and high-strength pancreatic enzymes. *Lancet* 1994;343:85–86.

Snyder CL, et al. Operative therapy of gallbladder disease in patients with cystic fibrosis. *Am J Surg* 1989;157:557–561.

Stern RC, et al. Treatment and prognosis of rectal prolapse in cystic fibrosis. *Gastroenterology* 1982;82:707–710.

Stern RC, Rothstein FC, Doershuk CF. Treatment and prognosis of symptomatic gallbladder disease in patients with cystic fibrosis. *J Pediatr Gastroenterol Nutr* 1986;5:35–40.

Stern RC, et al. Symptomatic hepatic disease in cystic fibrosis: incidence, course, and outcome of portal systemic shunting. *Gastroenterology* 1976;70(Pt 1): 645–649.

Vinocur CD, et al. Gastroesophageal reflux in the infant with cystic fibrosis. *Am J Surg* 1985;149:182–186.

Chest and Respiratory System

Corey R, Hla KM. Major and massive hemoptysis: reassessment of conservative management. *American Journal of the Medical Sciences* 1987;294:301–309.

Kesten S. Pulmonary rehabilitation and surgery for end-stage lung disease. *Clin Chest Med* 1997;18:173–181.

Penketh AR, et al. Management of pneumothorax in adults with cystic fibrosis. *Thorax* 1982;37:850–853.

Robinson DA, Branthwaite MA. Pleural surgery in patients with cystic fibrosis. A review of anaesthetic management. *Anaesthesia* 1984;39:655–659.

Smith MB, et al. Predicting outcome following pulmonary resection in cystic fibrosis patients. *J Pediatr Surg* 1991;26:655–659.

Steinkamp G, von der Hardt H, Zimmermann HJ. Pulmonary resection for localized bronchiectasis in cystic fibrosis. Report of three cases and review of the literature. *Acta Paediatr* 1988;77:569–575.

Genitourinary System

Hirsh AV, et al. Factors influencing the outcome of in-vitro fertilization with epididymal spermatozoa in irreversible obstructive azoospermia. *Hum Reprod* 1994; 9:1710–1716.

Liu J, et al. Birth after preimplantation diagnosis of the cystic fibrosis delta F508 mutation by polymerase chain reaction in human embryos resulting from intracytoplasmic sperm injection with epididymal sperm. *JAMA* 1994;272: 1858–1860.

10
Transplantation

LUNG

Despite the tremendously improved prognosis for patients with cystic fibrosis (CF), and the promise of new and more effective therapies afforded by the dramatic increase in our understanding of the molecular and cellular underpinnings of CF, it is still a profoundly life-shortening disorder, with the median age of survival of just over 30 years. Eighty-five percent of CF patients die of their lung disease. The ability to perform lung transplantation for someone with respiratory failure and irreversibly damaged lungs is appealing, and the science and art of lung transplantation have improved steadily since the first lung transplant was performed in 1982 and the first such procedure for a patient with CF in 1983. The science and art have not yet been perfected, however, as reflected by the fact that transplant complications have now replaced liver disease as the second most common cause of death among CF patients. In this chapter, we review the current understanding of lung transplantation in patients with CF, against the background that this is a rapidly changing field. We emphasize the approach to the potential-transplant, pretransplant, and posttransplant patient outside the transplant center. This chapter is not intended to provide detailed information on exactly how to perform a transplant, but rather it should help physicians manage a patient who will have or has had a transplant.

Indications and Contraindications

Indications

In theory, it is easy to list indications for lung transplantation in CF: extensive and irreversible lung damage and severe compromise of pulmonary function, exercise tolerance, and life quality below what is tolerable for the patient (Table 10–1). In practice, particularly given the shortage of donor organs, the system for determining organ distribution, the length of time required on the waiting list, and an only moderate long-term success rate, this decision is considerably more challenging (see later).

TABLE 10–1. *Indications and Contraindications for Lung Transplantation in CF*

Indications	Contraindications*
FEV_1 <30% predicted	Previous pleural ablation (chemical or surgical)
24-hour oxygen requirement	Poorly controlled diabetes
Rapidly progressive, irreversible lung disease	Steroid doses >10 mg prednisone every other day
Intolerable quality of life because of lung disease	HIV infection
	Malignancy
	Renal failure
	Severe liver disease; hepatitis B, hepatitis C
	Colonization with multiply resistant organisms
	Bloodstream infection
	Patient healthy
	History of noncompliance with medical regimen
	Current cigarette smoking
	Opiate/chemical dependency, drug abuse
	Psychiatric disorders
	Inadequate finances
	Lack of social support

*Some of these contraindications are relative, and others are absolute, differing by transplant center.
HIV, human immunodeficiency virus.

Contraindications

The list of contraindications for lung transplantation has shrunk considerably over the past decade as surgeons and medical transplant physicians have gained more experience and expertise. Previous surgery involving the pleura, particularly those procedures in which the goal has been the establishment of extensive pleural adhesions (e.g., chemical or surgical pleurodesis used in the treatment of pneumothorax), makes removing the native lungs difficult and bloody, and is considered by some transplant centers to be an absolute contraindication, a relative contraindication by others, and a mere nuisance by still others. Diabetes is made worse by antirejection medications after transplant and complicates wound healing and postsurgical recovery. Consequently, diabetes is at least a relative contraindication. Corticosteroids complicate wound healing, and so their use is discouraged before transplant. Any other organ system that is seriously diseased reduces the recipient's chance for a full recovery. Liver disease is the most common of these complicating conditions among patients with CF, and serious liver dysfunction is considered a contraindication by most centers. However, a few centers have performed successful lung-liver (or heart-lung-liver) transplants. Of 14 CF patients who underwent lung transplantation at the Seattle center, four had liver disease with portal hypertension (but not synthetic dysfunction), and all did well. Serious renal dysfunction is also a problem, because the current centerpieces of most immunosuppressive regimens, cyclosporine A and tacrolimus (FK506), have substantial nephrotoxic potential. Many centers consider creatinine clearance below 35 mg/min/1.73 m^2 to be at least a relative contraindication to transplantation.

Organ Distribution

The system that determines distribution of cadaveric lungs in the United States is relatively simple but controversial. Once a donor is identified, usually in an intensive care unit (ICU), most often after trauma and brain death, the organs are offered to the person on the waiting list with the same blood type and chest size as the donor, and with the longest time on the list, regardless of disease severity. The organs are made available first to patients and centers within 500 miles of the donor. If there is no suitable recipient within 500 miles, the organs are next made available to the entire country. Waiting times are more than 2 years in many U.S. centers, and as many as 60% of CF patients on lung transplant waiting lists die before donor lungs become available. It is largely because of this cadaveric donor organ shortage that the use of living lobar donation is increasing rapidly (see later).

Timing of Referral

Because of the long wait for a donor, most patients should be evaluated before they are terminally ill. Various guidelines have been used to help physicians and families decide on the timing of these steps. Because there are still many complications of transplantation, with considerable morbidity and mortality, patients should not undergo the procedure too soon; however, since many people die on the waiting list, they should not go on the list too late either. Some physicians have used oxygen requirement as a criterion indicating a reasonable time for evaluation and placement on the transplant waiting list. Pulmonary function is the other frequently used criterion. In one large study (Kerem, 1992), patients were found to have a greater than 50% 2-year mortality if their forced expired volume in one second (FEV_1) was less than 30% predicted, and thus, many patients are referred for evaluation when their FEV_1 reaches 30% predicted. In this study, younger patients had a higher mortality rate for a given low FEV_1 than older patients, probably because reaching an FEV_1 of 30% predicted in 10 years indicates more relentlessly progressive disease than taking 30 years to reach that low point. More recent studies do not support a 30% FEV_1 cut-off, and suggest that the rate of decline of FEV_1 is more important than any absolute value.

The penalty for going onto the waiting list too late is death while waiting; there is almost no penalty for going on the list too early: If someone has worked his way to the top of the list and organs become available but the patient feels too healthy (or not ready for any reason), the patient and family can decline the transplant without penalty. If they decline twice, the patient is taken off the active list but does not lose any of the time already accrued. When the patient, family, and physician subsequently agree that the patient is nearing readiness to undergo transplantation, the patient can be "reactivated" without losing the time accrued before the inactivation. Taking these factors into account has led most experts to advise evaluation a little too early rather than too late. This process has meant that the physician is often in the position of discussing a transplant when the patient feels much too healthy for transplantation. "I can't believe I'm that sick" is a very common patient reaction to the physician's suggestion of transplant evaluation.

The workings of the list are such that it probably makes sense for every patient to be evaluated, with the exception of the rare patient who is absolutely certain that he or she will never want to consider transplantation or has too many irreversible contraindications. Timing of the referral for transplant evaluation varies among patients and their physicians, but a useful rule of thumb is to consider referral when a patient's FEV_1 reaches 30% predicted, or when the FEV_1 has fallen faster than 1.5% predicted per year over the preceding years. Oxygen dependence is an even stronger sign that evaluation is appropriate.

In some patients, deterioration is so rapid, or the decision to undergo transplantation made so late, that it seems unlikely that the patient will be able to survive the 2 years that might be required for cadaveric lungs to become available. In these cases, living lobar transplantation could be considered (see later).

Transplantation Evaluation

The evaluation is usually conducted at the transplant center, after it receives data sent by the referring CF center. Those data usually include a clinical synopsis, pulmonary function test results (PFTs) and PFTs from 1 year prior (to give an idea of how rapidly the patient's lung function is worsening), chest roentgenograms, computed tomograms when available (more to help evaluate the lung volume and the pleural space than the degree of endobronchial or parenchymal disease), recent respiratory tract cultures and antibiotic susceptibility tests, and serum chemistries, particularly as they relate to liver and kidney function. At the transplant center, the center personnel and patient and family get to know each other, an important part of the process. Evaluations are conducted by the CF physicians, transplant surgeons, transplant coordinators, and specialists in cardiology, infectious diseases, perhaps otolaryngology, and psychiatry. Some studies may be repeated, and others obtained afresh: These include tests noted earlier, plus serologic studies for cytomegalovirus (CMV) exposure, hepatitis, blood type, human immunodeficiency virus (HIV), blood sugar and glycosylated hemoglobin, and Epstein-Barr virus (EBV) exposure. Age- and sex-appropriate cancer screening should be carried out. Pulmonary function testing, electrocardiogram, and echocardiogram are carried out. Exercise testing is performed at some transplant centers. Some centers have otolaryngologists perform a formal evaluation, perhaps including sinus computed tomography (CT), and a few centers have patients undergo functional endoscopic sinus surgery (FESS) before the transplant procedure.

Care While Awaiting Transplant

Patient and family education about transplantation begins during the evaluation visit. After the patient is accepted and placed on the list, he is given a pager, and transportation arrangements are made. The patient must arrive at the transplant center within 4 hours of being called. Many centers require that families live closer to the center when the patient is near the top of the list. Most centers also require aggressive nutritional supplementation, perhaps including nighttime gastrostomy feeds for the patient whose weight is substantially below the normal for height. This is based on the observation that nutritional status seems to be related to patient survival after transplant. Some centers also institute an exercise program, theorizing that patients with greater exercise tolerance may withstand the perioperative and postoperative challenges better.

The goals of pretransplant CF care are similar to those of general CF care, but there are some differences. In common with standard CF care, a goal is to keep the patient as healthy for as long as possible. In this case, health refers to pulmonary health, nutritional status, and exercise tolerance. Referring and transplant centers work out different approaches to achieve these goals. Almost all use aggressive intravenous antibiotic regimens for recognized exacerbations, and some programs schedule courses of intravenous antibiotics even in clinically stable patients. The aggressive use of intravenous antibiotics in CF patients, particularly those whose airways are already colonized with multiply-resistant organisms, raises the issue of antibiotic resistance and the specter of a worse outcome for those who harbor such organisms before the transplant. There are several approaches: one is the aggressive approach that dictates that the patient first of all must survive to receive a transplant and deserves the best care possible while awaiting transplant. Half of all patients on the waiting list die before donor organs become available; certainly their care should not be compromised to make them better transplant candidates. Therefore, if someone needs the antibiotics to survive, he or she should get them. Proponents of this approach point to the Chapel Hill experience. Their patients with panresistant *Burkholderia cepacia* did have a significantly higher mortality rate than their CF transplant population as a whole, but their patients with panresistant *Pseudomonas aeruginosa* fared just as well during and after the transplant procedure as their patients without resistant organisms.

The alternative approach is to worry that panresistant organisms can cause trouble in any patient, not just those who received a lung transplant and are being treated with immunosuppressive drugs. While using no antibiotics is not an attractive approach to the CF patient who is sick enough to be on the transplant list, a different approach might work: Twenty patients with panresistant *P. aeruginosa* were given twice-daily administration of colistin (75 mg) by aerosol, while intravenous antibiotics were discontinued (Bauldoff, 1997). All 20 patients (100%) became colonized with antibiotic-sensitive organisms in a mean of 45 days, whereas only 3 of 10 comparable patients not treated with colistin experienced emergence of sensitive organisms.

Patients on the waiting list are scheduled for periodic visits to the transplant center, usually every 3 to 6 months. In the meantime, care continues at the referring center, with full communication with the transplant center. The transplant center might have suggestions for treatment if newly resistant organisms emerge, if the patient develops a pneumothorax (see later), or if the patient develops diabetes or other complications either related or unrelated to CF. Certainly, the transplant center needs to know immediately if the patient dies or otherwise becomes ineligible for transplantation (e.g., he or she decides not to get one).

Pneumothorax

Because the cumulative incidence of pneumothorax in CF is 10% to 25% and pneumothorax is more likely to occur in patients with severe lung involvement, it is not uncommon among patients on the transplant waiting list. The approach to pneumothorax has been altered with the advent of lung transplantation. In the pretransplant era, treatment usually took into account the fact that—without preventive treatment—the recurrence rate for (ipsilateral) pneumothorax in a patient with CF was 50% to 100%. Therefore, treatment was directed at preventing a recurrence, as well as resolving the current episode. The preventive treatment consisted of procedures to ablate the pleural space, either with surgery and manual pleural stripping and pleural abrasion, or with tube thoracostomy and chemical sclerosing (e.g., with quinacrine, tetracycline, talc), or a combination of these approaches. However, ablating the pleural space by creating extensive adhesions makes removing the lungs more difficult; and extensive bleeding has caused some intraoperative and perioperative deaths. Some centers now believe that with better operative technique, with less use of cardiopulmonary bypass during surgery, and with the use of aprotinin, the risk of serious bleeding is considerably less than it used to be. Therefore, in some transplant centers, prior pleural procedures are less of a contraindication than they once were. Nonetheless, some centers still consider pleural ablative procedures to be at least a relative, or even an absolute, contraindication to lung transplantation, and they never should be undertaken lightly. The prior use of talc, with its potential for diaphragm "freezing," is especially like to give surgeons pause. It is for these reasons that a new, stepwise approach is now being followed in many CF centers for treating pneumothorax in the CF patient who may possibly be a future transplant candidate: The first step is tube thoracostomy drainage of the extrapleural air. If a chest tube alone brings about resolution of the leak, no further treatment is undertaken. If there continues to be an air leak, or in the event of a recurrence, the next step is to perform thoracoscopy, with identification and sewing (stapling) of any leaks or even nonleaking blebs that can be found. No pleural stripping or abrasion is attempted. If the first two steps have not succeeded, and the air leak continues or recurs, the definitive procedure, including pleural stripping or chemical pleural abrasion, is carried out.

Sinus Disease

The relevance of sinus disease to the outcome of patients with CF after lung transplant is unclear. The reason for concern, however, is quite clear: The sinuses are not removed with the old lungs and remain colonized with CF organisms, with direct access to the relatively pristine yet also relatively unprotected new lungs. Some centers have advocated sinus surgery and repeated antibiotic lavage of the sinuses for all CF patients who are transplant candidates. Others point to the lack of success of these procedures in sterilizing the sinuses and believe that until prospective controlled studies show a benefit from sinus surgery before the transplant procedure, it cannot be advocated for all patients.

Respiratory Failure

The approach to the CF patient with respiratory failure has changed more profoundly than any other aspect of care with the advent of lung transplantation. In the past, the standard of care for a patient who was at the end of a gradual but steady, inexorable decline ending in respiratory failure (as opposed to the patient who had been relatively stable, and suffered an acute event), was to provide for comfort and avoid mechanical ventilation, given the small likelihood of recovery. With the advent of transplantation, there is a tendency to keep the patient alive until donor lungs become available. Hence, mechanical ventilation is being used in some centers for patients awaiting transplantation. The most popular mode of ventilation is noninvasive ventilation, as with bilevel positive airway pressure (BiPAP). This form of ventilation is administered through a face mask and allows patients to eat, talk, and even walk. Some physicians advocate its use as a bridge to transplantation. Others argue that it simply prolongs the dying process, and although it is not as invasive as tracheal intubation and standard mechanical ventilation, it still is uncomfortable. In any case, no form of mechanical ventilation should be used as a bridge to transplantation for a patient for whom the wait for donor organs is likely to exceed a few weeks. It is wise for patient, family, and physicians to agree at the outset on an outside limit (e.g., 4 weeks) for how long mechanical ventilation will be used.

The Operation

The first procedure employed for replacing lungs in patients with CF was en bloc removal and replacement of heart and lungs together, with donor organs coming from patients who were brain dead (cadaveric donor organs). This procedure has largely been replaced by bilateral single lung transplantation, with bibronchial anastomoses, instead of a single tracheal anastomosis. A newer and more controversial procedure, namely, living donor lobar transplantation, has gained ever wider acceptance and application (see later). Single lung transplantation has been successful in patients with nonsuppurative lung diseases but cannot be considered in patients with CF because of the virtual certainty that infection from the remaining native lung would quickly overwhelm the newly transplanted lung, which has compromised defenses (no cough reflex in denervated lungs, diminished trafficking of immune competent cells to fight infection, and decreased mucociliary transport). However, single lung transplant after double pneumonectomy has been performed.

In what is now the standard bilateral single lung transplant procedure, the chest is opened with a so-called clamshell incision (transthoracic, through the fourth intercostal space). This approach affords the surgeon excellent access—including visual—to the pleural cavities, an important aid in identifying adhesions and other potential sources of bleeding, which are numerous in CF patients because of long-standing pleural inflammation. The mainstem bronchus of the patient's better lung is intubated and ventilated, while the worse lung is removed and replaced. The new lung is then intubated and ventilated while the remaining lung is replaced. This approach allows most transplants to be carried out without cardiopulmonary bypass and its attendant difficulties (especially anticoagulation). Aprotinin has been useful in helping control intraoperative bleeding in those patients with extensive adhesions, and in anticoagulated patients.

Living Lobar Transplant

In recent years, the technique of transplanting a single lobe from each of two living donors (usually relatives of the patient, thus the original term living-related lobar transplantation) has been introduced and has proven to be as successful in the short term as the traditional bilateral single lung transplant. The advantages of this approach include the possibility of scheduling the procedure and having it performed under well-controlled conditions (instead of being performed when a donor has died, perhaps in a distant location), not having to wait months or years for cadaveric organs to become available, less ischemic time for the donor organs, and the opportunity to screen the donor more completely for infectious diseases. Disadvantages include the risk to the donors (probably less than 1% mortality rate for lobectomy), the common occurrence of asynchronous rejection in the donor lobes (one donor lobe is rejected, while the other is not rejected), the possibility for undue pressure on potential donors (coercion), and in the case of families with more than one affected member, using the available donor lobes for one child that will then not be available for the other child or children.

IMMEDIATE POSTOPERATIVE (HOURS-TO-DAYS) CARE

Immunosuppression

Standard immunosuppression is based on three-drug therapy, with cyclosporine or tacrolimus (FK506), methylprednisolone, and azathioprine. The cyclosporine or tacrolimus is begun intraoperatively, as a continuous intravenous infusion (2.5 mg/kg/day or 0.05 mg/kg/day, respectively). These infusions are continued until the patient can tolerate oral feedings, after which the drugs can be administered orally. Achieving adequate and consistent blood levels of these lipophilic substances has proven difficult in patients with CF, and most protocols call for their administration with food and pancreatic enzymes. However, preliminary data from a small study suggest that absorption is not improved by pancreatic enzymes. One small study has suggested that the addition of diltiazem may help patients achieve good levels. Doses are adjusted to achieve acceptable blood levels. For cyclosporine, this means a random whole blood level of 500 to 700 ng/mL and, for tacrolimus, a trough whole blood level of 10 to 15 ng/mL. Methylprednisolone is given in a single intraoperative dose of 10 mg/kg, and then for the next 3 days is given in three divided doses for a total of 7 mg/kg/day. Once the patient tolerates oral medication, prednisone is initiated at 2 mg/kg/day, tapering over the next few weeks to 0.1 to 0.3 mg/kg/day, if there is no evidence of rejection. In recent years, several centers have tapered the prednisone dose more quickly in CF patients than in non-CF patients, because of the perceived higher risk of (and mortality from) infection in CF lung recipients. Azothioprine is given within the first few days after transplantation, starting with a dose of 1 to 2 mg/kg/day, and then at doses adequate to keep peripheral white blood cell counts above 3,000/mm^3. Some centers have omitted the azothioprine in CF patients, in order to decrease the risk of infection.

Antimicrobials

Intravenous antibiotics (usually clindamycin, ceftazidime, and an aminoglycoside) are given intraoperatively. The choice of antibiotics may be changed depending on the patient's preoperative respiratory tract culture results. In the first 2 weeks after transplantation, intravenous antibiotics are continued, with the choice of antibiotics based on the patient's clinical status and postoperative respiratory tract cultures. All CF patients are given intravenous amphotericin B for at least 48 hours after transplant. Treatment with amphotericin continues in those from whom aspergillus has been cultured recently.

Pneumocystis carinii prophylaxis with trimethoprim/sulfamethoxazole (TMP/SMZ), 5 mg of trimethoprim/kg body weight three times each week, is initiated within the first month after transplant. Dapsone or aerosolized pentamidine can substitute in TMP/SMZ-allergic or intolerant patients. Mycostatin mouthwash (swish and swallow) is begun shortly after transplant and continued indefinitely, to prevent candida colonization and infection. CMV infection is thought to increase morbidity, either directly with pneumonia, or with its association with chronic rejection and obliterative bronchiolitis. Therefore, CMV prophylaxis is given to all recipients who are seropositive for CMV, and for those CMV-seronegative recipients who receive lungs from seropositive donors. CMV prophylaxis consists of intravenous ganciclovir at 10 mg/kg/day for 14 days, followed by 5 mg/kg/day for two more weeks, followed, in turn, by oral acyclovir for 3 months, at a dose of 650 mg/m^2, with downward adjustments if dictated by the patient's creatinine clearance. High-titer anti-CMV immunoglobulin (CytoGam) may have a role in prevention or treatment of CMV disease.

General Care

Airway clearance techniques (chest PT, Flutter) need to be instituted very soon after surgery. The new lungs are denervated, and there is an absent cough reflex below the anastomotic sites. Surgeons, intensivists, and ICU nurses often need gentle reminders that the CF patient who has just received a new pair of lungs still has CF in the rest of his or her body. Distal intestinal obstruction syndrome is distressingly common in the CF lung recipient in the weeks after transplant. Pancreatic enzymes must be given as oral feeds start, even in the early stages of feeding. (The time-honored progression of feeds from "clear fluids," or just "clears," to "soft mechanical" to "full diet" makes little sense in CF patients: "Clears" usually include chicken broth—loaded with fat—and gelatin—loaded with protein (enzymes need to be given), while a potato, with neither fat nor protein, is not permitted until a soft mechanical diet has been reached.)

Hypomagnesemic seizures and hypochloremic alkalosis are also relatively common in care units not used to addressing CF electrolyte problems.

Longer Term Care After the Transplant Procedure (Days to Weeks and Beyond)

In the days, weeks, and years after transplant, compulsive navigation is required to avoid the Scilla and Charybdis of complications, namely, organ rejection and infection. And although acute infection is much more often life-threatening than acute rejection, chronic rejection, which is manifest as obliterative bronchiolitis, is probably the main obstacle to long-term survival. After the transplant procedure, patients are followed very closely, with clinic visits, pulmonary function testing, measurement of tacrolimus or cyclosporine levels, and kidney function. Most transplant centers send patients home after transplant with portable electronic spirometers for daily use. If forced vital capacity (FVC) or FEV_1 falls more than 10%, the patient contacts the center. Bronchoscopy, with bronchoalveolar lavage (BAL) and transbronchial biopsy are the most useful tools for diagnosing infection, rejection, and several other posttransplant complications (Table 10–2). This procedure is usually scheduled for 1 to 2 weeks after transplant, 1 and 2 months after transplant, and then every 3 months for the first year. After the first year, bronchoscopic examination with BAL and biopsy have been performed about every 4 months in clinically stable patients, but recently, the need for such surveillance biopsies has been called into question, because it appears that unsuspected infection or rejection is relatively uncommon. Patients who develop cough, fever, shortness of breath, or infiltrates on radiographs are usually evaluated at the transplant center. In most of these instances, bronchoscopy with BAL and transbronchial biopsy are part of the evaluation. Although in certain circumstances, bronchoscopy and transbronchial biopsies may be performed by skilled bronchoscopists in the patient's home center to obviate the need to travel to the transplant center, it is absolutely essential that the slides are interpreted by pathologists experienced in transplantation pathology, because some findings of infection and rejection can

TABLE 10–2. *Complications After Lung Transplantation in Patients with Cystic Fibrosis*

Infection**
Bacterial, especially *Pseudomonas aeruginosa, Burkholderia cepacia*
Viral, especially Cytomegalovirus
Fungal, especially Aspergillus species
Parasitic, especially *P. carinii*
Rejection–
Acute
Chronic (obliterative bronchiolitis)
Posttransplant lymphoproliferative disease (PTLD)**
Airway dehiscence (especially early after transplant)
Bronchial stenosis
Diaphragmatic paresis
Vocal cord paresis
Hypertension**
Renal failure**
Distal intestinal obstruction syndrome
Osteopenia, perhaps with fractures⁻
Psychosocial
Narcotic dependence
Financial stress

Items followed by a superscript are those thought or known to be associated with too much (**) or too little (–) immunosuppressive drug. (Modified from Noyes BE, et al. Experience with pediatric lung transplantation. *J Pediatr* 1994;124:261–268.)

be subtle and confused for each other. The results of major changes in immunosuppressive therapy based on an incorrect reading of tissue can be devastating.

Acute rejection of grade II or worse, as defined by Yousem's criteria, is usually treated with methylprednisolone, given as a single intravenous dose of 10 mg/kg each day for 3 days. After this treatment, bronchoscopy, BAL, and transbronchial biopsy are repeated in 2 to 4 weeks. In the event of rejection that does not respond to the methylprednisolone, the choices are limited. Lympholytic therapy with OKT3 or rabbit or horse antithymocyte globulin may be attempted. Aerosolized cyclosporine is being evaluated as a possible tool in the treatment of refractory rejection, and photophasis is also being evaluated.

If infection is diagnosed, antimicrobials or antiviral agents are begun, based on cultures of sputum or BAL fluid, and susceptibility testing of the recovered organisms. Bacterial infection is a constant threat in lung transplant recipients, especially those with CF, who have native trachea and sinuses intact, along with whatever organisms reside there, in close proximity to the transplanted—immune compromised—lung. Two viral infections deserve special mention. The first is CMV, which is thought to play a role in chronic rejection. So among the therapeutic challenges in the transplant patient is this: too little immunosuppression leads to rejection; and repeated episodes of rejection presage chronic rejection; yet too much immunosuppression may lead to infection, including infection with CMV, and CMV infection may lead to chronic rejection. CMV activity is reflected in the PP65 level measured in serum; this test can help guide decisions regarding the necessity for further evaluation and treatment in the transplant recipient at high risk for CMV disease (especially those who were CMV-negative before the transplant procedure and received organs from a CMV-positive donor). If CMV pneumonitis is diagnosed, acyclovir 5 to 10 mg/kg/day, with or without high-titer anti-CMV immunoglobulin, is administered for 2 weeks. The other virus that can cause especially troublesome disease after transplant is Epstein-Barr virus (EBV). EBV can cause a relatively mild mononucleosis-like disease that requires no treatment. It can also cause posttransplant lymphoproliferative disease (PTLD), a lymphoma that can affect the transplanted lungs, regional or distant lymph nodes, and other visceral organs in as many as 20% of transplant recipients. The diagnosis is often suggested by nodular disease on chest roentgenograms or CT and is confirmed by transbronchial or open lung biopsy. Morbidity and mortality rates are substantial. Treatment consists largely of decreasing immunosuppression (stopping prednisone and azothioprine; decreasing tacrolimus or cyclosporine doses).

Other complications are listed in Table 10–2. Bronchial stenosis, nearly always at the anastomosis, can be severe, requiring balloon dilatation or endobronchial stent placement. Complications of the immunosuppressive agents themselves, in addition to infection seen with too much immunosuppression, include hypertension, renal dysfunction (including frank nonreversible renal failure necessitating kidney transplantation), and diabetes.

Psychosocial Considerations

Undergoing transplant evaluation and the procedure itself requires tremendous emotional energy. Patients and families are forced to make difficult decisions based on minimal data. The knowledge that some CF patients do extremely well for many years after transplantation whereas others do dreadfully and our inability to predict the course beforehand make the decision to undergo the procedure wrenching. Patients must often spend prolonged periods at the transplant center, often far removed from home, family, friends, and pets. The possible benefit from transplantation is almost impossible for patients and families to resist, even if they are not emotionally equipped to undergo the hardships and even when the mortality figures are not terribly different for those undergoing transplantation and those awaiting transplantation. Indeed, patients, families, and medical professionals often also fall prey to the urge to "do something" in what appears to be a hopeless situation. Already, physicians have been sued for not providing liver or heart transplants for patients; the day cannot be too far off when this will occur for lungs. Although most centers of which we are aware are very careful to list the dangers and the unknowns of transplantation, some patients and families are not able to hear this message, and enter into the endeavor expecting everything to be made right. For these patients, it is especially difficult when the nearly inevitable episode of infection or rejection occurs.

There are even psychological hurdles for those patients who do very well from a pulmonary point of view. It is not uncommon for patients who had been severely debilitated to have difficulty getting used to their newfound energy and no longer needing supplemental oxygen. They may have trouble letting go of the sick role and going forward with their lives. Patients and families must be amazingly strong (and most are!) to undergo the roller coaster–like ups and downs of transplantation.

Prognosis

The outcome for lung transplant recipients, including those with CF, has improved over the past decades, with one large series now reporting 84% 1-year and 61% 3-year survival rates (Mendeloff et al., 1998). Some patients do spectacularly well, whereas some do abysmally. The factors determining which group a given patient will fall into are not yet understood. Some factors have been identified that correlate with better or worse survival, and of these, some are modifiable: Sharples discovered that seven of eight CF patients who died after lung transplant were below 80% predicted weight for height. Many transplant centers now insist that their patients have aggressive nutritional repletion, including enteral tube feedings, before the transplant procedure. *B. cepacia* cultured from respiratory secretions is a poor prognostic sign. Panresistant *P. aeruginosa*, at least in one center, did not have quite the ominous implication as did *B. cepacia*.

Most surviving patients have improved pulmonary function, exercise tolerance, and a high quality of life. There are still obstacles to surmount, however, because only 43% of those 3-year survivors were free of bronchiolitis obliterans, and exercise tolerance—while it increased in the first year after transplant—decreased in years 2 and 3 after transplant. A recent analysis of survival benefit of lung transplantation for different underlying diagnoses based on all patients listed for transplantation in the United States from 1992 to 1994 (Hosendpud, 1998) concluded that in CF, as contrasted with emphysema and interstitial fibrosis, the statistics pointed to a favorable risk of transplantation (relative risk of transplantation versus continued waiting = 0.61, p<0.008). However, the survival curves in that paper show 50% survival at 3 years, for both the qualifications of "after transplantation" and "on waiting list." Lung transplantation is a relatively new procedure, and the outcome of the procedure is clearly improving. Perhaps as time goes on, fewer patients will need transplants, and those who do will have improved chances of survival.

LIVER

Liver abnormalities are relatively common in patients with CF, with as many as 30% having elevated serum transaminases, usually with no other sign or symptom of liver disease, and with autopsy series showing as many as 25% of CF subjects with focal biliary fibrosis. In many of these patients, there was no indication of liver disease during life. In fact, symptomatic liver disease is fairly unusual. In 1997, 2.1% of patients in the U.S. national patient registry had "liver disease requiring a GI consult." Liver disease ranks a distant third (1.5%) behind cardiorespiratory disease (84.5%) and "transplant complications" (12.3%), as the primary cause of death among CF patients reported in the U.S. Cystic Fibrosis Foundation's Patient Registry. However, its presence on the list at all indicates that in those few patients, liver disease is a very important problem. With the possible exception of ursodeoxycholic acid (see Chapter 5), there are few medical options available to treat progressive hepatic disease in CF. By 1998, there were 98 living CF patients in the United States who had received a liver transplant, from as recently as a few months to as long as 13 years before.

Indications and Contraindications

There are three indications for liver transplantation in CF (Table 10–3). These are (1) progressive liver failure with severely impaired synthetic function, (2) recurrent esophageal variceal hemorrhage that is uncontrollable with variceal banding or sclerosing, and (3) uncontrolled ascites. Liver transplants have been carried out for other reasons, but we believe that with few exceptions, these three criteria are the only justifiable ones, because CF liver disease is usually a very slowly progressive disorder and transplantation still carries a significant mortality rate (see later). Contraindications are not very different from those for lung transplantation, with malignancy, bloodstream infection, and other organ failures leading the list. It is not clear what degree of lung disease should disqualify one for liver transplantation. The early fear that CF patients' lungs would deteriorate dramatically after liver transplantation, because of immunosuppression, has not been borne out. In fact, in most series, pulmonary function has actually improved in those CF patients who received new livers. Yet, there clearly are patients whom most physicians would consider "too sick" for isolated liver transplantation. There have been cases of successful combined lung and liver transplantation, as well as of heart, lung, and liver in patients with CF. As

TABLE 10–3. *Indications and Contraindications for Liver Transplantation in Cystic Fibrosis*

Indications	Contraindications*
Progressive failure or hepatic synthetic function	Poorly controlled diabetes
Bleeding from varices that is uncontrollable with sclerosing or banding procedures	Bacterial sepsis
Uncontrollable ascites	Steroid doses >10 mg prednisone every other day
	HIV infection
	Malignancy
	Renal failure
	Severe lung disease†
	Patient healthy
	History of noncompliance with medical regimen
	Psychiatric disorders
	Inadequate finances
	Lack of social support
	Opiates/chemical dependency, drug abuse

*Some of these contraindications are relative, and others are absolute, differing by transplant center.

†Although severe lung disease is a contraindication to isolated liver transplantation, some centers have performed lung–liver transplants or heart–lung–liver transplants.

HIV, human immunodeficiency virus.

yet, there are no guidelines to help decide which CF patients with liver failure and clinically important lung disease should undergo isolated liver transplantation, with the hope that their pulmonary function will improve afterward, and which should be considered for combined liver-lung transplants.

Timing of Referral

Organ allocation in liver transplantation is different from lung transplantation in several ways. First, waiting time is not the sole determinant of one's place on the list; rather, disease severity is the most important determinant, with a ranking system from status 1 (in an ICU, on a ventilator) to status 4 (stable, not hospitalized). Livers preferentially go to status 1 patients. Second, there is a wider range of possible donors for liver transplantation than for lung transplantation because the liver is less sensitive to whatever disease or trauma has killed the donor, and because the liver can be preserved longer than the lungs. This means that a donor liver can be transported over a longer distance to the transplant center, and that the patient need not be as close to the center when the call comes. There are pros and cons to this allocation system, as there will always be when there are more people who need organs than there are organs available. In the case of liver transplantation, on occasion, patients have been admitted to an intensive care unit in order to move them higher on the list, even when their medical condition might not have merited intensive care. Another feature of the allocation system complicates matters: a patient deemed to require a multiorgan transplant (liver and heart, for example) automatically moves to the top of the list. Several years ago, there was a public outcry when the governor of Pennsylvania received a heart-liver transplant (for amyloidosis) the day after he was put on the list, while many people believed that they were languishing on the heart or liver transplant list. Fair or not, it was probably the governor's physicians' decision that he needed two organs that got him moved to the top of the list, not his lofty political status.

Sudden acute deterioration of hepatic function is relatively unusual, so the need to get onto the liver transplant list is not as pressing as the need to be listed for lungs. In fact, survival of more than 10 years after the diagnosis of cirrhosis has been the prevalent feature of CF liver disease. We recommend evaluation and listing only when a patient's liver synthetic, metabolic, or excretory function has been deteriorating steadily for months and is causing unacceptable morbidity and is an imminent threat to life—either directly or indirectly (by aggravating lung disease) or when a patient has uncontrollable ascites or uncontrollable bleeding from varices, despite attempted variceal banding or sclerosing. A single variceal bleed is not justification for liver transplantation.

Care While Awaiting Transplant

Standard care should continue while the patient awaits liver transplantation, with an emphasis on maintaining good pulmonary health.

Periodic visits to the transplant center should be scheduled. Episodes of variceal hemorrhage should be treated as before, with stabilization of hemodynamic state and with attempts to control the bleeding, as outlined in Chapters 5 and 9, for example, with endoscopic variceal banding or sclerosis. If portal hypertension becomes uncontrollable, with variceal bleeds or hypersplenism, portosystemic shunting may be indicated. Because the standard open operative procedure for portosystemic shunting is extensive it creates the potential for widespread adhesions, and makes a subsequent liver transplant procedure especially challenging. The newer procedure of transjugular intrahepatic portosystemic shunting (TIPS) has been a major innovation. With deterioration in hepatic metabolic function, in the patient's overall health, or both, transfer to the transplant center for hospitalization, including placement in an ICU if indicated, facilitates patient care and moves the patient higher on the waiting list.

Care After Liver Transplantation

Patients are maintained on treatment with immunosuppression, usually based on cyclosporine or tacrolimus (FK506). Although levels required for adequate immunosuppression are generally lower than those required after lung transplantation, they may still be difficult to achieve consistently in CF patients, probably at least in part because of pancreatic insufficiency and fat malabsorption. As with lung transplant recipients, with liver recipients, there is the constant concern of too much versus too little immunosuppression. Although the liver itself is not at especially high risk for infection, the lungs are still affected by CF and are already infected. The initial concern that lung function would deteriorate soon after liver transplant in CF patients because of immunosuppression and worsening lung infection has proved unfounded. Nonetheless, vigilance is important. Airway clearance techniques and aggressive use of antibiotics for signs of increased airways infection must be employed.

Frequent visits to the transplant center and even more frequent checks of cyclosporine or tacrolimus levels and liver function tests are required. Almost any increase in liver function test values prompts a transcutaneous liver biopsy to rule out rejection. On occasion, particularly with low blood levels of whichever immuno-suppressive agent the patient is using, a minute change in the liver function tests will prompt instead an empiric trial of higher-dose immunosuppression.

Prognosis

Liver transplantation has become more successful, with 10 of 14 patients in one series surviving from 2 months to 7.5 years after transplantation. Survival for CF patients is about the same as that for other liver transplant recipients.

REFERENCES

General

Cystic Fibrosis Foundation. *Cystic Fibrosis Foundation patient registry annual data report 1997.* Bethesda, MD: Cystic Fibrosis Foundation, 1998.

Frederiksen B, et al. Improved survival in the Danish center-treated cystic fibrosis patients: results of aggressive treatment. *Pediatr Pulmonol* 1996;21:153–158.

Lung

Aris RM, et al. The effects of panresistant bacteria in cystic fibrosis patients on lung transplant outcome. *Am J Respir Crit Care Med* 1997;155:1699–1704.

Armitage JM, et al. Post-transplant lymphoproliferative disease in thoracic organ transplant patients: ten years of cyclosporine-based immunosuppresson. *J Heart Lung Transpl* 1991;10:877–886.

Armitage JM, et al. Pediatric lung transplantation: expanding indications, 1985 to 1993. *J Heart Lung Transpl* 1993;12(Pt 2):S246–S254.

Barbers RG. Cystic fibrosis: bilateral living lobar versus cadaveric lung transplantation. *American Journal of the Medical Sciences* 1998;315:155–160.

Bauldoff GS, et al. Use of aerosolized colistin sodium in cystic fibrosis patients awaiting lung transplantation. *Transplantation* 1997;64:748–752.

Busschbach JJ, et al. Measuring the quality of life before and after bilateral lung transplantation in patients with cystic fibrosis. *Chest* 1994;105:911–917.

Caine N, et al. Survival and quality of life of cystic fibrosis patients before and after heart-lung transplantation. *Transplant Proc* 1991;23:1203–1204.

Ciriaco P, et al. Analysis of cystic fibrosis referrals for lung transplantation. *Chest* 1995;107:1323–1327.

Couetil JP, et al. Combined lung and liver transplantation in patients with cystic fibrosis. A 4 1/2-year experience. *J Thorac Cardiovasc Surg* 1995;110: 1415–1422; discussion 1422–1423.

Couetil JP, et al. Combined heart-lung-liver, double lung-liver, and isolated liver transplantation for cystic fibrosis in children. *Transpl Int* 1997;10:33–39.

Cropp G, et al. Heart-lung transplantation in cystic fibrosis. *Cystic Fibrosis Club Abstracts* 1984;25:117.

Dark JH. Lung: living related transplantation. *Br Med Bull* 1997;53:892–903.

Davis PB, di Sant'Agnese PA. Assisted ventilation for patients with cystic fibrosis. *JAMA* 1978;239:1851–1854.

Dennis CM, et al. Heart-lung-liver transplantation. *J Heart Lung Transpl* 1996;15: 536–538.

Forty J, et al. Single lung transplantation with simultaneous contralateral pneu-monectomy for cystic fibrosis. *J Heart Lung Transpl* 1994;13:727–730.

Griffith BP, et al. Anastomotic pitfalls in lung transplantation. *J Thorac Cardiovasc Surg* 1994;107:745–754.

Griffith BP, et al. A decade of lung transplantation. *Ann Surg* 1993;218:310–318; discussion 318–320.

Hodson ME, et al. Non-invasive mechanical ventilation for cystic fibrosis patients—a potential bridge to transplantation. *Eur Respir J* 1991;4:524–527.

Hosenpud JD, et al. Effect of diagnosis on survival benefit of lung transplantation for end-stage lung disease. *Lancet* 1998;351:24–27.

Keller C, Frost A. Fiberoptic bronchoplasty. *Chest* 1992;102:995–998.

Kerem E, et al. Prediction of mortality in patients with cystic fibrosis. *N Engl J Med* 1992;326:1187–1191.

Klima LD, et al. Successful lung transplantation in spite of cystic fibrosis-associ-ated liver disease: a case series. *J Heart Lung Transpl* 1997;16:934–938.

Koutlas TC, et al. Pediatric lung transplantation—are there surgical contraindica-tions? *Transplantation* 1997;63:269–274.

Kurland G, Orenstein DM. Complications of pediatric lung and heart lung trans-plantation. *Curr Opin Pediatr* 1994;6:262–271.

Madden BP, et al. Intermediate-term results of heart-lung transplantation for cys-tic fibrosis. *Lancet* 1992;339:1583–1587.

McLaughlin RJ, et al. Pneumothorax in cystic fibrosis: management and outcome. *J Pediatr* 1982;100:863–869.

Mendeloff EN, et al. Pediatric and adult lung transplantation for cystic fibrosis. *J Thorac Cardiovasc Surg* 1998;115:404–413; discussion 413–414.

Milla CE, Warwick WJ. Risk of death in cystic fibrosis patients with severely com-promised lung function. *Chest* 1998;113:1230–1234.

Nixon PA, et al. Exercise tolerance and quality of life in paediatric lung transplant recipients. In: Armstrong N, Kirby B, Welsman J, eds. *Children and exercise,* Vol XIX. London: E & FN Spon, 1997:31–36.

Noyes BE, Griffith BP, Kurland G. Lung transplantation. In: Orenstein DM, Stern RC, eds. *Treatment of the hospitalized cystic fibrosis patient.* New York: Marcel Dekker, Inc., 1998:341–355. Vol. 109 of *Lung Biology in Health and Disease.* Ed. C Lenfant.

Noyes BE, et al. Experience with pediatric lung transplantation. *J Pediatr* 1994; 124:261–268.

Noyes BE, DM Orenstein. Treatment of pneumothorax in cystic fibrosis in the era of lung transplantation (Editorial). *Chest* 1992;101:1187.

Noyes BE, et al. *Pseudomonas cepacia* empyema necessitatis after lung transplantation in two patients with cystic fibrosis. *Chest* 1994;105:1888–1891.

Ramirez JC, et al. Bilateral lung transplantation for cystic fibrosis. The Toronto Lung Transplant Group. *J Thorac Cardiovasc Surg* 1992;103:287–293.

Rothbaum RJ. Gastrointestinal complications. In: Orenstein DM, Stern RC, eds. *Treatment of the hospitalized cystic fibrosis patient,* 1st ed. New York: Marcel Dekker, Inc., 1998:135–173. Vol. 109 of *Lung Biology in Health and Disease*. Ed. C Lenfant.

Sarris GE, et al. Long-term results of combined heart-lung transplantation: the Stanford experience. *J Heart Lung Transpl* 1994;13:940–949.

Sharples L, et al. Prognosis of patients with cystic fibrosis awaiting heart and lung transplantation. *J Heart Lung Transpl* 1993;12:669–674.

Shennib H, Auger JL. Diltiazem improves cyclosporine dosage in cystic fibrosis lung transplant recipients. *J Heart Lung Transpl* 1994;13:292–296.

Snell GI, et al. *Pseudomonas cepacia* in lung transplant recipients with cystic fibrosis. *Chest* 1993;103:466–471.

Sonett JR, et al. Endobronchial management of benign, malignant, and lung transplant airway stenoses. *Ann Thorac Surg* 1995;59:1417–1422.

Spector ML, RC Stern. Pneumothorax in cystic fibrosis: a 26-year experience. *Ann Thorac Surg* 1989;47:204–207.

Starnes VA, Barr ML, Cohen RG. Lobar transplantation. Indications, technique, and outcome. *J Thorac Cardiovasc Surg* 1994;108:403–410; discussion 410–411.

Starnes VA, et al. Living-donor lobar lung transplantation experience: intermediate results. *J Thorac Cardiovasc Surg* 1996;112: 1284–1290; discussion 1290–1291.

Starnes VA, et al. Cystic fibrosis. Target population for lung transplantation in North America in the 1990s. *J Thorac Cardiovasc Surg* 1992;103:1008–1014.

Tan KK, et al. Altered pharmacokinetics of cyclosporin in heart-lung transplant recipients with cystic fibrosis. *Ther Drug Monit* 1990;12:520–524.

Tsang VT, et al. Cyclosporin pharmacokinetics in heart-lung transplant recipients with cystic fibrosis. Effects of pancreatic enzymes and ranitidine. *Eur J Clin Pharmacol* 1994;46:261–265.

Walter S, et al. Epidemiology of chronic *Pseudomonas aeruginosa* infections in the airways of lung transplant recipients with cystic fibrosis. *Thorax* 1997;52: 318–321.

Whitehead B, et al. Incidence of obliterative bronchiolitis after heart-lung transplantation in children. *J Heart Lung Transpl* 1993;12(Pt 1):903–908.

Yousem S, Berry G, Brunt E. A working formulation for the standardization of the nomenclature in the diagnosis of heart and lung rejection: Lung Rejection Study Group. *J Heart Lung Transplant* 1990;9:593–601.

Liver

Colombo C, et al. Hepatobiliary system. In: Yankaskas JR, Knowles MR, eds. *Cystic fibrosis in adults*. Philadelphia: Lippincott-Raven Publishers, 1999:309–324.

Couetil JP, et al. Combined lung and liver transplantation in patients with cystic fibrosis. A 4 1/2-year experience. *J Thorac Cardiovasc Surg* 1995;110: 1415–1422; discussion 1422–1423.

Couetil JP, et al. Combined heart-lung-liver, double lung-liver, and isolated liver transplantation for cystic fibrosis in children. *Transpl Int* 1997;10:33–39.

Dennis CM, et al. Heart-lung-liver transplantation. *J Heart Lung Transpl* 1996;15: 536–538.

Hultcrantz R, Mengarelli S, Strandvik B. Morphological findings in the liver of children with cystic fibrosis: a light and electron microscopical study. *Hepatology* 1986;6:881–889.

Kerns S, Hawkins I. Transjugular intrahepatic portosystemic shunt in a child with cystic fibrosis. *AJR Am J Roentgenol* 1992;159:1277–1278.

Mack DR, et al. Clinical denouement and mutation analysis of patients with cystic fibrosis undergoing liver transplantation for biliary cirrhosis. *J Pediatr* 1995;127: 881–887.

Mieles LA, et al. Liver transplantation in cystic fibrosis (letter). *Lancet* 1989;1: 1073.

Mieles L, et al. Outcome after liver transplantation for cystic fibrosis. *Pediatr Pulmonol* 1991;(Suppl A6):130–131.

Noble-Jamieson G, et al. Liver transplantation for hepatic cirrhosis in cystic fibrosis. *Arch Dis Child* 1994;71:349–352.

11
Adolescents and Adults

Cystic fibrosis (CF) used to be a baby killer, but as of 1998, 51.2% of patients seen in CF centers in the United States were teenagers or older, and 33.3% were 18 or older. Thirty years before, 8% of patients were adults. Obviously, CF is becoming of major concern to those who take care of adolescents and adults.

Although much of CF care is similar regardless of the patient's age, there are some important distinctions between children and older patients with CF. These distinctions apply to some specific CF medical problems; some non-CF medical problems of adolescents and adults, which do not spare CF patients; and psychosocial and financial considerations.

CYSTIC FIBROSIS–RELATED MEDICAL CONSIDERATIONS IN ADOLESCENTS AND ADULTS

Respiratory System

Upper Respiratory System. Although the upper respiratory system of adults is indistinguishable radiographically from that of younger patients, more adults than younger patients have symptomatic sinus disease. The treatment of symptomatic sinus disease is similar, regardless of patient age.

Lower Respiratory System. More adults than children have severe pulmonary disease (Table 11–1). Older patients are more likely to harbor antibiotic-resistant organisms and organisms associated with poorer prognosis, such as *Pseudomonas aeruginosa* and *Burkholderia cepacia.* The worsened pulmonary function and the more resistant organisms make the adolescent and adult more likely to need hospitalization and intravenous antibiotics: Thirty-four percent of patients

TABLE 11–1. *Pulmonary Function by Age*

Age (years)	FEV$_1$ percent predicted (mean)
5	103.3
10	85.9
15	75.2
20	62.3
25	56.5
30	55.3
35	51.1
40	54.3
45	52.1
50	52.7

(From Cystic Fibrosis Patient Registry, 1997; Annual Data Report, September, 1998.)

older than 17 years of age had one or two hospitalizations during 1994, compared with 24% of those 17 years of age or younger. More striking was the difference between younger and older patients with more than two hospitalizations in that same year (13.4% of adults; 5.3% of children).

Pulmonary Complications. Massive hemoptysis and pneumothorax are both more common in older patients than in younger patients (Table 11–2). The increased incidence of these complications is probably related to more severe underlying pulmonary obstruction, infection, and inflammation, but the role of time (e.g., longer exposure to inflammation) cannot be known for certain.

Mortality. Adolescents and adults are more likely than children to die. The mortality rate for 15- to 17-year-old patients in 1997 was 1.1%, while it was 3.9% for those 30–31 years old, with little

TABLE 11–2. *Pulmonary Complication Rate by Age in 1997*

Age (years)	Massive Hemoptysis	Pneumothorax
2–5	0	0.1
6–10	0.1	0.2
11–17	0.4	0.3
18–24	1.2	1.7
25–34	2.4	1.1
35–44	1.3	1.6

(From Cystic Fibrosis Patient Registry, 1997; Annual Data Report, September, 1998.)

TABLE 11–3. *Mortality Rate by Age Among Patients Under Care in Cystic Fibrosis Care Centers in the United States by 1997*

Age (years)	Annual Mortality Rate %
0–1	0.013
5–6	0.003
10–11	0.002
15–16	0.011
20–21	0.041
25–26	0.012
30–31	0.039
35–36	0.054
40–41	0.061

(From Cystic Fibrosis Patient Registry, 1997; Annual Data Report, September, 1998.)

increase over the ensuing 10-year age group (Table 11–3). However, it is important to note that the mortality rate for any given low pulmonary function value is higher for younger patients than older ones. For example, in one large study (Kerem et al., 1992) among patients with the same FEV_1, the risk of death in patients 10 years or younger was two times that of older patients. The same could be said of hypercapneic respiratory failure, which is a very ominous sign in children, yet which some adults can survive for years. Presumably what this reflects is that the patient whose FEV_1 has fallen to, for example, 30% predicted by age 9, or whose PCO_2 is elevated, must be in worse condition overall than someone whose lung function has taken 20 or 30 years to fall that low.

Gastrointestinal System

Pancreas. The incidence of pancreatic insufficiency may be as low as 50% at birth and rises to nearly 90% by midchildhood. Adults with CF and pancreatic insufficiency may have less troublesome symptoms from their pancreatic insufficiency than younger patients, possibly because they have simply learned better diet and enzyme control. On the other hand, among patients with pancreatic sufficiency, acute pancreatitis, which can be extremely debilitating, becomes more common (2.2% of all patients 45 years of age and older, compared with 1.2% of all patients 25 to 34 years of age and 0.2% of those 11 to 17 years of age, in 1997).

Intestines. From the National Cystic Fibrosis Patient Registry, distal intestinal obstruction syndrome (DIOS) rates seem to be relatively constant over the decades: 4.0% among those 0 to 1 year old, 3.0% of those 18 to 24 years old, and 3.9% in 35 to 40 year olds. Other sources (Rubenstein et al., 1994) suggest that approximately 27% of adults older than 30 years have DIOS at some point.

Rectal Prolapse. This complication is much more common in children than in adults. It most often has a benign course in youngsters, responding to relatively conservative measures of adjusting enzymes, but is more difficult to manage in adults. Adult caregivers have much less experience with this problem and are less comfortable treating it; additionally, it may be a more pernicious problem in adults. Adults with rectal prolapse should be instructed to push the prolapsed rectum in gently as soon as possible. Their enzyme doses should be adjusted, but if these simple steps do not prevent recurrent episodes, these patients should be referred early to a surgeon with experience in treating rectal prolapse.

Hepatobiliary System. It is perhaps surprising that liver disease is not more common and that it does not increase in incidence beyond the teenage years. Surprising or not, this seems to be the case: cirrhosis with portal hypertension was reported in 1.1% of patients older than 45 years, 1.1% of those 25 to 34 years old, 1.5% of those 18 to 24 years old, and 0.5% of those 6 to 10 years old.

Gallstones are reported much more commonly among older CF patients than younger ones (1.2% of those aged 25 to 34, and 0.1% among children 6 to 10 years old).

Endocrine and Metabolic Systems

CF-related diabetes mellitus is distinctly unusual in the first decade of life and becomes progressively more common in the ensuing decades. By one estimate, only 35% of adults with CF who are older than 25 years of age have normal glucose tolerance, whereas 33% have abnormal glucose tolerance and 32% have clinical diabetes.

Hyponatremic, hypochloremic dehydration and metabolic alkalosis are much more common in infancy than in later childhood and are distinctly uncommon in adulthood.

Musculoskeletal System

It appears anecdotally that skeletal complications such as hypertrophic pulmonary osteoarthropathy, pronounced thoracic kyphosis with back pain, and osteopenia with fractures, including vertebral compression fractures, are all more common in adults with CF than in children. Almost certainly, some of this increased incidence among older patients is attributable to their generally more severe pulmonary disease, but some may be related to age or to prolonged exposure to medications, for example, corticosteroids.

Reproductive System

Reproductive issues become relevant to CF patients as they approach and enter adulthood. First, entry into adulthood through the portal of puberty is often delayed, especially in those with severe lung or nutrition problems. Eventually, most patients do develop sexually, and for these patients, there are important reproductive issues. It makes good sense to introduce these issues to patients well in advance so that it will not be a rude shock, for example, for a young man with CF to discover on the eve of his wedding that he is likely to be sterile. Nearly all men with CF are sterile as a result of obstructive azoospermia, caused by an atretic or absent vas deferens. Sexual desire and functioning are otherwise completely normal. Male fertility is associated with genotype, at least to some degree. Most men homozygous for the ΔF508 mutation have bilateral atresia of the vas deferens, but there has been one report of an aborted fetus, homozygous for ΔF508, with an intact vas. The 3849 + 10 kb C→T mutation, with a worldwide incidence of 1.4%, is associated with male fertility, whether it occurs in the homozygous or heterozygous state. It is essential that patients know that, in the absence of semen analysis, CF cannot be assumed to confer adequate birth control. Of course, there is nothing about CF that protects against sexually transmitted disease.

Female sexuality, similarly, is normal, yet fertility is reduced. The reduction in fertility is attributable in part to thick cervical mucus, which is likely to be a physical barrier to sperm penetration. Nutrition deficiencies and severe lung disease may also interfere with fertility. Despite these impediments to fertility, there have been hundreds of pregnancies among women with CF, many carried to term. Women with good lung function seem able to maintain their health through and beyond their pregnancy. On the other hand, many of those with compromised lung function before pregnancy have a very difficult time throughout and beyond their pregnancy, with considerable maternal morbidity and mortality and an increased rate of preterm delivery.

Sex. With increasing pulmonary disease, sex drive (libido) and sex performance can be impaired, with potentially serious effects for the individual (a potential cause of depression) and for a couple (possibly even threatening a previously solid marital relationship). A woman may complain of the inability to sustain the weight of her partner during intercourse, decreased interest in sex, and inability to reach orgasm. The woman with CF may be able to be more successful, however, by using vigorous airway clearance before sex, adaptive positions (e.g., woman on top, or seated positions), supplemental oxygen, and decreased coital frequency. The man with advancing pulmonary disease may have more trouble with intercourse, because his performance is vital to intercourse itself. Nonetheless, he, too, can benefit from presex airway clearance, oxygen, and adaptive positions. Coughing paroxysms are not common during intercourse, and they can be prevented to some extent by presex airway clearance. The partner with CF may need to rest periodically, and the non-CF partner may need to keep himself or herself stimulated during these rests. As could be said of couples without CF, the success of the sexual relationship benefits greatly from understanding on the part of both members and willingness to adapt to each other's needs.

NON-CYSTIC FIBROSIS–RELATED MEDICAL CONSIDERATIONS IN ADOLESCENTS AND ADULTS

Adults with CF, for the most part, should receive the same health maintenance advice and surveillance as otherwise normal persons.

Some routine advice, such as avoidance of cigarette smoking, is even more important. However, some aspects of health maintenance are not the same. Dietary advice is one example. Patients with pancreatic insufficiency are unlikely to develop hyperlipidemia. They may not need to avoid saturated fat to the extent that non-CF persons do, and in fact, may continue to benefit from the higher calories of foods high in fat.

Cancer. For unknown reasons, CF adults have a higher incidence of gastrointestinal tract cancers. Given these data, routine surveillance colonoscopy could be indicated beginning at a relatively early age (e.g., 40 years). It is important that patients receive all other age-appropriate cancer screening procedures, for example, mammography, Papanicolaou smear, and prostate exam, in accordance with recommended guidelines.

PSYCHOSOCIAL AND FINANCIAL ISSUES

Independence vs. Dependence

Adolescence is the time when young people begin to establish their independence from their parents. This process is made more difficult by CF, because children have been dependent all of their young lives on their parents for health care procedures (e.g., chest physical therapy [PT]) in addition to the usual necessities of life. Reluctance to leave the safe haven competes with the desire to be independent, and this factor may worsen the common teenager-parent conflicts. Teenagers and young adults face the difficult decision of leaving home for college or for employment, or just for living away from home. Sometimes, young adults suddenly on their own for the first time (e.g., at college) let their CF care lag. These lapses, although very understandable and part of normal development, can have devastating and irreversible consequences. These issues need to be discussed frankly and fully with families and patients in advance.

Career selection may also be influenced by CF. Extended exposure to chemical fumes or dust can be harmful, and heavy physical labor may be difficult to sustain as health deteriorates.

Medical insurance needs to be a major consideration as patients consider career possibilities, and insurance is becoming an increasingly difficult issue. More and more insurance companies are limiting patients' access to specialized CF care, much to the detriment of their health. This problem is even more pronounced among adult patients. We have received calls from physicians in the community asking what to do for a CF patient on a ventilator—patients who had been denied care at CF centers familiar with CF care. It is essential that patients and families fight for their right to continued CF care.

REFERENCES

Cystic Fibrosis Foundation. *Cystic Fibrosis Foundation patient registry annual data report 1997.* Bethesda, MD: Cystic Fibrosis Foundation, 1998.

Davis PB. Special considerations for the hospitalized adult. In: Orenstein DM, Stern RC, eds. *Treatment of the hospitalized cystic fibrosis patient.* New York: Marcel Dekker, Inc., 1998:319–340. Vol. 109 of *Lung Biology in Health and Disease.* Ed. C Lenfant.

Kerem E, Reisman J, Corey M, et al. Prediction of mortality in patients with cystic fibrosis. *N Engl J Med* 1992;326:1187–1191.

Langg S, et al. Glucose tolerance in cystic fibrosis. *Arch Dis Child* 1991;66: 612–616.

Orenstein, DM. *Cystic fibrosis: a guide for patient and family,* 2nd ed. Philadelphia: Lippincott-Raven, 1997.

Rubenstein S, Moss R, Lewiston N. Constipation and meconium ileus equivalent in patients with cystic fibrosis. *Pediatrics* 1994;78:473–479.

Yankaskas JR, Knowles MR, eds. *Cystic fibrosis in adults.* Philadelphia: Lippincott Williams & Wilkins, 1999.

12
Terminal Care

Although life expectancy has increased tremendously for patients with cystic fibrosis (CF) over the past decades, it is still a life-shortening disease, and almost all CF patients die from their disease. Care for these patients at the end of their lives is among the most important tasks or responsibilities that CF caregivers are entrusted with. It is also one that many patients focus on for years. Many patients' parents have confided to us that the first chapter they turned to on purchasing a family guide to CF was the one entitled "Death and Cystic Fibrosis." Despite the importance of this phase of care, it is rarely emphasized in physician or nurse training. It is difficult and frequently unpleasant, and therefore, it is not surprising that staff members often distance themselves from dying patients and their families.

Yet, despite the undeniable difficulties, terminal care can be tremendously rewarding as well, and the physician and care team who focus on this aspect of care make an invaluable contribution to patient and family comfort. The goals of such care should be to maintain the maximum comfort—physical and emotional—for patient and family, while at the same time allowing for the chance of improvement, as long as it remains a possibility. A delicate sense of balance is required between treatments that can give maximum chance of extending life and allowing improvement and those that give maximum comfort, because some of these approaches can be in direct conflict with each other. Perhaps the most obvious example is endotracheal intubation and mechanical ventilation, a procedure that might extend life yet seldom provides physical comfort. At the other extreme is withholding all treatments, which might provide some relief over the short term but clearly does nothing to enhance a patient's chances of recovering from a serious health setback. Taking away all treatment says clearly that the medical team has given up, which never enhances family and patient emotional well-being. There can always be hope for recovery or—lacking that—at least maximum comfort. At the same time that it is wrong to take away all hope, it is cruel to hold out unrealistic hope for recovery. Doing so denies the patient and family the opportunity to deal with the issues surrounding death, and perhaps to put their affairs in order.

PREDICTING THE TIME OF DEATH

It is very difficult to predict accurately when someone with CF will die. Studies have helped define a few factors that correlate with survival among groups of patients with CF. The strongest correlate found to date has been cardiopulmonary fitness. In one large center, patients in the upper third for fitness measured on a maximal exercise test were three times more likely to survive than those in the lowest third. This study tracked survival over an 8-year period. Strong as this correlation is, it does not help at all in predicting time of death in the individual patient.

Several studies have tried to hone in on factors that might help predict mortality over a shorter time than 8 years. Most of these studies have picked pulmonary function, which at face value, seems to make the most sense, because most patients die from failure of the respiratory system. Kerem and colleagues calculated that a forced expired volume in one second (FEV_1) of less than 30% predicted was associated with about 50% 2-year mortality rate. Although this figure could not be used to advise a family to call loved ones in from out of town to say a last good-bye, it did seem to give a rough milestone for timing the initiation of evaluation and listing for lung transplant (because in many transplant centers, the waiting time is about 2 years). Two subsequent studies (Doershuk and Stern, 1999; Milla and Warwick, 1998), however, have cast some doubt on the ominous guideline of 2 years with FEV_1 less than 30%. In one center, survival with FEV_1 less than 30% predicted averaged 3.9 years, whereas in another center, it was more than 4.5 years. These investigators have pointed out that the rate of decline is probably more important than any given level of pulmonary function, with a rapid decline almost always being a more ominous finding than a much slower fall to the same level. These studies were for large groups of patients, and there is large interindividual variation in survival, even over a short period. An exception to the rule of "a faster decline in pulmonary function portends death more clearly than a slow decline" is the patient who has had an extremely precipitous deterioration, as for example with an acute viral illness or with forced immobility after a calamitous automobile accident. Patients with acute deterioration from these causes often have a much better chance for recovery than those who have deteriorated steadily over months or years. Still, there remains a large element of unpredictability. Most experienced CF clinicians have seen individual patients who were not expected to survive until morning go on to live reasonably active lives for months or even years and others in relatively good health who died in a few weeks after contracting a serious viral infection or after stopping self-care because of depression.

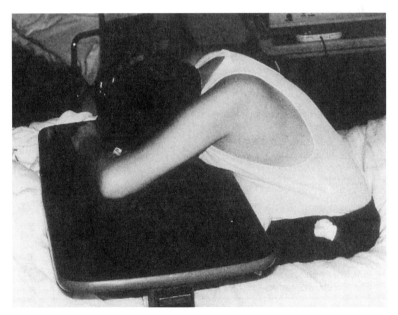

FIG. 12–1. Characteristic posture adopted by patients in the final days of life. (From Orenstein DM. Terminal care. In: Orenstein DM, Stern RC, eds. *Treatment of the hospitalized cystic fibrosis patient.* New York: Marcel Dekker, Inc., 1998;360. Volume 109 of *Lung Biology in Health and Disease* (Enfant C, ed.), with permission.)

There are some features that frequently mark the final days of patients dying with CF lung disease. They have little appetite, frequently sleep well past noon, are difficult to arouse even then, and have little energy while awake. The shortest of trips out of bed (even in a wheelchair) may be exhausting. There may be gurgling with respirations which is audible without a stethoscope. Patients may have

TABLE 12–1. *Signs and Symptoms of Altered Blood Gases*

Symptoms and Signs of Hypoxemia
  Respiratory
    Tachypnea (if severe, depression of respiration)
    Dyspnea, particularly with exertion (if severe, also occurs at rest)
  Cardiovascular
    Tachycardia
    Hypertension (with more severe disease, may have hypotension)
  Neuromuscular
    Headache
    Weakness
    Hyperreflexia
    Behavioral changes
    If more severe, visual disturbance, somnolence, coma
  Miscellaneous
    Sweating
    Panic
    Anxiety
Symptoms and Signs of Hypercapnia (elevated carbon dioxide levels)[1]
  Cardiovascular
    Flushed, hot hands and feet
    Bounding pulses
  Neurologic
    Headache
    Confusion
    Drowsiness (CO_2 narcosis)
    Muscular twitching (fine facial tremor, myoclonus, asterixis)
    (If more severe) engorged retinal veins, papilledema, coma
  Miscellaneous
    Sweating
    Gastrointestinal upset
    Electrolyte depletion

[1]The symptoms and signs of hypercapnia largely reflect vascular dilation and sympathetic activity. The severity of the symptoms depends more on the rapidity of the rise in $Paco_2$ than on the absolute level of CO_2.

(Adapted from Orenstein DM. Terminal care. In: Orenstein DM, Stern RC, eds. *Treatment of the hospitalized cystic fibrosis patient.* Vol. 109 of *Lung Biology in Health and Disease.* New York: Marcel Dekker Inc., 1998:364.)

a very difficult time raising very thick sputum and may be exhausted with hard coughing. Cough may actually decrease as the patient weakens. Patients frequently adopt a characteristic posture, sitting cross-legged in bed, leaning forward on pillows or a bedside table (Fig. 12–1).

Blood gas alterations fit into several main patterns in the terminally ill CF patient (Table 12–1). There is always hypoxemia, and often hypercapnia, but the degree to which each of these abnormalities influences the clinical picture differs from patient to patient. Hypercapnia is a particularly ominous sign in children with CF, unlike the situation in adult chronic obstructive pulmonary disease (COPD), in which it is not uncommon for patients to have numerous episodes of ventilatory failure (defined as elevated Pa_{CO_2}). In CF patients, Pa_{CO_2} greater than 55 mm Hg is associated with an 80% 2-year mortality rate. Carbon dioxide retention can be suggested by a patient's being difficult to arouse, although many sick CF patients with normal Pa_{CO_2} are slow to get started in the morning. Measurement of end-tidal carbon dioxide is noninvasive and can obviate the need for repeated arterial punctures.

MEDICAL CARE IN THE TERMINALLY ILL CYSTIC FIBROSIS PATIENT

Many aspects of standard CF care should continue through the terminal stages of the disease. If it appears likely that the patient is dying, the emphasis should be providing for patient (and family) comfort, while at the same time allowing for improvement if it is thought to be possible. If the patient is eating, pancreatic enzymes must still be given. Enteral tube feedings and parenteral nutrition are seldom helpful and are often inconvenient and uncomfortable for the terminally ill CF patient. Because there is certainly pulmonary infection, intravenous antibiotics should be continued, as should monitoring for toxicity from these agents. Aerosols and airway clearance treatments—be it chest physical therapy (PT), percussion vest, Flutter valve, positive expiratory pressure (PEP) mask, or other types—should also continue. At some point, any or all of these components of CF care may interfere unreasonably and inhumanely with patient comfort. If that becomes the case, the part of care that has become onerous should be stopped, even if doing so may hasten death. There are remarkable differences among patients regarding when and which treatments become unbearable. Some patients tolerate aerosols and chest PT but not venipuncture for monitoring drug toxicity, whereas for others, blood tests are hardly noticed, but eating or perhaps chest PT is intolerable. Standard treatment can be modified to fit a patient's tolerance. Perhaps chest PT can be done less frequently, and head-down positions can be skipped. The care team should work hard, with frequent revisions as needed, to find the most aggressive level of care that can be accomplished with minimal discomfort. Throughout the treatment, the patient and family should be able to define the level of care and discomfort that is acceptable, and their wishes should be respected.

Treating Dyspnea, Hypoxemia, and Hypercapnia

In terminally ill CF patients, blood gas abnormalities are universally present, and usually cause symptoms (Table 12–1). As one approaches the treatment of the blood gas abnormalities, it is important to keep in mind that other problems may underlie some of the symptoms attributed to the altered gas exchange. For example, dehydration from diminished oral intake (not just hypoxemia) can cause tachycardia, and hypomagnesemia (not just hypercapnia) can cause muscle twitching.

Treatment of the altered blood gases and associated symptoms differs somewhat depending on the clinical impact of these abnormalities. In some patients, hypercapnia and CO_2 narcosis dominate the picture, whereas in others, it is hypoxemia and air hunger that are more prominent. In the former case, the problem is its own solution, at least for patient comfort: patients may be difficult to arouse, but they are not uncomfortable. In stark contrast, the air hunger of profound hypoxemia is among the most distressing symptoms in all of clinical medicine and one of the most important to treat. The precise causes of dyspnea, the unpleasant sensation of difficulty with breathing, are poorly understood but probably include various combinations of (a) increased ventilatory demands, (b) increased effort in response to increased work of breathing, and (c) increased muscle force required to maintain normal ventilation. Patients with CF have all of these problems: increased ventilatory demands because of increased dead space; increased work of breathing because of the need to move air through airways narrowed by mucus, mucosal edema, or both; and increased muscle force needed both to overcome increased airway resistance and to compensate for the mechanical disadvantage imposed on the diaphragm by its being flattened by pulmonary overinflation.

Oxygen

Oxygen is the mainstay in the treatment of the hypoxemic terminally ill CF patient. The central role of oxygen is twofold: it is needed to prevent tissue damage, and it also relieves dyspnea. Despite these two obvious (and generally recognized) benefits of oxygen, it may be underutilized in the dying patient because of a misguided emphasis by many physicians on the possible dangers of suppression of hypoxic drive to breathe. Many physicians worry that the chronically hypercapneic patient maintains adequate ventilation because of hypoxic drive, and that relieving hypoxemia would take away the brain's reason to sustain breathing. The feared result would be further increases in carbon dioxide retention, with respiratory acidosis and perhaps CO_2 narcosis. This physiology is worth considering, and oxygen supplementation should be undertaken relatively cautiously. The dose of oxygen delivered through nasal cannulae can be increased by 1 liter per minute (LPM) every 30 minutes or so, while pulse oximetry and end-tidal (or, in the absence of an end-tidal capnometer, arterial) Pa_{CO_2} is monitored. A reasonable blood gas target is a Pa_{O_2} of 50 mm Hg or greater (ideally, it should be 60 mm Hg or greater, although this may not always be achievable), SaO_2 over 88%, and a Pa_{CO_2} that does not rise, or at least does not rise quickly. A slowly increasing Pa_{CO_2} allows for metabolic compensation for the respiratory acidosis.

Although these blood gas targets are reasonable, the primary goal should always be patient comfort rather than a particular number, if both comfort and a target number cannot be achieved. In fact, the target Pa_{O_2} may not always be achievable. Although oxygen delivery by nasal cannula is usually the most convenient method, because the cannulae do not interfere with eating, coughing, or talking, some patients prefer a face mask, and this preference should be honored. Some patients require very high flow rates for comfort and may continually ask for more oxygen, in some cases even when they have an apparently adequate PaO_2. In some of these patients, especially those with adequate PaO_2 who still ask for more flow, a fan directed toward the face may help relieve the dyspnea. In normal volunteers, cold air directed against the cheek decreases dyspnea caused by hypercapnia and breathing against increased resistance.

Despite the concern about hypercapnia, oxygen supplementation seldom actually results in worsened ventilatory failure. To the contrary, in adults with COPD and in patients with CF, oxygen administration most often results in little change in CO_2. In fact, improved ventilation (reflected in lower $PaCO_2$) is probably more common than worsened ventilatory failure after oxygen administration. This beneficial result suggests that impaired carbon dioxide removal in the terminally ill CF patient is more likely a result of obstructed airways and fatigued hypoxic ventilatory muscles than abnormal ventilatory drive. In those few patients in whom this result is not achieved and in whom ventilation is suppressed by even very cautiously increasing oxygen therapy, CO_2 narcosis at least provides transient comfort.

Other Drugs

β-2 Adrenergic Agonists. Most CF patients have less expiratory airflow obstruction after inhaling β-2 agonists, and these agents may help relieve dyspnea through that effect. Particularly if the dying patient has previously shown a benefit from β-2 agonists, these agents should be given in the terminal stages of the disease while the physician monitors the treatment to make certain that a detrimental effect does not occur (see later). There are reasons other than bronchodilation that β-2 agonists might help the dyspneic CF patient. Mucociliary transport rates and ventilatory muscle contractility and endurance may be enhanced. Also, in adults with COPD, β-2 agonists decrease dyspnea, even if they do not improve pulmonary function. However, β agonists have potential side effects in the terminal setting. About 10% of CF patients—almost exclusively those with the most severe disease—have a paradoxical worsening of obstruction with β agonist treatment, probably because some bronchiectatic airways require greater than normal resting motor tone from bronchial smooth muscle to maintain patency. Ventilation-perfusion relationships may be altered adversely, with worsening of hypoxemia. Also, β-2 agonists may adversely affect cellular chloride transport. Despite these real and theoretical problems with β agonists, the majority of terminally ill CF patients either benefit or are not adversely affected by them, and therefore, they should be tried.

Theophylline, like the β-2 agonists, can decrease dyspnea in adults with COPD, even while not providing measurable bronchodilation, perhaps through a beneficial effect on ventilatory muscles. Toxicity, particularly gastrointestinal, seems particularly common among patients with CF. Therefore, in the unusual case in which this drug is being considered for the dyspneic dying CF patient, dosing should begin at very low levels, with increases administered cautiously.

Psychoactive Treatment. Dyspnea and anxiety feed off each other, each making the other worse. Both are frequently present in dying CF patients, and each merits treatment. Skillful practitioners can be extremely helpful with the application and teaching of various interventions that help decrease dying patients' anxiety and panic attacks. These techniques include relaxation and hypnosis. In the relaxation approach, the patient focuses on decreasing muscle tension in different muscle groups, in rotation. In so doing, the patient diverts his or her attention away from the dyspnea. Hypnosis is most useful if the practitioner gives the patient the tools for self-hypnosis, to be used whenever it is needed, again to distract the focus of attention away from the unpleasant effort of breathing. These tools often include the repetition or thinking of specific words or images in a structured pattern. Sometimes, the patient is taught to tense and relax individual muscle groups in a particular sequence. Meditation, visual imagery, and biofeedback have been used with success in different institutions where there are skilled practitioners in a specific technique. Practitioners span the breadth of backgrounds, coming from pediatrics, psychiatry, psychology, family medicine, complementary medicine, nursing, and social work. Pastoral and spiritual care is sometimes comforting to some families at this stage.

Morphine. Morphine is one of the most important weapons in the fight against intractable dyspnea in the terminally ill CF patient. It unequivocally relieves breathlessness and anxiety. It also has potential for harm, including fatal respiratory depression from overdose. Smaller doses can cause distressing urinary retention, constipation, and vomiting. The potential for overdose is even greater in patients with CF dying of respiratory failure, because they are exquisitely sensitive to morphine. The reasons for this enhanced sensitivity are not fully understood, but may be explained in part by respiratory acidosis, which heightens sensitivity to opiates. Because of the heightened responsiveness to morphine, it is best to start treatment with what seems like an exceedingly low dose. We recommend a starting intravenous dose of 0.1 mg. We emphasize that this is not a per-kilogram dose, but a total dose, and it will be effective in some patients. If it is not effective, the dose can be doubled every 5 to 15 minutes until an effective dose is reached. If the physician prefers continuous dosing, start with 0.2 mg/hour, with infusion rates increased as needed by 0.1 mg/hour. Changes can be made after reevaluation every 30 minutes. Nebulized opioids (morphine and fentanyl) have been employed, with varying results, in other conditions for the non-sedating relief of dyspnea, but they have not been adequately studied in CF.

Other Psychotropic Drugs. Lorazepam (Ativan) has proved helpful for some patients with agitation (pediatric dose, 0.05 mg/kg/dose every 4 to 8 hours; adult dose, 2 to 6 mg/day in two to three divided doses). The choice of other anxiolytic agents depends on the experience of the physician and, in the terminal stages, should be made largely on the basis of their effectiveness for relieving anxiety. Possible respiratory depression should be considered but should not preclude any drug from being used.

Mechanical Ventilation

Except in several unusual circumstances, mechanical ventilation is unlikely to be helpful in patients with CF. The exceptions include cases in which respiratory failure has developed suddenly in a patient who had been stable at a reasonable level of health. Such circumstances have been reported in infants with acute respiratory events, patients with severe viral pneumonia, and some patients with trauma. It may occur uncommonly after surgery. Most CF patients with respiratory failure have reached this situation gradually, over months and years, and have little reserve. They are unlike the adult with COPD who may be able to deal with a respiratory exacerbation temporarily with mechanical ventilation multiple times.

Some centers consider endotracheal intubation and mechanical ventilation acceptable in patients awaiting lung transplantation. Most others do not, given the difficulty of predicting organ availability and therefore the difficulty of forecasting the time that would be required on the ventilator. Many physicians also recognize that the "stay alive at all costs to await transplantation" approach interferes with the patient's and family's ability to prepare for death with equanimity.

Bilevel positive airway pressure ventilation (BiPAP), delivered through a face mask or (less commonly) nasal prongs can be a less invasive mechanical means of supporting ventilation, and has been used with some success both as a bridge to maintain the life of the patient until a transplant operation can be performed and for comfort care in hypoxemic, hypercapneic air-hungry patients. Treatment can be delivered continuously or only during sleep. Its success has not been universal, however. In some patients, the tight mask creates a claustrophobic reaction. In all patients, the mask interferes with cough, airway clearance, and the ability to talk. Many institutions now have respiratory therapists who are experienced in helping patients adjust to this therapy. Their help and attention to detail can make the difference between success and failure. The many variables that influence the comfort and usefulness of BiPAP include mask size and shape; padding for the nasal bridge, with frequent checking for pressure sores; FIO_2; expiratory pressure; inspiratory pressure; and timing.

AFTER THE PATIENT'S DEATH

Talking With the Family. In most cases, the physician has been talking regularly with the family throughout the patient's life and terminal illness. There are several issues of particular importance surrounding the patient's death, including an overview of the patient's life and final weeks, autopsy, organ donation, funeral arrangements, and family (especially siblings') reactions.

It is not uncommon for families to voice concern (or to harbor it silently) that if only they had done more or done things differently, the patient would have lived longer, been happier, or been healthier. It is important to be alert to such feelings, because in most cases, families have done a remarkable job of helping the patient live a good, full, and fulfilling life despite the ravages of a merciless diagnosis and disease. When this has been the case, it is worth reaffirming that fact to the family.

Autopsy. It may be possible, even in some cases of apparently typical CF life and death, to learn something about the person's disease course from a postmortem exam. Many families are reluctant to grant permission for such exams, believing that the process is mutilating and precludes the possibility of an open casket funeral. It is not uncommon to hear that "he (she) has been through too much already." Yet the autopsy may offer information and solace to the family. Some families may consent to limited exams, for example, thorax only. Many families who are otherwise opposed to autopsy will be in favor of the removal of tissue for use in basic CF research. It should be a goal of all who care for patients with CF to try to facilitate research that may one day bring a cure, and—before that time— better treatment. Part of that research effort still depends on having CF tissue. In virtually every case, organs (especially trachea and bronchi) are acceptable for basic CF research. Information on which programs use or need CF tissue, whom to contact, and so on can be obtained from the Medical Affairs Department, Cystic Fibrosis Foundation at 1-800-FIGHT-CF (1-800-344-4823).

Organ Donation. Most patients and families are aware of organ donation for transplantation and might have considered such a transplant procedure for themselves or even have been on a waiting list. Many will be eager to help by becoming organ donors themselves. In some cases, this will be possible. Eyes, skin, and bones may be acceptable, and kidneys, heart valves, and the heart itself may be acceptable under certain circumstances. Unfortunately, the procedure for harvesting heart and kidneys makes donating these organs difficult from patients dying from CF lung disease. For a heart to be viable, it must be removed while it is beating. In the usual non-CF setting, the donor is brain dead, usually after head trauma. The family can say its good-byes while the patient is on the ventilator. The patient then is taken to the operating room, where the heart is removed. For kidneys, the requirements are nearly as demanding: They need not be removed while the heart is beating, but their removal must be within 15 minutes of cardiac arrest. A CF patient rarely experiences brain death, but rather dies from cardiorespiratory causes, for which the timing is not predictable with precision, making these organ harvesting procedures challenging or impossible. Local organ procurement organizations have teams on call if a death and donation are imminent. For skin, eyes, and heart valves, harvesting can be accomplished anytime within 12 hours of cardiorespiratory arrest. For information about the organ procurement process in various geographic areas, the United Network for Organ Sharing (UNOS) can be contacted at 1-800-24-DONOR (1-800-243-6667).

Funeral Arrangements

Most families have thought about and perhaps have even made funeral arrangements before the patient dies, and the physician seldom needs to help. In some cases, families need a little guidance. In most hospitals, mortuary personnel contact the family's chosen funeral home to work out details. If an open casket service is planned, families may need to know if an autopsy will interfere with those plans. It almost never does.

Questions sometimes arise about whether young siblings should attend the funeral. The preponderance of expert opinion is that, difficult though this will be, it is often less difficult for the young child to go to the funeral than to be excluded from this important family ceremony and farewell. In many cases, center staff may choose to attend viewings, wakes, or the funerals of beloved patients.

Family Reactions

The reactions of any family when one of its members has died are complex and different from family to family. Yet there are certain themes that repeat themselves among families of CF patients. They frequently ask the question, "Could I or we have done more?" The dying is usually a long, drawn-out process, and therefore there is frequently relief when death finally releases the patient and family from the travails of the past days, weeks, months, and years. Yet, many families feel guilt at that feeling of relief. It can be helpful for the physician to explore these feelings and to let the family know that it is very common and normal to have these feelings, and that feeling some sense of relief is not evil or uncaring. In more unusual circumstances, one or, rarely, more family members may be so distraught that they may want sedatives or anxiolytics. In most cases, it is not wise for the patient's physician to prescribe such drugs. Sedatives may dull the normal reactions that need to take place in order for the person to achieve resolve and peace; additionally there is a finite medical risk in prescribing psychoactive drugs for a family member whose medical history is not known. In some cases, giving a family member who will not be driving a small dose (5 mg) of diazepam may be justifiable.

The physician and family may take some comfort and even joy from going over high points of the patient's life and personality. The physician should acknowledge how painful the loss is and should never urge the family to "get over it." It can be useful to point out that with time, the very sharp, deep pain the family feels will lessen, making it easier to take solace in the many good memories. It may also be somewhat reassuring and supportive to point out that they will doubtless never stop missing this unique individual who was such an important part of their lives.

It may be helpful to warn the family of a common cause of family stress in the months after a child has died. Family members will likely have good days and bad days intermixed, without warning as to which kind of day is scheduled for today. Also, different family members may experience their ups and downs asynchronously. Parents of a child who has died should be prepared for this eventuality so they can more easily keep from criticizing or feeling cut off from each other. Rather, the one having a good day should be patient with the one who is having a rough time, realizing that their roles may well be reversed the next day. Similarly, the person feeling low should not think that the partner who is having a relatively good day just does not care.

Siblings' reactions, especially if the siblings are very young, deserve mention in discussions with the family. If the sibling has CF, it is worth stressing what is different about that child from the dying (or dead) sibling, and perhaps what is different about CF care now that might make the outcomes different. It may also be helpful to address openly that it is perfectly normal for a surviving sibling to have had so-called selfish feelings and worries mixed in with positive feelings for the dead brother or sister. If the sibling does not have CF, a particularly common (nearly universal) experience is a dual feeling of (a) gladness that the sibling who has stolen much of the parents' time (and apparent affection) during the prolonged illnesses and hospitalization is finally gone, and (b) guilt at feeling that way. In the very young child, so-called magical thinking might result in the child's believing that he or she is to blame for the sibling's death by having had the occasional wishes that the offending sibling was dead. The possibility of siblings having these thoughts should be addressed explicitly even if those thoughts have not been voiced. It is worth pointing out that all children sometimes wish their siblings out of existence, that this is not evil or naughty, and that in any case, the thoughts did not cause the illness or death. At the same time, it is worth recalling the ways that the siblings were special to each other.

Outside of the immediate family, there are others who have been touched by the dying patient and who need to know about his or her death. This might include other patients, with CF or otherwise, who have shared hospital times and stories. It may be appropriate for a member of the staff to find out from the family which other patients the family would like notified. Staff members themselves may grieve a well-known and loved patient. It is sometimes helpful for the physician to talk with hospital staff, to acknowledge their help and grief, and allow them to express their feelings about the patient, the illness, and the patient's care.

REFERENCES

Davis P, di Sant'Agnese P. Assisted ventilation for patients with cystic fibrosis. *JAMA* 1978;239:1851–1854.

Doershuk CF, Stern RC. Timing of referral for lung transplantation for cystic fibrosis: overemphasis on FEV_1 may adversely affect overall survival. *Chest* 1999; 115:782–787.

Erbland M, Ebert R, Snow S. Interaction of hypoxia and hypercapnia on respiratory drive in patients with COPD. *Chest* 1990;97:1289–1294.

Gift A, Plaut S, Jacox A. Psychologic and physiologic factors related to dyspnea in subjects with chronic obstructive pulmonary disease. *Heart Lung* 1986;15: 595–601.

Jardim J, Farkas G, Prefaut G, et al. The failing inspiratory muscles under normoxic and hypoxic conditions. *Am Rev Respir Dis* 1981;124:274–279.

Kerem E, Reisman J, Corey M, et al. Prediction of mortality in patients with cystic fibrosis. *N Engl J Med* 1992;326:1187–1191.

Milla CE, Warwick WJ. Risk of death in cystic fibrosis patients with severely compromised lung function. *Chest* 1998;113:1230–1234.

Nixon P, Orenstein D, Kelsey S, Doershuk C. The prognostic value of exercise testing in patients with cystic fibrosis. *N Engl J Med* 1992;327:1785–1788.

Noyes BE, Orenstein DM. Treatment of pneumothorax in cystic fibrosis in the era of lung transplantation [Editorial]. *Chest* 1992;101(5):1187–1188.

Schwartzstein R, Lahive K, Pope A, et al. Cold facial stimulation reduces breathlessness in normal subjects. *Am Rev Respir Dis* 1987;136:58–61.

Wagener J, Taussig L, Burrows B, et al. Comparison of lung function and survival patterns between cystic fibrosis and emphysema or chronic bronchitis patients. In: Sturgess J, ed. *Perspectives in cystic fibrosis.* Mississauga, Ontario: Imperial Press, 1980:236.

Appendix A
Organization of Patient Care

Because of the complexity of disease manifestations and the life-long medical and psychosocial needs of individuals with cystic fibrosis (CF), they are best followed in a specialized CF care center in conjunction with their primary care physician. Survival of patients followed at such centers is significantly longer than for patients not followed at centers. At these centers, a multidisciplinary team approach can be provided by physicians, nurses, respiratory and physical therapists, nutritionists, social workers, and genetic counselors who have expertise and experience in managing the broad range of patients with CF. Patients should receive their care in an age-appropriate setting. The overwhelming majority of patients with CF have the diagnosis established by 5 years of age (mean age 4 years, median age 7 months), and in 1980, median survival was only 18 years. Because of this factor, most CF care in the United States has been delivered by specialists with training in pediatrics. However, in recent years, median survival has increased to 31 years and at least a third of patients now followed at U.S. CF centers are adults. Because of this shift, there is now increased involvement of adult pulmonologists in the treatment of patients with CF. Physicians with primary training in internal medicine and its subspecialties are better able to address the psychosocial issues faced by adults and the adult-onset second illnesses that accumulate over the patient's lifetime. Until quite recently, most physicians trained in adult pulmonology have not had extensive experience with CF-specific complications, especially those of organ systems other than the lungs. Fortunately, in most major academic centers, this factor is changing, and increasing numbers of adult pulmonologists are becoming superb CF specialists. Adult CF care can be provided in a number of different settings: (a) at a single CF center staffed by both adult and pediatric professionals, (b) at a separate adult CF center, and (c) at a pediatric CF center with care provided by an appropriately trained adult medicine physician. The decision as to which model works best is a local one based on geography, number of adult patients needing services, and the availability of age-appropriate personnel and resources. Based on these considerations, the Cystic Fibrosis Foundation now recommends that on reaching adulthood, CF patients be transferred to adult care providers. The success of this approach rests on having adequate numbers of well-trained and experienced physicians who are committed to leading a multidisciplinary CF care team.

Although the frequency of visits to a CF care center vary based on severity of illness, it is recommended that for most patients, the optimal visit interval is 2 to 3 months. The components of each visit include

1. An interval history, which focuses on overall clinical status, nutrition, gastrointestinal and respiratory tract status, reproductive issues, CF-related complications, and current medications and respiratory therapies. It is important that all findings be compared with previous evaluations.
2. A physical examination relevant to the nutritional, gastrointestinal and respiratory manifestations of CF. Weight should be measured at all visits on all patients, and weight and height should be measured and plotted on a growth grid for all patients younger than 18 years. Tanner staging can help monitor pediatric patients' development.
3. A nutrition assessment should be carried out at each visit and should focus on qualitative dietary history (by recall), changes in appetite or eating patterns, and use of nutrition supplements and enteral feeds. Midarm circumference and triceps skin-fold thickness should be measured by a registered dietician annually on all patients younger than 18 years, or more frequently as indicated. Calculation of weight as a percentage of ideal weight for height and classification as to nutrition status should be completed annually by a registered dietician. A 3-day quantitative dietary history performed by a registered dietician is recommended for

patients who have suboptimal nutrition status or growth, defined as weight less than 90% of ideal body weight, height less than 5th percentile, lack of weight gain in 6 months in patients younger than 18 years of age, or in those patients who have increased nutrition needs.

4. Functional and psychosocial issues should be addressed at each visit, and a complete psychosocial assessment should be performed annually by a social worker or psychologist. Issues to be addressed include changes in family structure and coping (supports, stressors, risk factors, divorce, and death), school or work performance, participation in age-appropriate activity, developmental and emotional issues, compliance with treatment regimen, financial issues related to provision of health care, vocational training, family planning, concerns about CF care, and understanding of disease manifestations and treatments.

5. Patient and family education should be addressed at each visit. Topics to be covered include dietary education, review of airway clearance techniques, understanding of CF manifestations and treatments, use of respiratory therapy equipment, exercise, medication administration and complications, genetic counseling, and new CF therapies and clinical trials.

6. Recommended laboratory and imaging procedures are outlined in Appendix B.

7. It is important that all patients with CF have an identified primary care provider and that there be ongoing communication between the primary care provider and the CF care center team. Regular interim check-ups, including administration of all immunizations, should be carried out by the primary care provider in accordance with the guidelines of the American Academy of Pediatrics, American College of Physicians, and other advisory boards. In some instances, it may be more convenient to have the annual influenza vaccination administered at the CF center. The visits to the primary care provider should cover recommended age-appropriate screening procedures including, but not limited to, audiology, developmental assessment for pediatric patients, vision, cancer screening (cervical, breast, prostate, and gastrointestinal), blood pressure, and cholesterol. The primary care provider can also play an important

role in the evaluation and management of intercurrent respiratory tract infections and exacerbations, and patient and family counseling, support, and advocacy.

8. Many centers have found value in regular discussions of all patients with the entire CF clinical team. At these meetings, the team is updated on the current status of the patient, including growth and nutrition status; pulmonary status (based on pulmonary function tests, physical examination, radiologic findings, respiratory tract microbiology); psychosocial and functional status; intercurrent illnesses and complications; and changes in therapy, home care, and educational needs. Each patient's overall change in clinical status during the previous 12 months is reviewed. A database that follows and graphically displays pulmonary function test results and weight and height (for patients younger than 18 years of age) over the previous year is very helpful. At the end of the clinical review, the team should develop recommendations for management in the coming year, and these recommendations should be discussed with the family and conveyed to the patient's primary care provider.

REFERENCES

Bosworth DG, Nielson DW. Effectiveness of home versus hospital care in the routine treatment of cystic fibrosis. *Pediatr Pulmonol* 1997;24:42–47.

Clinical practice guidelines for cystic fibrosis: Cystic Fibrosis Foundation. Bethesda, MD: Cystic Fibrosis Foundation, 1997.

Consensus conference: Cystic Fibrosis Foundation. Bethesda, MD. Microbiology and infectious disease in cystic fibrosis. 1994;5:1–26.

The Cystic Fibrosis Foundation Center Committee and Guidelines Subcommittee. Cystic Fibrosis Foundation guidelines for patient services, evaluation, and monitoring in cystic fibrosis centers. *Am J Dis Child* 1990;144:1311–1312.

Pond MN, Newport M, Joanes D, Conway SP. Home *versus* hospital intravenous antibiotic therapy in the treatment of young adults with cystic fibrosis. *Eur Respir J* 1994;7:1640–1644.

Ramsey BW, Wentz KR, Smith AL, et al. Predictive value of oropharyngeal cultures for identifying lower airway bacteria in cystic fibrosis patients. *Am Rev Respir Dis* 1991;144:331–337.

Schidlow DV, Fiel SB. Life beyond pediatrics: Transition of chronically ill adolescents from pediatric to adult health care systems. *Med Clin North Am* 1990;74: 1113–1120.

Stern RC. The primary care physician and the patient with cystic fibrosis. *J Pediatr* 1989;114:31–36.

Appendix B
Recommendations for Laboratory Testing, Imaging, and Pulmonary Function Monitoring

GENERAL GUIDELINES

Recommendations for routine monitoring of all patients and monitoring of patients on specific drugs or with diabetes mellitus are shown in Tables B1–B3. All laboratory testing, including cystic fibrosis (CF) mutation analysis, should be carried out in a Clinical Laboratory Improvement Amendment (CLIA)–approved laboratory. Respiratory tract cultures and antibiotic susceptibility testing should be performed in a laboratory that is capable of speciating unusual gram-negative organisms and identifying *Burkholderia cepacia,* mycobacteria, *Aspergillus fumigatus,* and mucoid variants of *Pseudomonas aeruginosa.* The laboratory should be able to perform or have access to a reference laboratory that is capable of performing synergy studies on multiply-resistant organisms. Pulmonary function tests (PFTs) should be performed according to American Thoracic Society (ATS) guidelines by personnel who have expertise in age-appropriate testing. Chest radiography should be performed at an age-appropriate facility with expertise in the interpretation of radiographs of patients with CF.

TABLE B-1. Schedule for Routine Monitoring

Test	Purpose	Frequency
Mutation analysis (with genetic counseling)	To identify cystic fibrosis mutations	**At diagnosis**
Posterior-anterior (PA) and lateral chest radiograph	To monitor progression of lung disease	**Every 2 years** in patients with stable clinical status; annually in patients with frequent infections or declining lung function
Asparatate transaminase (AST), alanine transaminase (ALT), gamma glutamyl transferase (GGT), alkaline phosphatase	To screen for liver disease	**Annually** (in pancreatic insufficient patients)
Complete blood count and red blood cell indices	To screen for anemia	**Annually**
Random (casual) blood glucose	To screen for diabetes	**Annually,** and at time of intravenous antibiotic therapy for pulmonary exacerbation, and at times of other stress
Retinol (vitamin A) and alpha-tocopherol (vitamin E) levels in blood	To monitor compliance with and response to vitamin supplementation	**Annually** (at least), in patients with pancreatic insufficiency (more frequently in patients with suboptimal nutrition status or poorly controlled malabsorption, or change in clinical status resulting in increased caloric need)
Respiratory tract culture (oropharyngeal, sputum)	To assess microbial flora and antibiotic susceptibility; to detect onset of pseudomonas colonization	**Every 6 months,** and at times of respiratory tract exacerbations in patients who are culture positive for *P. aeruginosa;* **every 2–3 months** in patients who have been culture negative for *P. aeruginosa.*

		Every 2–6 months
Spirometry*	To monitor pulmonary function	**As indicated** by symptoms or elevated random blood glucose
Fasting blood glucose	To screen for diabetes	
Oral glucose tolerance test	To screen for diabetes	**As indicated** in patients with failure to gain weight despite nutritional intervention; failure to grow; delayed puberty; unexplained chronic decline in pulmonary function, and during the first trimester of pregnancy
Prothrombin time	To monitor vitamin K status and hepatic synthetic function	**As indicated** in patients on long-term antibiotic therapy, those with nutritional failure or liver disease, and those undergoing surgery
72-hour stool fat study	To assess degree of steatorrhea and response to enzyme supplementation	**As indicated** in patients with apparent ongoing steatorrhea or growth failure; in some patients at diagnosis
25-OH-vitamin D level	To screen for vitamin D status	**As indicated** in high-risk patients, such as those on chronic steroid therapy, and those with suboptimal nutrition status

*In patients with decline in respiratory status, spirometry before and after use of a bronchodilator, measurement of oxyhemoglobin saturation, arterial blood gases and lung volumes, and exercise testing should be considered.

TABLE B–2. *Monitoring of Patients on Specific Drugs*

Drug	Test	Frequency
Aminoglycosides (intravenous)	Peak (30 minutes after a 30-minute infusion) and trough (just before infusion) serum concentrations	Around third, fourth, or fifth dose of each course
	Urinalysis, BUN, serum creatinine	Before each course and then weekly while on therapy
Aminoglycosides (aerosolized)	Urinalysis, BUN, creatinine	After 180 cumulative days of therapy
	Creatinine clearance	If a doubling of serum creatinine concentration is documented on two occasions at least a week apart
	Audiogram (500- to 800-Hz range)	After 180 cumulative days of therapy
Chloramphenicol	CBC, differential, and reticulocyte count	Every 2–4 weeks
Ibuprofen (long-term high-dose)	Pharmacokinetics	Initially, then every 2 years, or after >25% weight gain
	BUN and serum creatinine	Initially, then every 6–12 months
Prednisone (>3 months on drug)	Oral glucose tolerance test	Every 6 months
	Ophthalmologic exam	Annually
	Blood pressure	Every visit
	Growth parameters	Every visit for pre-pubertal patients
	Vitamin D, calcium, phosphorus, DEXA scan	As clinically indicated (remembering that alternate-day dosing does not protect against osteopenia)
Trimethoprim-sulfamethoxazole	CBC, differential, and reticulocyte count	Every 6 months
Vancomycin (intravenous)	Peak level	After initiation of each course

TABLE B–3. *Monitoring Patients with Diabetes Mellitus*

Test/Procedure	Frequency
Blood glucose	Before meals and bedtime daily; early morning (1–3 a.m.) monthly
Hemoglobin A1c	Every 3 months
Urine evaluation for microalbuminuria	Annually
Fasting lipid profile	At diagnosis, after metabolic control is achieved
Blood pressure	Every visit
Ophthalmologic exam	Annually

RADIOGRAPHY AND IMAGING

Standard Radiographs

Chest

Standard chest radiographs are only minimally invasive (there is very little radiation exposure when they are properly done), and patient cooperation, although helpful, is not essential. Radiologic evidence of deterioration (e.g., overinflation and so-called peri-bronchial cuffing) can precede clinical signs and symptoms, especially in infants. At all ages, routine chest films can also detect large lesions (e.g., lobar atelectasis and mucus plugs), which may cause few or even no symptoms or signs. Considering the relatively uncomplicated operation of the equipment (and its almost universal availability), the minimal radiation risk, and the reasonable chance that an otherwise undetected treatable abnormality will be found, the standard chest film is a logical procedure for routine interval screening (in asymptomatic stable patients, perhaps ideally performed every 2 years; each year in those with frequent infections or declining lung function), and more frequently as indicated in patients to evaluate acute changes. With regard to research, many scoring systems, which can be used by both radiologists and non-radiologists for standard radiographs of the chest, have been devised, standardized, and validated. Chest radiographs can sometimes be useful in the setting of a pulmonary exacerbation. New findings help confirm the clinical impression of exacerbation (although frequently pulmonary exacerbations occur with no radiographic changes) and follow-up films can be useful in gauging the extent of the response to treatment.

Abdomen

Routine abdominal films are probably unnecessary. Flat and upright films (so-called obstruction series) can be useful for CF patients who complain of abdominal pain as an adjunct in the diagnosis of distal intestinal obstruction syndrome (DIOS), constipation, and nephrolithiasis. However, many asymptomatic CF patients have large amounts of solid stool throughout the large bowel, making such a finding of limited value for the diagnosis of constipation. However, a normal film helps rule out significant constipation or DIOS.

Upper gastrointestinal and small bowel follow-through examinations can be helpful in investigating possible complications of meconium ileus surgery. Contrast enemas, usually with hydrophilic agents (e.g., Gastrografin) can diagnose and treat DIOS (especially for patients who cannot tolerate oral intestinal lavage). Contrast enemas can diagnose and treat intussusception, and can diagnose the fibrosing colonopathy that occasionally is associated with high doses of pancreatic enzymes.

Sinuses

Routine sinus films are not helpful because virtually all CF patients have radiographic evidence of pansinusitis (i.e., opacification of all the paranasal sinuses) all the time. The majority of patients have no symptoms suggestive of sinusitis and do not require treatment. For this reason, if clinically important sinus disease is suspected in CF patients (e.g., because of frontal headache, postnasal drip, or visual disturbance), computed tomography (CT) is preferable in that it gives more useful information about the integrity of the sinus walls (to determine if there is an expanding mucocele) and the presence of polyps. A single coronal computed tomography CT view of the sinuses has now almost replaced the traditional plain film sinus series at institutions where both are easily obtained. The cost is little different from the conventional sinus series, and the CT approach provides a far superior study. For patients with symptoms suggestive of an expanding mucocele, perhaps with bone erosion (associated with very severe headache and visual disturbance), a traditional multicut CT sinus examination may be indicated.

Bone Films

Plain films of the long bones (especially of the lower extremity) are often obtained to diagnose hypertrophic pulmonary osteoarthropathy.

Imaging

Chest

Computed Tomography and Magnetic Resonance Imaging Scans. Although scans can detect some lesions before they become apparent on plain chest films, they are still too expensive for routine use, and for young children, the need for sedation is often an added problem. Even with spiral CT, which allows extremely rapid scans (thus occasionally obviating the need for sedation), the usefulness of the scans is often limited by the lack of patient cooperation. CT scans are useful for specific indications (to evaluate the patient before a proposed lobectomy; intake evaluation for lung transplant eligibility; evaluation of possible second pulmonary disease, e.g., hemangioma). CT scans have been used (with various grading systems) for research studies. CT is usually superior to magnetic resonance imaging (MRI) for investigation of CF-related abnormalities.

Ventilation/Perfusion Scans. Ventilation/perfusion V̇/Q scans are useful before proposed lobectomy (an uncommonly performed operation) or pneumonectomy (extremely rare) to assess the percentage of total ventilation, and—especially important—pulmonary blood flow going to the area under consideration for resection. Perfusion scans are theoretically useful in patients with active hemoptysis as a method of localizing the origin of the bleeding, but as a practical matter, they are not usually used for this purpose.

Arteriography and Venography. Bronchial artery contrast is needed for embolization treatment of hemoptysis. The bronchial arteries can be identified in preparation for embolization. The origin of the spinal arteries can be determined so that the risk of inadvertently embolizing them (resulting in catastrophic neurologic complications) can be minimized. Pulmonary artery angiography (e.g., for diagnosis of pulmonary embolus) is rarely needed for CF patients.

Venography is sometimes needed (usually if Doppler ultrasound is not conclusive) to investigate extensive thrombus formation in patients who have implantable venous access devices. It can also be used to assist in the insertion of percutaneously inserted central catheters.

Head

Total head scans (with and without contrast), mainly to rule out brain abscess, are indicated for patients with very severe (especially nonfrontal) headache, prolonged fever of unknown origin, and for the investigation of localizing neurologic findings that are not precipitated by paroxysmal cough.

Abdomen

Computed Tomography Scan. Although there is no indication for routine use, CT scans of the abdomen are often needed when various CF complications are suspected. Common indications are (a) investigation of possible pancreatitis, pancreatic pseudocyst, or suspected pancreatic cancer in patients with abdominal pain; (b) evaluation of abdominal lymph nodes in patients with fever of unknown origin; (c) suspected appendiceal disease; and (d) suspected volvulus.

Ultrasound Examinations. Ultrasound examinations are more commonly used than CT, mainly because of the frequency of complaints that could indicate cholelithiasis or cholangitis. Ultrasound is used to evaluate the presence and severity of ascites in patients with suspected CF-related liver disease and for evaluation of appendicitis or one of its complications (subphrenic or other intraabdominal abscess) in patients with fever of unknown origin or unexplained abdominal pain.

Doppler ultrasound can be used to assess the direction of blood flow in the portal system to determine if severe portal hypertension is present. Similarly, this procedure can help assess the status of a transplanted liver.

Bone Density

Because of the increased incidence of osteopenia and osteoporosis, a screening dual-energy x-ray absorptiometry (DEXA) scan is indicated in adult patients.

PULMONARY FUNCTION TESTING

The primary function of the lungs is to provide sufficient gas exchange to meet the metabolic demand for oxygen supply and carbon dioxide removal, while maintaining normal acid–base status. Considerable CF-related pulmonary disease (destruction and fibrosis plus obstruction) must be present before the ability to perform these functions is seriously compromised. Once this point is reached, however, worsening disease is usually obvious to both the patient and the physician, and can easily be documented by objective tests.

The ideal PFTs for the management of patients with CF would yield quantitative information (across the entire range of disease severity) on the rate of destruction of pulmonary parenchyma, the rate of formation of pulmonary fibrosis, the severity of airway obstruction, and the status of the lungs with regard to the efficiency of gas exchange and amount of parenchyma that has been lost or irretrievably damaged. This information would indicate the need for a change in treatment (and could assess the efficacy of treatment after it was instituted) and the overall prognosis, and would provide the ideal outcome measure or measures for studies of new treatments. Unfortunately, no such tests exist. No accurate markers (e.g., substances that could be measured in blood or urine) of pulmonary destruction or fibrosis have been identified.

Conventional PFTs do not become abnormal until there has been considerable anatomic change, and at least in the early stages of disease progression, short-term changes in PFT results are not reliably related to actual changes in lung status. Also, PFTs are expensive, time consuming, effort dependent, and for patients with moderate to severe disease, may be unpleasant and stressful. Furthermore, PFT options in infants, at best, are qualitatively different and, because patient cooperation cannot be achieved, inferior compared to those performed by older children and adults. Also, because sedation is required, they are not risk free (see below). Nonetheless, standard PFTs, when conducted by skilled technicians with cooperative and motivated patients, often provide the best objective data available for assessing clinical pulmonary disease severity, need for intensified treatment, response to such treatment, prognosis, and research study outcomes. Because test results may begin to decline before a patient or family notices a change in symptoms, they play a major role in the management of most patients older than 6 or 7 years of age.

Standard Pulmonary Function Tests

Standard Spirometry and Plethysmography

Standard spirometry and plethysmography are the most useful and most easily obtained PFTs. Spirometry (i.e., measured breathing) is the simplest PFT. It involves recording the volume of air breathed in and out, and plotting these volumes against time, giving important measurements such as forced vital capacity (FVC), that is, the amount of air exhaled in a maximal forced exhalation after a maximal inspiration, and the forced expired volume in 1 second (FEV_1). Both measures depend on the size of the lungs and the patency of the larger airways. FEV_1 is the most universally employed single PFT parameter in CF clinical trials. Expiratory flow rates are other useful measurements derived from spirometry, with mathematical manipulation of the volume of air moved and time (volume/time) at various parts of a single maximal breath. Flow rates after the very early proportion of a forced exhalation are thought to reflect the caliber of the smaller, more peripheral, airways. For example, $Vmax_{25}$ (maximal flow in the last 25% of an FVC maneuver), $Vmax_{50}$ (forced expired flow at the midway point of an FVC maneuver), and FEF_{25-75} (forced expired flow between 25% and 75% of the FVC) are all used as measures of small airway patency. There is greater variability among the small airway measurements than with FVC and FEV_1, yet they are relatively less dependent on patient effort than the FVC or FEV_1 (Fig. B–1). Although optimal results require sophisticated equipment and an experienced technician who is a combination equipment operator and coach, there is increasing interest in more limited but self-administered tests that can be performed at home. Plotting flow at each lung volume against the volume gives the so-called flow-vol-

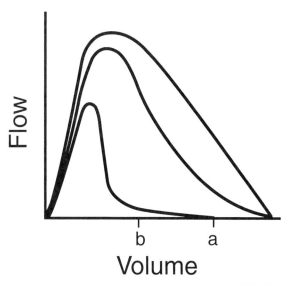

Fig. B–1. Expiratory flow-volume loop tracing (schematic). Flow is plotted on the vertical axis for each point of a forced expiration, from full inspiration (total lung capacity) at the left end of the volume (horizontal) axis, through full exhalation [with the remaining volume being residual volume (RV)], at the right end of the volume axis. The curves represent normal (outermost), mild, and severe obstruction. In the "obstructive" curves, there is "scooping," or concavity of the flow-volume curve towards the volume axis, representing lower flow for a given volume, with this tendency especially pronounced towards the end of the expiratory effort (a) because of peripheral, smaller, airway obstruction; but in the severely obstructed curve, it is also evident earlier in expiration (b).

ume loop with recognizable shapes, characteristic of various normal and pathologic conditions. The flow-volume loop (which includes measurement of the FVC and the FEV_1), is probably sufficient for usual patient care. However, the slow vital capacity (also a spirometric measure) and static lung volumes (including the thoracic gas volume measured with plethysmography) can add useful information. Ideally, spirometry should be obtained at every visit, especially on patients who are relatively healthy. In these patients, a decrease in FEV_1 or FEF_{25-75} can indicate the need for intensification of treatment before the patient is able to discern (or is willing to admit) any functional decline. Early disease progression in CF is marked by swollen airways and expiratory obstruction, resulting in air trapped within the lung. One of the most sensitive tests to detect this condition is the residual volume (RV) or the RV to TLC ratio (in which RV is defined as the amount of air remaining in the lung after a maximum expiratory effort, and TLC is total lung capacity). The RV and TLC can be measured with a body plethysmograph. Because of uneven ventilation of various portions of the lung in CF patients, helium dilution techniques underestimate the amount of trapped gas and should not be used.

Infant Pulmonary Function Studies

Because the pulmonary pathophysiology of CF usually begins very early in life, a method of assessing pulmonary function in infants and young children that could detect early worsening could be very useful in determining the need for antimicrobial or antiinflammatory treatment, or for more invasive procedures (e.g., bronchoscopy). There has been some research progress in this area (particularly to obtain an approximation of the FVC [by chest compression after an artificial maximal inspiration]), but because of technical limitations, infant PFTs are not widely used. Even if this technique were widely accepted and available, it is not clear that it is more sensitive in assessing the patient's response to treatment than the already available bronchoalveolar lavage fluid analysis.

Pulse Oximetry

Pulse oximetry (normal arterial saturation in room air generally accepted as 95% to 100%) allows intermittent or continuous noninvasive determination of arterial oxygen saturation. It is very useful for (a) roughly estimating the severity of pulmonary disease (and is therefore considered a vital sign in some clinics and hospitals); (b) continuous monitoring of unstable patients who are receiving or who may need supplemental oxygen; (c) testing of arterial saturation during sleep to determine the need for (or the dose) of supplemental oxygen at night; and (d) monitoring patients during exercise testing to detect desaturation with exercise (as a diagnostic test) and to ensure that dangerous desaturation does not occur (as a safety measure). Pulse oximetry cannot give an accurate determination of the actual partial pressure of oxygen or any information about arterial carbon dioxide tension, and so it is not useful for (a) assessment for hypercapnic respiratory failure, (b) tests that involve administration of 100% oxygen, or (c) an accurate determination of arterial oxygen tension.

Arterial Blood Gases

The ultimate question of pulmonary function is whether the lung can supply adequate oxygen and remove sufficient carbon dioxide (including participation in blood pH regulation) as dictated by the varying metabolic demands of everyday life. Arterial blood gas measurements assess this function directly and allow accurate determination of oxygen dose and, for some patients, the adjustment of mechanical ventilation or noninvasive assisted ventilation. However, blood gas measurements alone do not provide information on the work of breathing or on how long chronic hypoxemia has been present. For usual CF patient care, arterial blood gas measurements are used for (a) precise assessment of the need for supplemental oxygen (for many patients, this can also be accomplished using a noninvasive method, pulse oximetry), (b) determination and demonstration of hypercapnia, (c) documentation of hypoxemia to justify (for some insurers) the prescription of supplemental oxygen, (d) investigation of symptoms (e.g., headache or dizziness) that could be due to hypercapnia or hypoxemia, (e) quantitative demonstration of deterioration or improvement to justify hospitalization or to indicate readiness for discharge, and (f) research purposes. Arterial puncture is discussed in Chapter 8.

EXERCISE TESTING

Rationale for Exercise Testing

Exercise intolerance is one of the most common and troublesome consequences of CF, especially with advancing pulmonary disease. Possible causes include more severe airways obstruction with greater ventilatory muscle activity needed to overcome this obstruction, exercise-induced asthma (EIA), and deconditioning because of low levels of habitual activity. The exercise test can often isolate the various factors in exercise intolerance.

Further, cardiopulmonary fitness as measured on an exercise test has proved to be the factor with the highest correlation with survival in CF patients—higher than resting pulmonary function, higher than nutrition status.

Finally, exercise test values can be useful in patient management: finding the exercise intensity at which a patient with severe disease desaturates or tracking responses to various interventions, whether they are exercise programs, hospitalizations for treating pulmonary exacerbations, or intensive nutritional supplement programs.

Types of Tests

Tests can be carried out on cycle ergometers (also known as exercise bikes), treadmills, steps, or in measured lengths of hallway. The tests can be maximal tests, with workloads made progressively more difficult as time goes on (most commonly increasing in difficulty each minute or two), and ending when the subject can no longer maintain the set pace of cycling, walking or stepping. Alternatively,

TABLE B-4. *Exercise Tests Used in Cystic Fibrosis*

Test	Apparatus	Outcome measures	Validated in Cystic Fibrosis	Useful for before and after intervention?	$
Progressive test to exhaustion, with gas analysis	Treadmill; cycle ergometer; requires expensive gas analysis equipment	Physical working capacity; $\dot{V}O_2$, $\dot{V}CO_2$; $\dot{V}_E$; SaO_2	Yes	Yes	$$$
Test for exercise-induced asthma	Treadmill, cycle ergometer; hallway	FEV_1, FEF_{25-75} before and at 3–5 minute intervals after exercise	No	Limited	$-$$
Submaximal	Various	Various, including SaO_2; HR; breathlessness	Yes	Yes	$-$$
2-, 6-, 12-minute walk tests	Hallway	Various, including distance walked, SaO_2; HR; breathlessness	Yes	Yes	$
Shuttle walk tests	Hallway or lab	Various, including distance walked, SaO_2; HR; breathlessness	Prelim	Yes	$
GOS (Great Ormond Street) 3-minute step test	Anyplace	SaO_2; HR; breathlessness	Yes	Limited	$
Strength tests, e.g., 1-RM*	Free weights (barbells, with variable weights)	Muscle strength	Prelim	Yes	$
Wingate anaerobic test	Specially equipped cycle	Muscle power; muscle fatigue	Yes	Yes	$$

Modified from Orenstein DM. Exercise testing in cystic fibrosis. (Editorial). *Pediatr Pulmonol* 1998;25:223–225.
*1-RM: greatest weight liftable at a single time.

a submaximal test can be used. These tests are most often carried out over a set time, for example, the 2-, 6-, or 12-minute walk test (seeing how far the subject can walk in the allotted time), or conducted until a predefined end-point has been achieved. The most common end-points are a target heart rate, for example, 150 beats per minute (with more fit subjects able to accomplish a higher workload at this heart rate than less fit subjects), or an oxyhemoglobin desaturation. Strength tests have also been employed, measuring how much weight can be lifted using different maneuvers (e.g., bench press, biceps curl, and squat). The particular test that is indicated varies depending on the reason the test is being done. Table B–4 lists various tests, with information about apparatus, outcome measures, validation in CF, when useful, and cost.

If the purpose is to track overall health over time, several different tests could suffice, including progressive tests to maximum (the gold standard, both in terms of validation and in terms of the amount of gold required) and standard submaximal tests (e.g., 6-minute walk tests, step tests, or shuttle tests), with the test repeated at intervals (e.g., annually). If the test is being performed to delineate what factors limit exercise tolerance, the progressive test to exhaustion, with gas analysis, remains the gold standard.

Progressive Tests to Maximum, With Gas Analysis

These tests can measure peak work capacity (PWC), maximum oxygen consumption ($\dot{V}_{O_2MAX}$), carbon dioxide production ($\dot{V}_{CO_2}$), and minute ventilation ($\dot{V}_E$) while heart rate and oxyhemoglobin saturation are monitored. PWC and $\dot{V}_{O_2MAX}$ can be compared with normal values to compare patients' fitness with that expected for healthy subjects. $\dot{V}_E$ can be compared with resting maximal voluntary volume (MVV) to determine if ventilation is the factor limiting exercise, as it is with many CF patients (see Chapter 7). Most healthy subjects employ an $\dot{V}_E$ of less than 70% of their resting MVV, even at exhaustion, whereas many CF patients, who are forced to employ a large minute ventilation to make up for large dead space ventilation have $\dot{V}_E$/MVV ratios of 90%, 100%, or even 110%. This often happens before the heart has been pushed toward its limit, and CF patients may register maximum heart rates of 150 beats per minute or less (compared with the expected 200 or more). Simply put, the lungs have reached their limit (in terms of ability to move air) before the heart has been pushed to its limit. In other words, the ventilatory capacity is the limiting factor. During these progressive tests to maximum, oxyhemoglobin saturation can be monitored, and if a patient desaturates, the heart rate at which this happens can be noted, in order to advise the patient to exercise at lower heart rates or to exercise with supplemental oxygen.

Submaximal Tests

Submaximal tests of several types can provide valuable information, including degree of desaturation, heart rate response to a standardized workload, and distance walked in 6 minutes. These tests can be used to follow disease progression and response to interventions such as supplemental oxygen and antibiotics.

Testing for Exercise-induced Asthma

The standard laboratory test for EIA in a non-CF setting includes 6 to 8 minutes of exercise, usually on a treadmill, that is intense enough to elevate the heart rate above 180 beats per minute. PFTs, especially FEV_1 or FEF_{25-75}, are performed before and at 3- to 5-minute intervals after exercise, until 20 minutes after. This test is followed by a bronchodilator inhalation, with a final PFT after the bronchodilator. The best and worst PFTs are compared, and if there is more than a 20% difference, the patient probably has reactive airways. Because patients with CF may have trouble maintaining a heart rate of 180 beats per minute, and patients in a worse condition may be unable to pedal at any workload for 6 minutes, their EIA testing may have to be modified. In both non-CF and CF subjects, the best test for EIA is frequently a therapeutic trial of albuterol or sodium cromolyn just before exercise.

MICROBIOLOGY

Respiratory Tract Cultures: Bacterial Pathogens

Rationale for Obtaining Cultures

Although there may be an intrinsically heightened pulmonary inflammatory state and a tendency for a prolonged inflammatory reaction after disappearance or resolution of the precipitating cause, infection plays a pivotal role in the course of CF lung disease. Inflammation in CF patients cannot be fully controlled while infection persists. Furthermore, the severity of infection seems to correlate with the severity of inflammation. Thus, control of infection, as an antiinflammatory measure, is a critically important goal of treatment.

In addition to aggravating inflammation, some pulmonary pathogens, including *P. aeruginosa,* may behave differently when present in high density (e.g., by making more or different exotoxins). It is also clear that the invading pathogens themselves (including the nucleic acids of dead bacteria) contribute to the viscosity of pulmonary secretions. Treatment of infection may thus be important to suppress the number of pathogens, even if the organism cannot be eradicated. Microbiology data help in determining the need to treat, in guiding the duration of treatment, and in assessing the prognosis. For patients who are recently infected with *P. aeruginosa,* aggressive therapy can occasionally accomplish eradication, which if documented by follow-up cultures, constitutes an unequivocal reason to stop antibiotic treatment.

Culture Specimen

The gold standard for culture is lung tissue obtained at thoracotomy (or at thoracoscopy). Such a sample ensures that all recovered organisms originated in the lung (i.e., were free of contamination with nasopharyngeal secretions) and allows the sample to be collected (and cultured) anaerobically and aerobically. Lung tissue is rarely available, but lung biopsy for culture should be considered if a patient with puzzling or inconsistent microbiology data happens to be undergoing thoracic surgery for another reason.

Percutaneous lung puncture and aspiration would yield accurate data as well, but the risk of pneumothorax is too high to justify the procedure (unless the patient is known to have dense adhesions). Furthermore, lung puncture entails a risk of bronchopleural fistula formation. Transtracheal cultures are technically feasible (and avoid the problem of oral contamination and the risk of pneumothorax), but the risk of bleeding is high enough to preclude this procedure in most patients, and the risk of a tracheocutaneous fistula must be considered. Furthermore, transtracheal cultures are not optimal for recovery of anaerobic pathogens.

Bronchoalveolar lavage (BAL) fluid is almost as accurate as lung tissue for identification of pathogens and has some advantages. Flexible fiberoptic bronchoscopy is used to obtain BAL fluid and is less invasive than thoracotomy. By subjecting repeated BAL samples from the same area to quantitative cultures, longitudinal information on the severity of infection can be obtained for research or for clinical care. However, some contamination by mouth flora is unavoidable. The invasiveness of BAL makes it inappropriate for routine use, yet its safety makes it useful when a patient (especially one who does not raise sputum) has a disappointing response to treatment.

Sputum samples (proven by cytologic examination to contain macrophages) are more useful in CF than in other pulmonary infections, but organisms that are present in the lung can be missed. For routine use, especially in older symptomatic patients, sputum is generally adequate. Furthermore, antibiograms obtained on organisms recovered from sputum samples have good correlation to similar studies on lung and sputum isolates.

Throat and deep pharyngeal swabs have a sufficient, albeit not perfect, correlation to pulmonary flora to be clinically useful. Pathogens isolated from throat cultures in CF patients can be assumed to be of pulmonary origin, but a negative oropharyngeal culture cannot be taken as proof that there are no pathogens in the lower respiratory tract.

Summary of specimen selection for routine cultures:

Infants and young children: gagged oropharyngeal cultures
Older children, adolescents, and adults: sputum
For nonroutine cultures in symptomatic patients with inadequate
    response to therapy, especially in those who do not produce spu-
    tum: BAL
In all patients who will be undergoing thoracotomy or thoracoscopy
    (for whatever reason): culture of cut surface of lung.

Specimen Transport

Specimens should be transported promptly to the laboratory
(preferably in less than 3 hours) and processed on receipt. If this is
not possible, specimens should be stored at 4°C until processing. To
ensure special processing (e.g., *B. cepacia* medium), specimens
should be clearly identified as having come from a CF patient. In
unusual circumstances, specimens may be mailed to the laboratory,
with acceptable results. These circumstances include the sending of
isolates to reference laboratories for special studies (antibiotic synergy testing of *P. aeruginosa* at the laboratory of Dr. Lisa Saiman
(650 West 168th Street, Black Building 4-427, New York, NY
10032; 212-305-1991; e-mail: synergy@columbia.edu; website:
http://cpmcnet.columbia.edu/dept/synergy); speciation of *B. cepacia,* including confirmation that the specimen is, in fact, *B. cepacia*
and genomovar designation among recognized species of *B. cepacia,*
at the laboratory of Dr. John Lipuma (*B. cepacia* Research Laboratory, 1150 W. Medical Center Drive, 8323 MSRB III, Box 0646, Ann
Arbor, MI 48109-0646; (734) 936-9767; fax: (734) 764-4279; email:
jlipuma@umich.edu); and situations in which patients are at a far
distance from the CF center and are unable to deliver the specimens
in person.

Specimen Processing

All sputum and BAL specimens should be gram stained for the
presence of neutrophils and for presumptive identification of organisms.

Acceptable culture media:

Staphylococcus aureus: mannitol salt agar; automated systems are reliable.

P. aeruginosa: routine media, i.e., MacConkey, are acceptable; automated systems are reliable.

B. cepacia: selective PC or OFPBL agar is required: may require 48 to 72 hours for detectable growth; automated (commercial) identification systems are not reliable; isolates should be confirmed by a reference laboratory.

Mycobacterium species: specimen should be digested and decontaminated with NaOH and additional decontamination with 5% oxalic acid.

Haemophilus influenzae: horse blood or chocolate agar with the addition of bacitracin or anaerobic incubation.

Susceptibility Testing

P. aeruginosa, B. cepacia, and other gram-negative nonfermenters should be tested for antibiotic susceptibility using Kirby-Bauer disc diffusion. This system is based on measuring zones of growth inhibition around discs containing antibiotics that diffuse into the agar. Automated systems should not be used, because results may be inaccurate due to slow growth of the isolates. *H. influenzae* isolates should be tested for β-lactamase production, and *S. aureus* isolates should be tested for oxacillin resistance.

Specialized susceptibility and synergy testing (see above for information on special laboratories) is indicated in the following circumstances:

1. Presence of multiply-resistant strains
2. Drug allergy
3. Failure to respond to conventional antibiotic regimens
4. Before and after a lung transplant procedure

The following questions should be asked of the laboratory processing CF respiratory tract specimens:

1. Is there a specific protocol for processing CF specimens?
2. Are sputum and BAL specimens screened by gram stain to determine the adequacy of the specimen?

3. Are recommended media for CF pathogens being used, that is, mannitol salt for *S. aureus,* PC or OFPBL for *B. cepacia,* and horse blood or chocolate agar with bacitracin for *H. influenzae?*
4. Is the Kirby-Bauer disc diffusion system used for susceptibility testing?
5. Does the laboratory report the mucoid phenotype for *P. aeruginosa* isolates?
6. Does the laboratory understand that the presence of *P. aeruginosa* in a throat culture is important?
7. Does the laboratory understand the significance to the patient of a *B. cepacia* isolate?

In order to enhance microbial detection and identification, there should be on-going communication between the clinician and the laboratory.

Interpretation of Results

When *P. aeruginosa* is recovered from a patient who was previously culture negative, an immediate repeat culture is generally advisable (unless the patient is deemed too sick to wait for the results) before an aggressive attempt to eradicate the organism is undertaken. Asymptomatic infants are probably transiently colonized with many gram-negative organisms during the first year of life. The recovery of *Escherichia coli, Klebsiella pneumoniae, Alcaligenes xylosoxidans,* and others may not require treatment if the patient is asymptomatic and the organism is no longer present on the repeat culture. Recovery of *S. aureus* is more difficult to interpret in both infants and older patients because it can be present in the throat without being in the lung.

Antibiograms on pathogens recovered when the patient is symptomatic are a key consideration when treatment is prescribed (see Chapter 4).

Respiratory Tract Cultures: Mycobacteria and Fungi

Mycobacterium tuberculosis infection is not particularly common in CF, but colonization with atypical mycobacteria is common.

Mycobacteria cultures should be considered on sputum from inpatients, all BAL specimens (inpatients or outpatients), and depending on the circumstances, some outpatient sputum samples. Clinically significant infection with atypical mycobacteria (worthy of specific treatment) does occur, but colonization is far more common. The decision to treat the patient who has a positive smear (and, presumably, positive cultures as well) should be based on careful evaluation of the entire clinical picture. Patients with positive cultures but negative smears usually do not merit treatment unless there is strong clinical suspicion that the organism is acting as a pathogen.

Fungal cultures should be considered on patients who are sick enough to require intravenous (IV) antibiotics and on any outpatient suspected of having allergic aspergillosis (see Chapter 4). All BAL specimens should be cultured for fungus. Patients from whom yeast is consistently recovered from respiratory cultures should occasionally be considered for specific treatment, especially if no other pathogen can be isolated and the patient's pulmonary status is deteriorating.

Serologic Tests

Total Gamma Globulin. Elevated serum levels of gamma globulin are a non-specific indicator of long-standing infection. The absolute gamma globulin (if high) and the albumin/globulin ratio (if low) may be useful as an indicator of a poor prognosis, but they do not specifically suggest one organism (or group of organisms).

IgE Levels. Slight (up to three to four times normal) elevation of serum total IgE is a nonspecific finding of an allergic diathesis but does not identify specific allergies. However, a very high level (five times the normal local institutional value or higher) is strongly suggestive of allergic bronchopulmonary aspergillosis (ABPA; see Chapter 4). Specific IgE titers to aspergillus, alone or in conjunction with specific IgG levels (i.e., to aspergillus), can be very helpful in assessing the patient for ABPA.

Specific Antibody Titers. Very high acute titers or rising titers in convalescent serum samples can be diagnostic for a number of acute respiratory infections (e.g., influenza, Legionnaire's disease, and *Mycoplasma pneumoniae* infection). Confirmation of the diagnosis may not be necessary for treatment but may be epidemiologically and prognostically useful.

Specific pseudomonas antibody levels can provide therapeutically useful evidence for *P. aeruginosa* infection before the organism is recovered from respiratory cultures (and thus support a decision to perform bronchoscopy to attempt to recover the organism from the lung), but this test is not routinely available in hospital laboratories. Many specific antibody titers (e.g., Epstein-Barr virus [EBV], hepatitis, toxoplasmosis, and cytomegalovirus [CMV]) are used to investigate fever of unknown origin, but this is standard infectious disease practice and beyond the scope of this appendix.

Varicella antibody titers are specifically indicated in CF patients who are not known to have had the disease during childhood, and who are being evaluated for lung transplant. A low titer (indicating susceptibility) would be an indication for varicella vaccine. Routine varicella immunization is now recommended by the American Academy of Pediatrics as part of well child care. CF should not interfere with this recommendation. Several specific antibody titers (e.g., EBV, toxoplasmosis, hepatitis, and CMV) are performed as part of pretransplant evaluations.

Appendix C
Care Centers

ALABAMA

Birmingham

UAB Cystic Fibrosis Center
The Children's Hospital
University of Alabama at Birmingham
1600 7th Avenue, South, Suite 620ACC
Birmingham, AL 35233

Appointments: (205) 939-9583

Center Director:
Raymond Lyrene, M.D.
(205) 934-3574 or
(205) 939-9583
Fax: (205) 975-5983
Rlyrene@peds.uab.edu

Mobile

USA Children's Medical Center
P.O. Drawer 40130
1504 Spring Hill Avenue
Mobile, AL 36640-0130

Appointments: (334) 343-6848

Center Director:
Lawrence J. Sindel, M.D.*
(334) 343-6848
Fax: (334) 343-5708
Lsindel@zebra.net

Preferred Mailing Address:
Pulmonary Associates of Mobile, P.A.
3732A Dauphin Street
Mobile, AL 36608

ALASKA

See Children's Hospital and Regional
Medical Center, Seattle, Washington.

ARIZONA

Phoenix

Cystic Fibrosis Center
Phoenix Children's Hospital
909 E. Brill Street
Phoenix, AZ 85006

Appointments: (602) 239-6925

Center Director:
Peggy J. Radford, M.D.
(602) 239-5778
Fax: (602) 239-2469
Jrad333@aol.com

Adult Program Director:
Gerald D. Gong, M.D.
(602) 239-5778
Fax: (602) 239-2469
Ggong@phxchildrens.com

Tucson

Tucson Cystic Fibrosis Center
St. Luke's Chest Clinic
Arizona Health Sciences Center
1501 N. Campbell Avenue, Room 2332
Tucson, AZ 85724

Appointments: (520) 694-7450

Center Director:
Wayne J. Morgan, M.D.
(520) 626-7780
Fax: (520) 626-6970
Wmorgan@resp-sci.arizona.edu

ARKANSAS

Little Rock

Arkansas Cystic Fibrosis Center
Arkansas Children's Hospital
800 Marshall Street
Little Rock, AR 72202-3591

Appointments: (501) 320-1006

Center Director:
Astryd Menendez, M.D.
(501) 320-1006
Fax: (501) 320-3930
Menendezastryda@exchange.uams.edu

Adult Program:
University of Arkansas for Medical
  Sciences
Pulmonary/Clinical Care Medicine
4301 West Markham, Slot 555
Little Rock, AR 72205

Director:
Paula Anderson, M.D.

(501) 686-5525
Fax: (501) 686-7893
Andersonpaulaj@exchange.uams.edu

CALIFORNIA

Long Beach

Cystic Fibrosis Center
Miller Children's at Long Beach
  Memorial Medical Center
2801 Atlantic Avenue
P.O. Box 1428
Long Beach, CA 90801-1428

Appointments: (562) 933-8000
Fax: (562) 933-8569

Center Director:
Eliezer Nussbaum, M.D.
(562) 933-8740
Fax: (562) 933-8744
Enussbaum@memorialcare.net

Los Angeles

Cystic Fibrosis Comprehensive Center
Children's Hospital of Los Angeles
4650 Sunset Boulevard
Mail Stop #83
Los Angeles, CA 90027-6016

Appointments: (323) 669-2287 (direct
  line)
(323) 660-2450 (hospital)

Center Director:
C. Michael Bowman, M.D., Ph.D.
(323) 669-2101
Fax: (323) 664-9758 or
(323) 666-6563
mbowman@chla.usc.edu

Adult Program:
University of Southern California
Ambulatory Health Care Center
1355 San Pablo Street
Los Angeles, CA 90033

Appointments: (213) 342-5100

Director:
Bertrand Shapiro, M.D.
(213) 342-5100
Fax: (213) 342-5110

Affiliate Programs:
Kaiser-Permanente Southern California
13652 Cantara Street, VC103
Panorama City, CA 91402

Appointments: (818) 375-2909

*(Ask for Joan Franco. Open to
members of the Kaiser-Permanente
Health Plan only.)*

Director:
Allan S. Lieberthal, M.D.
(818) 375-2909
Fax: (818) 375-4073
Allan.s.lieberthal@kp.org
Ventura County Medical Center
3400 Loma Vista Road, Suite 1
Ventura, CA 93003

Appointments: (805) 652-6124

Director:
Chris Landon, M.D.
(805) 289-3333
Fax: (805) 289-3310
Landon@rain.org

Outreach:
Cedars Sinai Medical Center
8700 Beverly Boulevard
Los Angeles, CA 90048

Appointments: (310) 855-4433

Co-Directors.
C. Michael Bowman, M.D., Ph.D.
(children)
Andrew Wachtel, M.D. (adults)
Fax: (310) 967-0145

Outreach:
UCLA Medical Center
10833 Leconte Avenue
Los Angeles, CA 90094

(310) 267-1199
Fax: (310) 206-4855

Director:
C. Michael Bowman, M.D., Ph.D.

Oakland

Kaiser-Permanente Medical Care
Program
Attention: Gail Farmer, M.S., R.D.
Department of Pediatrics
280 West MacArthur Boulevard
Oakland, CA 94611

Appointments: (510) 596-6906
(ask for Gail Farmer)
gail.farmer@ncal.kaiperm.org

Center Director:
Gregory F. Shay, M.D.
(510) 596-6596
Fax: (510) 596-7054
Greg.shay@ncal.kaiperm.org

Adult Program:
Kaiser-Permanente Medical Care
Program
Pulmonary Medical Division
2025 Morse Avenue
Sacramento, CA 95825

Director:
John Lutch, M.D.
(916) 973-5858
Fax: (916) 973-5828
John.lutch@ncal.kaiperm.org

Oakland

Pediatric Pulmonary Center
Children's Hospital - Oakland
747 52nd Street
Oakland, CA 94609

Appointments: (510) 428-3305

Center Director:
Nancy C. Lewis, M.D.
Fax: (510) 428-3123
Cho.rt.ei@cho.org

Orange

Children's Hospital of Orange County
455 South Main Street
Orange, CA 92868

Appointments: (714) 532-8317

Center Director:
David A. Hicks, M.D.
(714) 532-8622
Fax: (714) 289-4072
Pcapstraw@choc.com

Palo Alto

Pediatric Pulmonary Division
Stanford University Medical Center
701 Welch Road, #3328
Palo Alto, CA 94304-5786

Appointments: (650) 497-8841
    (scheduling)
(650) 723-5191 (message for doctor)

Center Director:
Richard Moss, M.D.
(650) 723-5191
Fax: (650) 723-5201
md.mosri@/pch.stanford.edu

Adult Program Director:
John A. Wagner, M.D., Ph.D.
(650) 723-5191
Fax: (650) 723-5201
Wagner@leland.stanford.edu

Affiliate Program:
California Pacific Medical Center
Department of Pediatrics
2340 Clay Street, Room #325
San Francisco, CA 94115

Director:
Karen A. Hardy, M.D.
(415) 923-3434
Fax: (415) 923-3506
Khardyanp6@aol.com

Sacramento

Cystic Fibrosis and Pediatric
    Respiratory Diseases Center
University of California at Davis
    Medical Center
Department of Pediatrics
2516 Stockton Boulevard
Sacramento, CA 95817

Appointments: (916) 734-3112

Center Director:
Ruth J. McDonald, M.D.
(916) 734-3189
Fax: (916) 734-4757
Peds.cfpulmo@ucdmc.ucdavis.edu

Adult Program:
University of California
Davis Medical Center
4150 V Street, Suite 3400
Sacramento, CA 95817

Director:
Carroll Cross, M.D.
(916) 734-3564
Fax: (916) 734-7924
Cecross@ucdavis.edu

San Diego

San Diego Cystic Fibrosis and
 Pediatric Pulmonary Disease Center
UCSD Medical Center
200 West Arbor Drive
Mail Code 8448
San Diego, CA 92103-1990

Appointments: (619) 294-6125

Center Director:
Michael J. Light, M.D.
(619) 294-6125
Fax: (619) 296-3758
Mlight@ucsd.edu

Adult Program:
UCSD Medical Center
200 West Arbor Drive
Mail Code 8448
San Diego, CA 92103-1990

Appointments: (619) 294-6125

Director:
Douglas J. Conrad, M.D.
Fax: (619) 296-3758
Dconrad@ucsd.edu

San Francisco

Cystic Fibrosis Center
University of California at San
 Francisco
505 Parnassus Avenue,
 Room M650
San Francisco, CA 94143-0106

Appointments: (415) 476-2072

Center Director:
Gerd J.A. Cropp, M.D., Ph.D.
(415) 476-2072
Fax: (415) 476-4009
Zigbod@itsa.uscf.edu

Adult Program:
University of California at San
 Francisco
505 Parnassus Avenue,
 Room M1093
San Francisco, CA 94143-0120

Director:
Michael S. Stulbarg, M.D.
(415) 476-0631
Fax: (415) 476-5712
Michael@itsa.ucsf.edu

Affiliation Program:
Valley Children's Hospital
Pediatric Pulmonary and Respiratory
 Care
9300 Valley Children's Place
Madera, CA 93638

Appointments: (209) 243-5550

Director:
R. Sudhakar, M.D.
(209) 243-5550
Fax: (209) 243-5587
Rlcsud@pol.net

COLORADO

Denver

The Children's Hospital
1056 East 19th Avenue
Box B-395
Denver, CO 80218-1088

Appointments: (303) 861-6300

Center Director:
Frank J. Accurso, M.D.
(303) 837-2522
Fax: (303) 837-2924
Accurso.frank@tchden.org

Adult Program:
University of Colorado Health Sciences
   Center
4200 East 9th Avenue
Box B-133
Denver, CO 80262

Director:
David Rodman, M.D.
(303) 315-4473
Fax: (303) 315-4871
David.rodman@uschsc.edu

Affiliate Program:
Billings Clinic
2825 8th Avenue, North
Billings, MT 59107

Appointments: (406) 238-2310

Director:
Robert Pueringer, M.D.

CONNECTICUT

Hartford

Cystic Fibrosis Center
Pediatric Pulmonary Division
Connecticut Children's Medical Center
282 Washington Street
Hartford, CT 06107

Appointments: (860) 545-9440

Center Director:
Michelle M. Cloutier, M.D.
(860) 545-9442
Fax: (860) 545-9445
Mclouti@ccmckids.org

New Haven

Cystic Fibrosis Center
Yale University School of Medicine
333 Cedar Street, Fitkin 511
New Haven, CT 06520-8064

Appointments: (203) 785-4081

Center Director:
Regina M. Palazzo, M.D.
(203) 785-2480
Fax: (203) 785-6337
Regina.palazzo@yale.edu

DELAWARE

Wilmington

Alfred I duPont Hospital for Children
1600 Rockland Road
P.O. Box 269
Wilmington, DE 19899

Appointments: (302) 651-4200

Center Director:
Raj Padman, M.D.
(302) 651-6400
Fax: (302) 651-6408
Vpellegr@nemours.org

Center Co-Director:
Aaron Chidekel, M.D.

DISTRICT OF COLUMBIA

Metropolitan D.C. Cystic Fibrosis
  Center for Care,
    Training and Research
Children's National Medical Center
111 Michigan Avenue, N.W.
Washington, DC 20010-2970

Appointments: (202) 884-2610

Center Director:
Robert J. Fink, M.D.
(202) 884-2644
Fax: (202) 884-3461
Rfink@cnmc.org

FLORIDA

Gainesville

Cystic Fibrosis and Pediatric
  Pulmonary Disease Center
University of Florida
1600 SW Archer Road
P.O. Box 100296
Gainesville, FL 32610-0296

Appointments: (352) 392-4458

Center Director:
Mary H. Wagner, M.D.

Fax: (352) 392-4450
Wagneam@peds.ufl.edu

Adult Program Director:
Arundhati Foster, M.D.
(352) 392-2666
Fax: (352) 392-0821
Sa96raa@nervm.nerdc.ufl.edu

Affiliate Program:
Joe DiMaggio Children's Hospital
Cystic Fibrosis Clinic
5305 SW 111th Terrace
Ft. Lauderdale, FL 33328

Appointments: (954) 986-6333

Director:
Morton N. Schwartzman, M.D.*
(954) 986-6333
Fax: (954) 961-7027

*Preferred Mailing Address:
3435 Hayes Street
Hollywood, FL 33021

Jacksonville

Nemours Children's Clinic
807 Nira Street
Jacksonville, FL 32207

Appointments: (904) 390-3788

Center Director:
Bonnie B. Hudak, M.D.
(904) 390-3676
Fax: (904) 390-3422
Bhudak@nemours.org

Miami

Mailroom Center for Child
  Development
University of Miami School of
  Medicine
1601 N.W. 12th Avenue
Miami, FL 33136

Appointments: (305) 243-6641

Center Director:
Giovanni Piedmonte, M.D.
(305) 243-3176
Fax: (305) 243-6708
Gpiedimo@mednet.med.miami.edu

Orlando

Cystic Fibrosis Center
The Nemours Children's Clinic
83 West Columbia Street
Orlando, FL 32806

Appointments: (407) 650-7366

Center Director:
David Geller, M.D.
(407) 650-7270
Fax: (407) 650-7277
Dgeller@nemours.org

St. Petersburg

Cystic Fibrosis Center
All Children's Hospital
880 Sixth Street South, Suite 390
St. Petersburg, FL 33701

Appointments: (727) 892-4146

Center Director:
Juan Martinez, M.D.

(727) 892-4146
Fax: (727) 892-4218
Martinez@allkids.org

Adult Program:
University of South Florida
Pulmonary Critical Care
12901 Bruce B. Downs Boulevard,
  Box 33
Tampa, FL 33612

Appointments: (727) 892-4146

Director:
Mark W. Rolfe, M.D.
(813) 974-7551
Fax: (813) 907-1060
Mwrolfe@aol.com

Affiliate Program:
St. Mary's Medical Center
P.O. Box 24620
901 45th Street
West Palm Beach, FL 33407

Appointments: (561) 840-6065

Director:
Sue S. Goldfinger, M.D.
(561) 881-2911
Fax: (561) 882-1078

Affiliate Programs:
Division of Pulmonology
Miami Children's Hospital
MOB #203, 3200 S.W. 60th Court
Miami, FL 33155

Appointments: (305) 662-8380

Director:
Carlos E. Diaz, M.D.
(305) 662-8380
Fax: (305) 663-8417

University of South Florida
Department of Pediatrics
17 Davis Boulevard, Suite 200
Tampa, FL 33606

Appointments: (813) 272-2799

Director:
Bruce M. Schnapf, D.O.
(813) 276-5520
Fax: (813) 272-2995
Bschnapf@com1.med.usf.edu

Outreach Clinics:
New Port Richey Specialty Care Clinic
5640 Main Street
New Port Richey, FL 34652

Sarasota Clinic
5881 Rand Boulevard
Sarasota, FL 34238

Tampa Clinic
12220 Bruce B. Downs Boulevard
Tampa, FL 33612

Lakeland Clinic
3310 Lakeland Hills Boulevard
Lakeland, FL 33805

Appointments: (727) 892-4146

GEORGIA

Atlanta

Emory University
Egleston Cystic Fibrosis Center
Department of Pediatrics
1547 Clifton Road, N.E.
Atlanta, GA 30322

Appointments: (404) 727-5728

Center Director:
Daniel B. Caplan, M.D.
Fax: (404) 727-4828
Rhondahickson@oz.ped.emory.edu

Augusta

Medical College of Georgia
Pediatric Pulmonary Section
1120 15th Street
Augusta, GA 30912-3755

Appointments: (706) 721-2635

Center Director:
Margaret F. Guill, M.D.
(706) 721-2635
Fax: (706) 721-8512
Mguill@mail.mcg.edu

Adult Care Provider:
John DuPre, M.D.
Medical College Section of Georgia
Pulmonary Medical Section
1120 15th Street
Augusta, GA 30912

(706) 721-2566
Fax: (706) 721-3069
Jdupre@mailmcg.edu

Affiliate Program:
Scottish Rite Children's Medical
    Center
1001 Johnson Ferry Road, N.E.
Atlanta, GA 30342

Director:
Peter H. Scott, M.D.
(404) 252-7339
Fax: (404) 257-0337

Outreach Clinic:
Ware County Health Department

Daisy Clinic
Waycross, GA 31501

Appointments: (706) 721-2635

HAWAII

See Tripler Army Medical Center, San
Antonio, Texas.

IDAHO

See Intermountain Cystic Fibrosis
Center, Salt Lake City, Utah.

ILLINOIS

Chicago

Cystic Fibrosis Center
Children's Memorial Hospital
Northwestern University
2300 Children's Plaza, Box 43
Chicago, IL 60614

Appointments: (773) 880-4382

Center Director:
Susanna A. McColley, M.D.
(773) 880-4382
Fax: (773) 880-6300
Smccolley@nwu.edu

Adult Program:
Northwestern Memorial Hospital
303 E. Superior Street, Suite 774
Chicago, IL 60611

Director:
Manu Jain, M.D.
(312) 908-2003
m-jain@nmu.edu

University of Chicago Children's
    Hospital
Department of Pediatrics
5841 South Maryland Avenue
Mail Code 4064
Chicago, IL 60637

Appointments: (773) 702-6178

Center Director:
Lucille A. Lester, M.D.
(773) 702-6178
Fax: (773) 702-4041
Lalester@peds.bsd.uchicago.edu

Loyola University Medical Center
Department of Pediatrics
2160 S. First Avenue
Maywood, IL 60153

Appointments: (708) 327-9117

Director:
Edward R. Garrity, Jr., M.D.
(708) 327-5864
Fax: (708) 327-2424
Egarri@luc.edu

Rush-Presbyterian-St. Luke's Medical
    Center
1725 West Harrison, Suite 306
Chicago, IL 60612

Appointments: (312) 563-2270

Center Director:
John D. Lloyd-Still, M.D.
Fax: (312) 563-2299

Park Ridge

Cystic Fibrosis Center
Lutheran General Children's Hospital
Victor Yacktman Children's Pavilion
1775 W. Dempster Street
Park Ridge, IL 60068

Appointments: (847) 318-9330

Center Director:
Jerome R. Kraut, M.D.
(847) 723-7700
Fax: (847) 723-2325
Jerome.kraut_md@advocatehealth.com

Center Co-Director:
Youngran Chung, M.D.
(847) 723-8409
Fax: (847) 723-2325
Youngran.chung_md@
  advocatehealth.com

Adult Program:
Lutheran General Hospital
6000 Touhy Street
Chicago, IL 60649

Director:
Arvey Stone, M.D.
(773) 594-1900
Fax: (773) 594-1067

Peoria

Cystic Fibrosis Center
Saint Francis Medical Center
Hillcrest Medical Plaza
420 N.E. Glen Oak Avenue, Suite 201
Peoria, IL 61603

Appointments: (309) 655-3889

Center Director:
Umesh C. Chatrath, M.D.*
(309) 655-4070 ext. 3889
Fax: (309) 655-7449

Preferred Mailing Address:
420 N.E. Glen Oak Avenue, Suite 204
Peoria, IL 61603

Springfield

See Washington University School of
  Medicine, St. Louis, Missouri.

Urbana

See Washington University School of
  Medicine, St. Louis, Missouri.

INDIANA

Indianapolis

Cystic Fibrosis and Chronic Pulmonary
  Disease Center
Riley Hospital for Children
Indiana University Medical Center
702 Barnhill Drive, Room 2750
Indianapolis, IN 46202-5225

Appointments: (317) 274-7208

Center Director:
Howard Eigen, M.D.
(317) 274-3434
Fax: (317) 274-3442
Heigen@iupui.edu

Adult Program:
Indiana University
1481 West 10th Street, Room A740
VA 111P
Indianapolis, IN 46202-2884

Director:
Veena Antony, M.D.
(317) 269-6313
Fax: (317) 267-8762
Vantony@indyunix.iupui.edu

Affiliate Program:
Lutheran Hospital
c/o Cystic Fibrosis and Pediatric
 Pulmonary Clinic
7950 West Jefferson Boulevard
Ft. Wayne, IN 46804-4160

Appointments: (219) 435-7123
Fax: (219) 435-6947

Director:
James Pushpom, M.D.
Clinic Coordinator:
Eva Fish, R.R.T.
Efish@lutheran-hosp.com

Outreach:
Deaconess Hospital
600 Mary Street
Evansville, IN 47747

Appointments: (812) 426-3217

South Bend

Cystic Fibrosis and Chronic Pulmonary
 Disease Clinic of St. Joseph's
 Regional Medical Center
720 E. Cedar Street, Suite 440
South Bend, IN 46617-1935

Appointments: (219) 239-6126
Figgl@sjmrc.com

Center Director:
James Harris, M.D.*
(219) 237-9216
Fax: (219) 239-1451
Jbharrismd@aol.com

Preferred Mailing Address:1
South Bend Clinic
211 N. Eddy Street
South Bend, IN 46617

Adult Care Provider:
Mattnew Koscielsk

IOWA

Des Moines

Cystic Fibrosis Center
Blank Children's Health Center
1212 Pleasant Street, Suite 300
Des Moines, IA 50309

Appointments: (515) 241-6000
Fax: (515) 241-8717

Center Director:
Veljko Zivkovich, M.D.
(515) 244-7229
Fax: (515) 244-7233
office@allergyasthma.com

Iowa City

Cystic Fibrosis Center
Pediatric Allergy and Pulmonary
 Division
Department of Pediatrics
200 Hawkins Drive

University of Iowa Hospitals and
  Clinics
Iowa City, IA 52242-1083

Appointments: (319) 356-2229

Center Director:
Miles M. Weinberger, M.D.
(319) 356-3485
Fax: (319) 356-7171
miles-weinberger@uiowa.edu

Center Co-Director:
Richard C. Ahrens, M.D.
(319) 356-4050
Fax: (319) 356-7171
richard-ahrens@uiowa.edu

Adult Program Director:
Douglas Hornick, M.D.
(319) 356-8266
Fax: (319) 353-6406
douglas-hornick@uiowa.edu

Affiliate Program:
McFarland Clinic
Mary Greeley Hospital
1215 Duff
Ames, IA 50010

Appointments: (515) 239-4482

Director:
Edward G. Nassif, M.D.

KANSAS

Kansas City

Cystic Fibrosis Center
Kansas University Children's Center
3901 Rainbow Boulevard
Kansas City, KS 66160-7330

Appointments: (913) 588-6377

Center Director:
Joseph Kanarek, M.D.
(913) 588-6377
Fax: (913) 588-6280
alieberg@kumc.edu

Center Co-Director:
Pam Shaw, M.D.
(913) 588-6917
Fax: (913) 588-6319
pshaw@kumc.edu

Adult Program:
University of Kansas Medical Center
3901 Rainbow Boulevard
Kansas City, Kansas 66160-7381

Appointments: (913) 588-6044

Director:
Steven Stites, M.D.
Fax: (913) 588-4098
sstites@kumc.edu

Wichita

Cystic Fibrosis Care and Teaching
  Center
Via Christi, St. Francis Campus
929 North St. Francis
Outpatient Clinic/CF Clinic
Wichita, KS 67218

Appointments: (800) 362-0070 x5040

Center Director:
Maria Riva, M.D.*
(316) 689-9264
Fax: (316) 689-9140
mariariva@pol.net

Preferred Mailing Address:
Wichita Clinic
3311 East Murdock
Wichita, KS 67208

KENTUCKY

Lexington

Cystic Fibrosis Center
University of Kentucky
Division of Pediatric Pulmonology
740 South Limestone
J410 Kentucky Clinic
Lexington, KY 40536-0284

Appointments: (606) 323-8023

Center Director:
Jamshed F. Kanga, M.D.
(606) 323-8023
Fax: (606) 257-7706
jfkk@pop.uky.edu

Adult Program Director:
Michael I. Anstead, M.D.

Louisville

Kosair Children's Cystic Fibrosis
  Center
University of Louisville
571 S. Floys Street, Suite 414
Louisville, KY 40202

Appointments: (502) 629-8830

Center Director:
Nemr S. Eid, M.D.*
(502) 852-3772
Fax: (502) 852-4051
nseid001@athena.louisville.edu

Preferred Mailing Address:
233 East Gray Street, #201
Louisville, KY 40202

LOUISIANA

New Orleans

Tulane University School of Medicine
Department of Pediatrics SL-37
1430 Tulane Avenue
New Orleans, LA 70112

Appointments: (504) 587-7625

Center Director:
Scott H. Davis, M.D.
(504) 588-5601
Fax: (504) 588-5490
sdavis@tmcpop.tmc.tulane.edu

Adult Program:
Tulane University School of Medicine
1430 Tulane Avenue, SL-9
New Orleans, LA 70112

Director:
Dean Ellithorpe, M.D.
(504) 588-2250
Fax: (504) 584-2774

Shreveport

Cystic Fibrosis and Pediatric
  Pulmonary Center
Louisiana State University Medical
  Center
1501 Kings Highway
P.O. Box 33932
Shreveport, LA 71130-3932

Appointments: (318) 675-6094

Center Director:
Bettina C. Hilman, M.D.
(318) 675-6094
Fax: (318) 675-7668
bhilma@lsumc.edu

MAINE

Portland

MMC Cystic Fibrosis Center
295 Forest Avenue, 2nd Floor
Portland, ME 04101

Appointments: (207) 828-8226

Center Director:
Anne Marie Cairns, D.O.*
(207) 828-8226
Fax: (207) 775-6024
cairna@mail.mmc.org

Preferred Mailing Address:
Maine Pediatric Specialty Group
295 Forest Avenue
Portland, ME 04101

Adult Care Provider:
Edgar J. Caldwell, M.D.
(207) 871-2770
Fax: (207) 871-4691
caldwe@mail.mmc.org

Affiliate Programs:
Cystic Fibrosis Clinical Center
Eastern Maine Medical Center
417 State Street, Suite 305
Bangor, ME 04401

Appointments: (207) 973-7559
Fax: (207) 973-7674

Director:
Thomas Lever, M.D.
(207) 947-0147
Fax: (207) 990-3365
tflever@pol.net

Affiliate Programs:
Central Maine Cystic Fibrosis Center
Central Maine Medical Center
300 Main Street
Lewiston, ME 04240

Appointments: (207) 795-2830
Fax: (207) 795-5679

Director:
Ralph V. Harder, M.D.
(207) 784-5489
Fax: (207) 777-7241

Associate Director:
David Baker, M.D.
(207) 795-5730
Fax: (207) 795-5679

Center Coordinator:
Shelly Jo Stone, R.N.C.
(207) 795-2630

MARYLAND

Baltimore

The Johns Hopkins Hospital
600 N. Wolfe Street, Park 315
Baltimore, MD 21287-2533

Appointments: (410) 955-2795

Center Director:
Beryl J. Rosenstein, M.D.
(410) 955-2795
Fax: (410) 955-1030
brosenst@welchlink.welch.jhu.edu

Center Co-Director:
Pamela L. Zeitlin, M.D., Ph.D.
(410) 955-2795
Fax: (410) 955-1030
pzeitli@welchlink.welch.jhu.edu

Adult Program Director:
Michael P. Boyle, M.D.
(410) 955-2035
Fax: (410) 955-1030
mboyle@welchlink.welch.jhu.edu

Bethesda

Cystic Fibrosis Center
National Institute of Diabetes and
    Digestive and Kidney Diseases
National Institutes of Health
Building 10, Room 8C438
Bethesda, MD 20892

Appointments: (301) 496-3434

Center Director:
Milica S. Chernick, M.D.
(301) 496-3434
Fax: (301) 496-9943
milica_chernick@nih.gov

MASSACHUSETTS

Boston

Cystic Fibrosis Center
Pulmonary Division
Children's Hospital
300 Longwood Avenue
Boston, MA 02115

Appointments: (617) 355-7881

Center Director:
Mary Ellen Wohl, M.D.
(617) 355-8630
Fax: (617) 355-6109
wohl_m@a1.tch.harvard.edu

Adult Care Provider:
Craig Gerard, M.D.
(617) 355-6953

Cystic Fibrosis Center
Massachusetts General Hospital
ACC 709
15 Parkman Street
Boston, MA 02114

Appointments: (617) 726-8707 or
(617) 726-8708

Center Director:
Allen Lapey, M.D.
(617) 726-8707
Fax: (617) 724-0581
lapey.allen@mgh.harvard.edu

Adult Program Director:
Marcy Ruddy, M.D.
(617) 726-3734
Fax: (617) 726-6878
ruddy.marcy@mgh.harvard.edu

Cystic Fibrosis Center
Tufts New England Medical
    Center
750 Washington Street, Box 343
Boston, MA 02111

Appointments: (617) 636-7917

Center Director:
Henry L. Dorkin, M.D.
(617) 636-7917
Fax: (617) 636-7760
henry.dorkin@es.nemc.org

Springfield

Baystate Medical Center
3300 Main Street, Suite 4A
Springfield, MA 01199

Appointments: (413) 794-0555

Center Director:
Robert S. Gerstle, M.D.
(413) 794-5077
Fax: (413) 794-7140
rgerstle@bhs.org

Worcester

University of Massachusetts
Medical Center
Pediatric Pulmonology
55 Lake Avenue North, Room S5-860
Worcester, MA 01655

Appointments: (508) 856-4155

Center Director:
Robert G. Zwerdling, M.D.
(508) 856-4155
Fax: (508) 856-2609

MICHIGAN

Ann Arbor

University of Michigan Health System
Department of Pediatric Pulmonology
200 East Hospital Drive
Medical Professional Building
Box 0718
Ann Arbor, MI 48109-0718

Appointments: (734) 764-4123
   (Pediatrics)
(734) 936-5580 (Adult)

Center Director:
Samya Nasr, M.D.
Fax: (734) 764-4123
snasr@umich.edu

Adult Program Director:
Richard H. Simon, M.D.*
(734) 764-4554
Fax: (734) 764-4556
richsimo@umich.edu

Preferred Mailing Address:
University of Michigan Medical Center
Division of Pulmonary and Critical
   Care
6301 MSRB-3, Box 0642
1150 West Medical Center Drive
Ann Arbor, MI 48109-0642

Detroit

Children's Hospital of Michigan
Cystic Fibrosis Care, Teaching and
   Resource Center
3901 Beaubien Boulevard
Detroit, MI 48201

Appointments: (313) 745-5541

Center Director:
Debbie Toder, M.D.
(313) 745-5541
Fax: (313) 993-2948
dtoder@med.wayne.edu

Adult Program:
Wayne State University
Harper Hospital
3990 John R. Street, 3 Hudson
Detroit, MI 48201

Appointments: (313) 745-9151
Fax: (313) 966-7178

Director:
Dana Kissner, M.D.
(313) 993-0562
Fax: (313) 993-0229
dkissner@intmed.wayne.edu

Providence Hospital
16001 Nine Mile Road
DePaul Center, 3 West
Southfield, MI 48075

Director:
Bohdan M. Pichurko, M.D.

Appointments: (248) 424-5718
Fax: (248) 424-5726

Affiliate Program:
Mott Children's Health Center
806 Tuuri Place
Flint, MI 48503

Appointments: (810) 257-9344
Fax: (810) 762-7308

Director:
Mohammed El-Ghoroury

Grand Rapids

Cystic Fibrosis Care Center of Grand
  Rapids
Helen De Vos Women and Children's
  Center
330 Barclay, N.E., Suite 200
Grand Rapids, MI 49503

Appointments: (616) 391-8890
Fax: (616) 391-8896
(Contact Person: Ann Truax, R.N. or
Barbara Schoenborn, R.N.)

Center Co-Director:
John N. Schuen, M.D.
(616) 391-2125
Fax: (616) 391-2131
jschuen@bw.brhn.org

Center Co-Director:
Susan L. Millard, M.D.
(616) 391-2125
Fax: (616) 391-2131
susan.millard@spectrum-health.org

Kalamazoo

Michigan State University
Kalamazoo Center for Medical Studies
1000 Oakland Drive
Kalamazoo, MI 49008

Appointments: (616) 337-6430

Center Director:
Douglas N. Homnick, M.D.
(616) 337-6430
Fax: (616) 337-6474
homnick@kcms.msu.edu

Lansing

Michigan State University Cystic
  Fibrosis Center
1200 East Michigan Avenue,
  Suite 145
Lansing, MI 48912-1811

Appointments: (517) 364-5440

Center Director:
Richard E. Honicky, M.D.
Fax: (517) 364-5413
honicky@pilot.msu.edu

MINNESOTA

Minneapolis

University of Minnesota
CF Center
420 Delaware Street, S.E.,
    Box 742
Minneapolis, MN 55455-0392

Appointments: (612) 624-0962

Center Director:
Warren J. Warwick, M.D.
(612) 626-4440
Fax: (612) 624-0696
warwi001@maroon.tc.umn.edu

Center Co-Director:
Carlos E. Milla, M.D., M.P.H.
(612) 626-2963
Fax: (612) 626-0696
milla-5@tc.umn.edu

MISSISSIPPI

Jackson

University of Mississippi Medical
    Center
Department of Pediatrics
2500 North State Street
Jackson, MS 39216-4505

Appointments: (601) 984-5205

Center Director:
Suzanne T. Miller, M.D.
Fax: (601) 984-5982
cmclellan@ped.umsmed.edu

MISSOURI

Columbia

Children's Hospital
University of Missouri Health Sciences
    Center
Department of Child Health
Division of Pulmonary Medicine and
    Allergy
One Hospital Drive
Columbia, MO 65212

Appointments: (573) 882-6921

Center Director:
Peter König, M.D., Ph.D.
(573) 882-6978
Fax: (573) 882-2742
konigp@missouri.edu

Outreach Clinic:
St. John's Specialty Clinic
Fremont Medical Building
1961 South Fremont Avenue
Springfield, MO 65804

Appointments: (573) 882-6978
Contact: Connie Fenton, R.N.,
    B.S.N.

Outreach Clinic:
Southeast Missouri Hospital
1701 Lacey Street
Cape Girardeau, MO 63701

Appointments: (573) 882-6978
Contact: Connie Fenton, R.N.,
    B.S.N.

Kansas City

The Children's Mercy Hospital
University of Missouri at
  Kansas City
Pediatric Pulmonology Section
2401 Gillham Road
Kansas City, MO 64108

Appointments: (816) 234-3066
Sweat Test Only: (816) 234-3230

Center Director:
Michael McCubbin, M.D.
(816) 234-3033
Fax: (816) 234-3590
mmccubbin@cmh.edu

St. Louis

Cystic Fibrosis and Pediatric
  Pulmonary Center
Cardinal Glennon Children's Hospital
St. Louis University School of
  Medicine
1465 South Grand Boulevard
St. Louis, MO 63104

Appointments: (314) 268-5663

Center Director:
Anthony J. Rejent, M.D.
(314) 268-6439
Fax: (314) 268-2798
rejentaj@slu.edu

Adult Program:
St. Louis University Health Sciences
  Center
3635 Vista Avenue at Grand
  Boulevard

P.O. Box 15250
St. Louis, MO 63110-0250

Director:
Mary Ellen Kleinhenz, M.D.
(314) 577-8856
Fax: (314) 577-8859
kleinhme@wpogate.slu.edu

Washington University School of
  Medicine
St. Louis Children's Hospital
Cystic Fibrosis Center
One Children's Place
St. Louis, MO 63110

Appointments: (314) 454-2694
(314) 362-9366 (adults)
(314) 454-6248 (sweat test only)
Fax: (314) 454-2515

Interim Center Director:
Steven D. Shapiro, M.D.
(314) 454-8373
Fax: (314) 454-8605
sshapiro@imgate.wustl.edu

Pediatric Coordinator:
Jane A. Quaute, R.N., B.S.
(314) 454-2694

Adult Program:
Washington University School of
  Medicine
Division of Pulmonary/Critical Care
  Medicine
660 South Euclid Avenue, Box 8052
St. Louis, MO 63110

Director:
Daniel Rosenbluth, M.D.
(314) 362-6904

Fax: (314) 362-1334
drosenbl@im.wustl.edu

Adult Coordinator:
Joan Zukosky, R.N., B.S.N.
(314) 362-9366

Affiliate Programs:
Southern Illinois University School of
　Medicine
P.O. Box 19230—MC 1311
Springfield, IL 62794

Appointments: (217) 782-0187
　ext. 2321
or (217) 788-3381

Director:
Lanie E. Eagleton, M.D.
(217) 782-0187
Fax: (217) 788-5543

Coordinator:
Joni Colle, R.N., R.R.T.
Carle Clinic Association
Department of Pediatrics
602 W. University Avenue
Urbana, IL 61801

Appointments: (217) 383-3100

Director:
Donald F. Davison, M.D.
(217) 383-3100
Fax: (217) 383-4468
donald.davison@carle.com

MONTANA

See Billings Clinic, Denver,
　Colorado.

NEBRASKA

Omaha

University of Nebraska Medical Center
985190 Nebraska Medical Center
Omaha, NE 68198-5190

Appointments: (402) 559-6275

Center Director:
John L. Colombo, M.D.
(402) 559-6275
Fax: (402) 559-7062
jcolombo@unmc.edu

NEVADA

Las Vegas

University of Nevada Las Vegas
Children's Lung Specialists, Ltd.
3838 Meadows Lane
Las Vegas, NV 89127

Appointments: (702) 598-4411

Center Director:
Ruben P. Diaz, M.D.
(702) 598-4411
Fax: (702) 598-1988
docdiaz@aol.com

NEW HAMPSHIRE

Lebanon

New Hampshire CF Program
Dartmouth Hitchcock Medical Center
1 Medical Center Drive
Lebanon, NH 03756

Appointments: (603) 650-6244
　(Lebanon) or
(603) 695-2560 (Bedford)

Center Director:
William E. Boyle, Jr., M.D.
(603) 650-5541
Fax: (603) 650-8601
william.e.boyle@hitchcock.org
lynn.m.feenan@hitchcock.org

Adult Program Director:
H. Worth Parker, M.D.
(603) 650-5533
Fax: (603) 650-4437
h.worth.parker@dartmouth.edu

NEW JERSEY

Newark

UMDNJ-New Jersey Medical
  School
185 South Orange Avenue
MSB Room F534
Newark, NJ 07103-2714

Appointments: (973) 972-4815

Center Director:
Nelson L. Turcios, M.D.
Fax: (973) 972-7597
turcionl@umdnj.edu

Long Branch

Cystic Fibrosis and Pediatric
  Pulmonary Center
Monmouth Medical Center
279 Third Avenue, Suite 604
Long Branch, NJ 07740

Appointments: (732) 222-4474

Center Director:
Robert L. Zanni, M.D.
(732) 222-4474
Fax: (732) 222-4472
rzanni@monmouth.com

NEW MEXICO

Albuquerque

University of New Mexico School of
  Medicine
Department of Pediatrics
Ambulatory Care Center
2211 Lomas Boulevard, N.E.,
  ACC 3rd Floor
Albuquerque, NM 87131-5311

Appointments: (505) 272-5464

Center Director:
Marsha M. Thompson, M.D., Ph.D.
(505) 272-5551
Fax: (505) 272-0329
mthompson@salud.unm.edu

Adult Program Director:
David S. James, M.D.
(505) 272-4751
Fax: (505) 272-8700
dsjames@medusa.unm.edu

NEW YORK

Albany

Pediatric Pulmonary and Cystic
  Fibrosis Center
Albany Medical College
Department of Pediatrics, Mail Code
  A-112

47 New Scotland Avenue
Albany, NY 12208

Appointments: (518) 262-6880

Center Director:
Robert A. Kaslovksy, M.D.
(518) 262-6880
Fax: (518) 262-6884
rkaslovsky@ccgateway.amc.edu

Adult Program Director:
Jonathan M. Rosen, M.D.
(518) 262-5196
Fax: (518) 262-5555
jmrosen@pol.net

Brooklyn

Long Island College Hospital
340 Henry Street
Brooklyn, NY 11201

Appointments: (718) 780-1025 or
(718) 780-1026

Center Director:
Robert Giusti, M.D.
(718) 780-1025
Fax: (718) 780-2989
giucfdoc@pol.net

Buffalo

Children's Lung and Cystic Fibrosis
    Center
Children's Hospital of Buffalo
219 Bryant Street
Buffalo, NY 14222

Appointments: (716) 878-7524
After hours: (716) 878-7000

Center Director:
Drucy Borowitz, M.D.
(716) 878-7561
Fax: (716) 888-3945
dborowitz@upa.chob.edu

Adult Program Director:
Colin McMahon, M.D.
(716) 878-7655
Fax: (716) 888-3945
cmcmahon@ubmedd.buffalo.edu

Appointments: (716) 878-7524
After hours: (716) 515-4580

New Hyde Park

Cystic Fibrosis Care and Teaching
    Center
Schneider Children's Hospital
Long Island Jewish Medical Center
Albert Einstein School of Medicine
269-01 76th Avenue
New Hyde Park, NY 11040

Appointments: (718) 470-3305

Center Director:
Jack D. Gorvoy, M.D.
(718) 470-3305
Fax: (718) 343-3578
gorvoy@lij.edu

Center Co-Director:
Joan K. DeCelie-Germana, M.D.
(718) 470-3305
Fax: (718) 343-3578
germana@lij.edu

New York City

Cystic Fibrosis and Pediatric
    Pulmonary Center
Mount Sinai School of Medicine

One Gustave L. Levy Place,
    Box 1202B
New York, NY 10029-6574

Appointments: (212) 241-7788

Center Director:
Richard J. Bonforte, M.D.

Children's Lung and CF Center
Babies and Children's Hospital of New
    York
Columbia Presbyterian Medical Center
630 West 168th Street, BHS-801
    NORTH
New York, NY 10032

Appointments: (212) 305-5122

Center Director:
Lynne M. Quittell, M.D.
(212) 305-6551
Fax: (212) 305-6103
1mq1@columbia.edu

Cystic Fibrosis, Pediatric Pulmonary
    and Gastrointestinal Center
St. Vincent's Hospital and Medical
    Center of New York
36 Seventh Avenue, Suite 509
New York, NY 10011

Appointments: (212) 604-8895 or
(212) 604-8898

Center Director:
Maria Berdella, M.D.
(212) 604-8895
Fax: (212) 604-3899

Co-Director:
Patricia Walker, M.D.

Rochester

University of Rochester Medical
    Center
Strong Memorial Hospital
Department of Pediatrics
601 Elmwood Avenue, Box 667
Rochester, NY 14642-8667

Appointments: (716) 275-2464

Center Director:
Karen Z. Voter, M.D.
Fax: (716) 275-8706
karen_voter@urmc.rochester.edu

Affiliate Program:
House of Good Samaritan Medical
    Center
Child and Adolescent Health
    Associates
199 Pratt Street
Watertown, NY 13601

Appointments: (315) 788-2211

Director:
Ronald Perciaccante, M.D.
(315) 788-2211
Fax: (315) 788-0956
pereocon@pol.net

Stony Brook

University Medical Center at Stony
    Brook
Department of Pediatrics
Health Sciences Center T11, Room 080
Stony Brook, NY 11794-8111

Appointments: (516) 444-7726

Center Director:
Clement L. Ren, M.D.
(516) 444-8340
Fax: (516) 444-6045
cren@mail.som.sunysb.edu

Syracuse

Robert C. Schwartz Cystic Fibrosis
   Center
SUNY Health Science Center
750 East Adams Street
Syracuse, NY 13210

Appointments: (315) 464-6323

Center Director:
Ran D. Anbar, M.D.
(315) 464-6323
Fax: (315) 464-6322
anbarr@hscsyr.edu

Valhalla

The Armond V. Mascia Cystic Fibrosis
   Center
The Children's Hospital and
   Westchester Medical Center
New York Medical College
Munger Pavilion, Room 106
Valhalla, NY 10595

Appointments: (914) 493-7585

Center Director:
Allen Dozor, M.D.
(914) 493-7585
Fax: (914) 594-4336
pedpulm@nymc.edu

NORTH CAROLINA

Chapel Hill

University of North Carolina at Chapel
   Hill
Department of Pediatrics, CB #7220
635 Burnett-Womack Building
Chapel Hill, NC 27599-7220

Appointments: (919) 966-1055
   (Pediatrics)
(919) 966-1077 (Adults-18 years &
   older)

Center Director:
Margaret W. Leigh, M.D.
(919) 966-1055
Fax: (919) 966-6179
mleigh@med.unc.edu

Center Co-Director:
George Retsch-Bogart, M.D.
grzb@med.unc.edu

Adult Program:
Cystic Fibrosis/Pulmonary Research
   and Treatment Center
University of North Carolina at Chapel
   Hill
7019 Thurston Bowles Building,
   CB# 7248
Chapel Hill, NC 27599-7248

Co-Directors:
Michael Knowles, M.D.
James R. Yankaskas, M.D.
(919) 966-1077
Fax: (919) 966-7524
knowles@med.unc.edu
pwsjry@med.unc.edu

Affiliate Program:
The Children's Hospital at Carolinas
    Medical Center
Children's Respiratory Center
1000 Blythe Boulevard
P.O. Box 32861
Charlotte, NC 28232-2861

Appointments: (704) 355-1130

Director:
William S. Ashe, M.D.
Fax: (704) 355-1155

Durham

Cystic Fibrosis and Pediatric
    Pulmonary Center
Duke University Medical Center
Bell Building, Room 302
P.O. Box 2994
Durham, NC 27710

Appointments: (919) 684-3364

Center Director:
Marc Majure, M.D.
Fax: (919) 684-2292
majur001@mc.duke.edu

Center Co-Director:
Thomas Murphy, M.D.
Adult Program:
Duke University Medical Center
Box 31166
Durham, NC 27710

Director:
Peter S. Kussin, M.D.
(919) 684-3202 or (919) 684-8049
Fax: (919) 681-7837
kussi001@mc.duke.edu

Affiliate Program:
Children's Respiratory Center
58 Bear Drive
Greenville, SC 29605

Director:
Jane V. Gwinn, M.D.
(864) 220-8000
Fax: (864) 220-8009
gwinncrc@pol.net

Winston-Salem

Wake Forest University Baptist
    Medical Center
Department of Pediatrics
Medical Center Boulevard
Winston-Salem, NC 27157

Appointments: (336) 716-4126

Center Director:
Michael S. Schechter, M.D.,
    M.P.H.
(336) 716-0512
Fax: (336) 716-9229
mschech@wfubmc.edu

Center Co-Director:
Bruce K. Rubin, M.D.

NORTH DAKOTA

Bismarck

Heart and Lung Clinic
St. Alexius Medical Center
311 North 9th Street
P.O. Box 2698
Bismarck, ND 58502

Appointments: (701) 224-7502

Center Director:
James A. Hughes, M.D.
(701) 224-7504
Fax: (701) 224-7560

Center Co-Director:
William Riecke, A.A.P.

OHIO

Akron

Lewis H. Walker Cystic Fibrosis
  Center
Children's Hospital Medical Center of
  Akron
One Perkins Square
Akron, OH 44308

Appointments: (330) 258-3249

Center Director:
Rajeev Kishore, M.D.
(330) 379-8545
Fax: (330) 258-3751
ebryson@chmca.org

Cincinnati

The Children's Hospital Medical
  Center
Pulmonary Medicine, OSB 5
3333 Burnet Avenue
Cincinnati, OH 45229-3039

Appointments: (513) 636-6771

Center Director:
Robert W. Wilmott, M.D.

(513) 636-6771
Fax: (513) 636-4615
wilmr0@chmcc.org

Adult Program Director:
Patricia M. Joseph, M.D.
University of Cincinnati
(513) 558-4831
Fax: (513) 558-0835

Cleveland

The Leroy Matthews Cystic Fibrosis
  Center
Rainbow Babies and Children's Hospital
Case Western Reserve University
Mail Code: RBC 6006
11100 Euclid Avenue
Cleveland, OH 44106

Appointments: (216) 844-3267

Center Director:
Michael W. Konstan, M.D.
(216) 844-3267
Fax: (216) 844-5916
mwk3@po.cwru.edu

Center Co-Director:
Carl F. Doershuk, M.D.
(216) 844-3267
Fax: (216) 844-5916
shf@po.cwru.edu

Adult Program:
Case Western Reserve University
829 Biomedical Research Building
10900 Euclid Avenue
Cleveland, OH 44106

Director:
Michael D. Infeld, M.D.

(216) 844-3267
Fax: (216) 368-4223
mdi@po.cwru.edu

Columbus

Cystic Fibrosis Center
Columbus Children's Hospital
Section of Pulmonary Medicine
700 Children's Drive
Columbus, OH 43205-2696

Appointments: (614) 722-4766

Center Director:
Karen S. McCoy, M.D.
(614) 722-4767
Fax: (614) 722-4755
kmccoy@chi.osu.edu

Dayton

Pediatric Pulmonary Center
The Children's Medical Center
One Children's Plaza
Dayton, OH 45404-1815

Appointments: (937) 226-8376

Center Director:
Michel E. Steffan, M.D.
(937) 226-8440
Fax: (937) 463-5390
cflab@cmc-dayton.org

Toledo

Children's Hospital of Northwest
  Ohio/The Toledo Hospital
2142 North Cove Boulevard
Toledo, OH 43606

Appointments: (419) 471-2207 or
(800) 227-2959

Center Director:
Pierre A. Vauthy, M.D.
(419) 471-4549
Fax: (419) 479-6092

Associate Director:
David Hufford, Jr., M.D.

OKLAHOMA

Oklahoma City

Children's Hospital of Oklahoma
University of Oklahoma Health
  Science Center
CF Center
940 N.E. 13th Street, Room 3316B
Oklahoma City, OK 73104

Appointments: (405) 271-6390

Center Director:
James Royall, M.D.
(405) 271-6390
Fax: (405) 271-5055
james-royall@ouhsc.edu

OREGON

Portland

Oregon Health Sciences University
  UHN 56
Cystic Fibrosis Center
3181 S. W. Sam Jackson Park Road
Portland, OR 97201-3098

Appointments: (503) 494-8023

Center Director:
Michael Wall, M.D.
(503) 494-8023
Fax: (503) 494-6670
wallm@ohsu.edu

Outreach Clinic:
Medford CF Clinic
Rogue Valley Hospital
Medford, OR

PENNSYLVANIA

Harrisburg

Cystic Fibrosis Center
Pinnacle Health at Polyclinic Hospital
2601 North 3rd Street
Harrisburg, PA 17110

Appointments: (717) 782-4105

Center Director:
Muttiah Ganeshananthan, M.D.
(717) 782-4105
Fax: (717) 782-2798
jstaufffer@pinnaclehealth.org

Philadelphia

Children's Hospital of Philadelphia
University of Pennsylvania
Abramson Research Center, Room
  402G
34th Street and Civic Center Boulevard
Philadelphia, PA 19104-4318

Appointments: (215) 590-3749/3510
(Mon. thru Fri. 8:30–4:30; evenings and
  weekends—ask for physician on call)

Center Director:
Thomas F. Scanlin, M.D.
(215) 590-3608
Fax: (215) 590-4298
scanlin@email.chop.edu

Adult Program:
Hospital of the University of
  Pennsylvania
Pulmonary Medicine/Critical Care
  Medicine
835 West Gates Building
3600 Spruce Street
Philadelphia, PA 19104-4283

Appointments: (215) 662-8766

Director:
Jonathan Zuckerman, M.D.
(215) 349-5478
Fax: (215) 823-5171
jonz@mail.med.upenn.edu

St. Christopher's Hospital for Children
Erie Avenue at Front Street
Philadelphia, PA 19134-1095

Appointments: (215) 427-5183

Center Director:
Daniel V. Schidlow, M.D.
(215) 427-4801
Fax: (215) 427-4805
schidlow@allegheny.edu

Adult Program:
Pulmonary/Critical Care Division
Medical College of Pennsylvania
  Hospital
3300 Henry Avenue
Philadelphia, PA 19129

Appointments: (215) 842-7748

Director:
Stanley Fiel, M.D.
(215) 842-7748
Fax: (215) 843-1705
fiel@allegheny.edu

Outreach Clinic:
St. Luke's Hospital
801 Ostrum Avenue
Bethlehem, PA 18015

Pittsburgh

Cystic Fibrosis Center
Children's Hospital of Pittsburgh
University of Pittsburgh School of
  Medicine
3705 Fifth Avenue at DeSoto Street
Pittsburgh, PA 15213

Appointments: (412) 692-5661

Center Director:
David M. Orenstein, M.D.
(412) 692-5184
Fax: (412) 692-6645
davido+@pitt.edu

Adult Program Director:
Joel Weinberg, M.D.
(412) 621-1200
Fax: (412) 621-9958

PUERTO RICO

San Juan

Cystic Fibrosis Center
University of Puerto Rico School of
  Medicine
Department of Pediatrics
GPO Box 365067
San Juan, PR 00936-5067

Appointments: (787) 754-8500
  ext. 1080 or 3010

Center Director:
Jose R. Rodriguez-Santana, M.D.
Fax: (787) 743-1917
josrodriguez@pol.net

RHODE ISLAND

Providence

Brown University Medical School
Cystic Fibrosis Center
Rhode Island Hospital Child
  Development Center
593 Eddy Street
Providence, RI 02903

Appointments: (401) 444-5685

Center Director:
Mary Ann Passero, M.D.
(401) 444-5685
Fax: (401) 444-6115
mary_passero@brown.edu

SOUTH CAROLINA

Charleston

Cystic Fibrosis Center
Medical University of South Carolina
Division of Pediatric GI/Nutrition
158 Rutledge Avenue
Charleston, SC 29403

Appointments: (803) 876-0444

Center Director:
Robert D. Baker, M.D., Ph.D.

(843) 792-7653
Fax: (843) 792-6472
bakerrd@musc.edu

Adult Program:
Medical University of South Carolina
Division of Pulmonary and Critical
  Care
171 Ashley Avenue, Room 812-CSB
Charleston, SC 29425

Director:
Patrick Flume, M.D.
(843) 792-9219
Fax: (843) 792-0732
flumepa@musc.edu

Columbia

Palmetto Richland Hospital
5 Medical Park
Columbia, SC 29203

Appointments: (803) 748-7555

Center Director:
Roxanne Marcille, M.D.
(803) 748-7555
Fax: (803) 748-9555
mn31ca@rmh.edu

Assistant Director:
Daniel Brown, M.D.

Greenville

See Duke University Medical Center,
  Durham, North Carolina.

SOUTH DAKOTA

Sioux Falls

South Dakota Cystic Fibrosis Center
Sioux Valley Hospital
1100 South Euclid Avenue
P.O. Box 5039
Sioux Falls, SD 57117-5039

Appointments: (605) 333-7188
krelle@siouxvalley.org

Center Director:
Rodney R. Parry, M.D.*
(605) 357-1309
Fax: (605) 357-1311
rparry@usd.edu

Center Co-Director:
James Wallace, M.D.
(605) 333-7199
Fax: (605) 333-1585

*Preferred Mailing Address:
University of South Dakota School of
  Medicine
1400 West 22nd Street
Sioux Falls, SD 57105-1570

TENNESSEE

Memphis

University of Tennessee College of
  Medicine
Le Bonheur Children's Medical Center
50 North Dunlap
Memphis, TN 38103-2893

Appointments: (901) 572-5222

Center Director:
Robert A. Schoumacher, M.D.
(901) 572-5222
Fax: (901) 572-3337
rschoumacher@utmeml.utmem.edu

Nashville

Vanderbilt Children's Hospital
Vanderbilt University
Medical Center, CF Center
S-0119 MCN
Nashville, TN 37232-2586

Appointments: (615) 343-7617

Center Director:
Dennis C. Stokes, M.D.
(615) 343-7617
Fax: (615) 343-7727
dennis.stokes@mcmail.vanderbilt.edu

Adult Program:
Vanderbilt University Medical Center
CF Center
T-1217 MCN
Nashville, TN 37232-2586

Appointments: (615) 322-2386

Director:
Bonnie S. Slovis, M.D.
(615) 322-2386
Fax: (615) 343-3749
bonnie.slovis@mcmail.vanderbilt.edu

Affiliate Programs:
East Tennessee Children's Hospital
Cystic Fibrosis Clinic
2018 Clinch Avenue
Knoxville, TN 37916

Appointments: (423) 541-8336

Director:
Donald T. Ellenburg, M.D.
(423) 525-2640
Fax: (423) 525-9536
pnoe@earthlink.net

Co-Director:
John S. Rogers, M.D.
(423) 541-8583
Fax: (423) 541-8629
T.C. Thompson Children's Hospital
910 Blackford Street
Chattanooga, TN 37403

Appointments: (423) 778-6505

Director:
Joel C. Ledbetter, M.D.
(423) 778-6501
Fax: (423) 778-6215
ledbetjc@erlanger.org

TEXAS

Dallas

Children's Medical Center of Dallas
Cystic Fibrosis Center
1935 Motor Street
Dallas, TX 75235

Appointments: (214) 456-2361 or
(214) 456-2362

Center Director:
Claude B. Prestidge, M.D.
(214) 456-2361
Fax: (214) 456-2563
npratt@childmed.dallas.tx.us

Adult Program:
St. Paul Medical Center
5939 Harry Hines Boulevard, Suite 711
Dallas, TX 75235

Director:
Randall Rosenblatt, M.D.
(214) 879-6555
Fax: (214) 879-6312
rosie@pol.net

Affiliate Programs:
Allergy Alliance of the Permian Basin
606B North Kent Street
Midland, TX 79701

Appointments: (915) 561-8183

Director:
John D. Bray, M.D.
(915) 561-8183
Fax: (915) 684-7003

Scott & White Clinic
2401 South 31st Street
Temple, TX 76508

Appointments: (254) 724-4950

Director:
Steven C. Copenhaver, M.D.
(254) 724-5504
Fax: (254) 724-1425
scopenhaver@bellnet.tamu.edu

Oklahoma University Pediatric Clinic
2815 South Sheridan Road
Tulsa, OK 74129

Appointments: (918) 838-4820
Fax: (918) 838-4822

Director:
John C. Kramer, M.D.
(918) 481-8100
Fax: (918) 481-8128

The University of Texas
Health Center at Tyler
P.O. Box 2003
Tyler, TX 75710

Appointments: (903) 877-7220

Director:
Robert B. Klein, M.D.
(903) 877-7226
Fax: (903) 877-7218

Fort Worth

Cystic Fibrosis Center
Cook Children's Medical Center
801 Seventh Avenue
Fort Worth, TX 76104

Appointments: (817) 885-4207

Center Co-Directors:
James C. Cunningham, M.D.
Nancy N. Dambro, M.D.
(817) 810-1621
Fax: (817) 885-1090
jccunningham@cookchildrens.org
ndambro@cookchildrens.org

Outreach Clinic:
Texas Tech University Health Sciences
   Center
1400 Coulter, Building E, Suite 703
Amarillo, TX 79106

Appointments: (806) 354-5704
Fax: (806) 354-5433

Co-Directors:
James C. Cunningham, M.D.
Maynard Dyson, M.D.

Houston

Baylor College of Medicine
One Baylor Plaza
Houston, TX 77030

Appointments: (713) 770-3013

Center Director:
Peter W. Hiatt, M.D.*
(713) 770-3300
Fax: (713) 770-3308
pwhiatt@texaschildrenshospital.org

Center Co-Director:
Dan Seilheimer, M.D.
dkseilhe@texaschildrenshospital.org

Preferred Mailing Address:
Texas Children's Hospital
6621 Fannin, MC 3-2571
Houston, TX 77030

Adult Program:
The Methodist Hospital
6550 Fannin, Suite 1236
Houston, TX 77030

Director:
Kathryn A. Hale, M.D.
(713) 790-2076
Fax: (713) 790-3648
khale@bcm.tmc.edu

Affiliate Program:
Seton Medical Center
1201 West 38th Street
Austin, TX 78705

Appointments: (512) 454-4545

Director:
Allan L. Frank, M.D.*
(512) 454-3387

Preferred Mailing Address:
Capital Pediatric Group Associates
1100 West 39 1/2 Street
Austin, TX 78756

San Antonio

Cystic Fibrosis-Chronic Lung Disease
   Center
Santa Rosa Children's Hospital
519 West Houston Street
P.O. Box 7330, Station A
San Antonio, TX 78207

Appointments: (210) 704-2193 or
(210) 704-2201

Center Co-Director:
Amanda Dove, M.D.*
(210) 224-6224
Fax: (210) 224-2132

Preferred Mailing Address:
343 W. Houston Street, Suite #502
San Antonio, TX 78205

Center Co-Director:
Humberto A. Hidalgo, M.D.*
(210) 567-5320
Fax: (210) 567-6921

Preferred Mailing Address:
Pulmonary Division, Department of
   Pediatrics
University of Texas Health Science
   Center at San Antonio
7703 Floyd Curl Drive
San Antonio, TX 78284-7815

Affiliate Program:
San Antonio Pediatric Pulmonary and
   Critical Care Associates

Methodist Plaza
4499 Medical Drive, Suite 255
San Antonio, TX 78229

Appointments: (210) 614-3403

Director:
Martha Morse, M.D.
Fax: (210) 615-7804

Tri-Services Military CF Center
Department of Pediatrics
Wilford Hall USAF Medical Center
2200 Bergquist Drive, Suite 1
59MDW / MMNP
Lackland AFB, TX 78236-5200

Appointments: (210) 292-7585

Center Director:
Dr. Stephen Inscore, COL, MC,
  USA
(210) 292-6843
Fax: (210) 292-3836 or 5238
inscore@whmc-lafb.af.mil

Assistant Director:
Dr. Kenneth M. Olivier, LTC, USAF,
  MC
(210) 292-3170
Fax: (210) 292-6180
olivier@whmc-lafb.af.mil

Affiliate Programs:
Naval Hospital San Diego
Department of Pediatrics
34800 Bob Wilson Drive
San Diego, CA 92134-5000

Appointments: (619) 532-6896

Director:
Henry Wojtczak, M.D.

(619) 532-6883
Fax: (619) 532-7721
hwojtcza@snd10.med.navy.mil

Tripler Army Medical Center
Department of Pediatrics
1 Jarrett White Road
Tripler AMC, HI 96859-5000

Appointments: (808) 433-9226
(808) 433-6697

Director:
Dr. Charles Callahan, COL, MC
(808) 433-6407
Fax: (808) 433-4837
charles_w.callahan@tamc.chcs.amedd.
  army.mil

National Naval Medical Center
Pediatric Clinic, Building 9, Room 123
8901 Wisconsin Avenue
Bethesda, MD 20889-5000

Appointments: (301) 295-4900

Director:
Dr. Donna R. Perry, CAPT, MC,
  USN
(301) 295-4915
Fax: (301) 295-6173
bth0drp@bth20.med.navy.mil

USAF (Kessler) Medical Center
81st MDOS/SGOCC
301 Fisher Street
Keesler AFB, MS 39534-2519

Appointments: (800) 700-8603

Director:
Dr. Louis Mizell, LTC, USAF

(228) 377-6304
Fax: (601) 377-6304
mizell_louis@keesler.af.mil

Portsmouth Naval Medical Center
620 John Paul Jones Circle
Portsmouth, VA 23708-2197

Appointments: (757) 953-7558

Director:
David E. Thomas, M.D., Ph.D.
(757) 953-7494
Fax: (757) 953-5964
det@mosaictech.com

Madigan Army Medical Center
Department of Pediatrics
Pediatric Pulmonary Medicine
Tacoma, WA 98431

Appointments: (800) 404-4506

Director:
Dr. Donald Moffitt, COL, MC, USA
(253) 968-1881
(253) 968-0384
Fax: (253) 968-0384
donaldrmoffitt@mamc.chcs.amedd.
  army.mil

UTAH

Salt Lake City

Intermountain Cystic Fibrosis Center
Department of Pediatrics
University of Utah Health Sciences
  Center
50 North Medical Drive, 2A120 SOM
Salt Lake City, UT 84132

Appointments: (801) 588-2621
  (pediatrics)
(801) 581-2410 (adults)

Interim Center Director:
Barbara A. Chatfield, M.D.
(801) 581-2410
Fax: (801) 581-4920
barbara.chatfield@hsc.utah.edu

Adult Program:
Intermountain Cystic Fibrosis Center
Department of Pediatrics
University of Utah Health Sciences
  Center
50 North Medical Drive, 711 Wintrobe
  Building
Salt Lake City, UT 84132

Center Co-Director:
Bruce C. Marshall, M.D.
(801) 581-7806
Fax: (801) 585-3355
bmarshall@med.utah.edu

Affiliate Programs:
Mercy Medical Center
745 South Progress Street
Meridian, ID 83642

Appointments: (208) 884-2943

Director:
Eugene M. Brown, M.D.
(208) 463-3000
Fax: (208) 465-4825
emb37@aol.com

CF Affiliate Program
500 S. 11th Avenue
P.O. Box 4730
Pocatello, ID 83205

Appointments: (208) 232-1443

Director:
Don McInturff, M.D.
(208) 232-1443
Fax: (208) 239-3434

CF Affiliate Program
890 Oxford Avenue
Idaho Falls, ID 83401

Appointments: (208) 523-3060

Director:
George H. Groberg, M.D.
Fax: (208) 523-0028

VERMONT

Burlington

Cystic Fibrosis and Pediatric
  Pulmonary Center
The Children's Specialty Center, FAHC
111 Colchester Avenue
Burlington, VT 05401

Appointments: (802) 862-5529

Center Director:
Donald R. Swartz, M.D.*
Fax: (802) 863-9674 or (802) 652-8947
donald.swartz@vtmednet.org

Preferred Mailing Address:
20 Kimbal Avenue, Suite 305
South Burlington, VT 05403

VIRGINIA

Charlottesville

Division of Respiratory Medicine
Department of Pediatrics, Box 386

University of Virginia Health System
Charlottesville, VA 22908

Appointments: (804) 924-2250

Center Director:
Robert F. Selden, Jr., M.D.
(804) 924-2250
Fax: (804) 924-0390
rfs6b@virginia.edu

Associate Center Director:
Deborah K. Froh, M.D.
Barringer Building, Room 5411
(804) 924-1820
Fax: (804) 243-6618
dkf2x@virginia.edu

Adult Program:
Department of Medicine
Division of Pulmonary and Critical
  Care Medicine
University of Virginia Health Science
  Center
Hospital Drive, Box 546
Charlottesville, VA 22908

Director:
Mark K. Robbins, M.D.
Barringer Building, Room 2461
(804) 924-9687
Fax: (804) 924-9682
mkr3j@virginia.edu

Norfolk

Eastern Virginia Medical School
Children's Hospital of the King's
  Daughters
601 Children's Lane
Norfolk, VA 23507

Appointments: (757) 668-7132

Center Director:
Thomas T. Rubio, M.D.
(757) 668-7238
Fax: (757) 668-8275
t-rubio@chkd.com

Associate Director:
Karl Karlson Jr., M.D.
Adult Care Provider:
Ignacio Ripoll, M.D.

Richmond

Cystic Fibrosis Program
Medical College of Virginia
9000 Stony Point Parkway
Richmond, VA 23235

Appointments: (804) 786-6282

Center Director:
David A. Draper, M.D.
(804) 560-8930
Fax: (804) 560-7347
lbridge@vdh.state.va.us
or grelliott@ruby.vcu.edu

WASHINGTON

Seattle

Cystic Fibrosis Center
Division of Pediatric Pulmonary
  Medicine
Children's Hospital and Regional
  Medical Center
P.O. Box 5371, CH-18
4800 Sand Point Way, N.E.
Seattle, WA 98105

Appointments: (206) 526-2101

Center Director:
Ronald Gibson, M.D., Ph.D.
(206) 526-2024
Fax: (206) 528-2639
rgibso@chmc.org

Associate Director:
Bonnie Ramsey, M.D.
bramsey@u.washington.edu

Adult Program:
Cystic Fibrosis Clinic
Division of Pulmonary and Critical
  Care Medicine
University of Washington Medical
  Center
Box 356522, Health Sciences Center,
  BB1253
Seattle, WA 98195

Appointments: (206) 548-4615

Director:
Moira Aitken, M.D.
(206) 685-8434
Fax: (206) 685-8673
moira@u.washington.edu

Associate Director:
Mark Tonelli, M.D.

Clinic Coordinator:
Gwen McDonald, R.N., M.S.
(206) 548-8446
Fax: (206) 548-2105
gwen@u.washington.edu

Affiliate Programs:
Anchorage Cystic Fibrosis Clinic
Providence Medical Center
3200 Providence Drive
P.O. Box 196604
Anchorage, AK 99519-6604

Appointments: (907) 561-5440

Director:
Dion Roberts, M.D.*
Fax: (907) 562-0412
dmroberts@mem.po.com

Preferred Mailing Address:
4001 Dale Street, Suite 210
Anchorage, AK 99508

Mary Bridge Children's Health Center
311 South L Street
Tacoma, WA 98405

Appointments: (253) 552-1469
Fax: (253) 552-4979

Co-Directors:
Lawrence A. Larson, D.O.
David Ricker, M.D.

Deaconess Medical Center
West 800 Fifth Avenue
P.O. Box 248
Spokane, WA 99210-0248

Appointments: (509) 458-7300
Fax: (509) 458-7986

Director:
Michael M. McCarthy, M.D.
(509) 458-7300
Fax: (509) 458-7986

WISCONSIN

Madison

University of Wisconsin
Cystic Fibrosis/Pediatric Pulomonary
  Center

Clinical Sciences Center—H4/430
600 Highland Avenue
Madison, WI 53792 4108

Appointments: (608) 263-8555

Center Director:
Michael J. Rock, M.D.
Fax: (608) 263-0510
mjrock@facstaff.wisc.edu

Adult Program:
University of Wisconsin
Adult Cystic Fibrosis Program
Clinical Sciences Center—
  H6/330
600 Highland Avenue
Madison, WI 53792

Appointments: (608) 263-7203

Director:
Guillermo A. doPico, M.D.
(608) 263-3612
Fax: (608) 263-3104
gad@parc.medicine.wisc.edu

Adult Nurse Coordinator:
Lorna Will, R.N., M.A.
(608) 263-8937

Affiliate Programs:
St. Vincent's Hospital
835 South Van Buren
Green Bay, WI 54301

Director:
Stuart Adair, M.D.
(414) 437-0431
Fax: (414) 436-1319

Marshfield Clinic
1000 North Oak Street
Marshfield, WI 54449

Director:
Bradley J. Sullivan, M.D.
(800) 782-8581
sullivab@mfldclin.edu

Milwaukee

Children's Hospital of Wisconsin
Medical College of Wisconsin
Cystic Fibrosis Clinic
9000 West Wisconsin Avenue,
    Box 1997
MS #777A
Milwaukee, WI 53201

Appointments: (414) 266-6730

Center Director:
Mark Splaingard, M.D.
(414) 266-6730
Fax: (414) 266-6742
splain@mcw.edu

Adult Program Director:
Julie A. Biller, M.D.
(414) 266-6730
Fax: (414) 266-2653
jbiller@post.itsmcw.edu

WYOMING

See The Children's Hospital, Denver,
    Colorado.

Subject Index

*Page numbers followed by f refer to figures; page numbers
followed by t refer to tables.*

for patients with diabetes mellitus,
287t
routine, schedule for, 284t–285t
Laparoscopic surgery
fundoplication as, 214, 214t
special considerations with, 222
Leukotriene receptor antagonists,
systemic, for inflammation,
70
Libido, 260
Life expectancy, 263
Linoleic acid deficiency, 107
Lipase therapy, for pancreatic
insufficiency, 98–100, 101f
Liver disease. *See also* Hepatobiliary
disease; specific disorders
in adolescents and adults, 33
neonatal, 26–27
Liver enzymes, elevated
concentration of, in infants
and children, 32
Liver transplantation, 246–251
care following, 250–251
care while awaiting, 249–250
indications and contraindications
to, 247–248, 248t
prognosis following, 251
timing of referral for, 248–249
Living lobar transplant, 238, 239
Lobectomy, for hemoptysis, 86
Lorazepam (Ativan), for anxiety, 272
Lung resection
for bronchiectasis, 212–213
for hemoptysis, 213
Lung tissue, as culture specimen,
300–301
Lung transplantation, 229–246
care while awaiting, 234–238
pneumothorax and, 236–237
respiratory failure and, 237–238
sinus disease and, 237
complications following, 242–244,
243t
contraindications to, 231
evaluation for, 233–234

immediate postoperative care for,
239–244
antimicrobials and, 240–242
immunosuppression and,
239–240
indications for, 230, 230t
living lobar transplant for, 238,
239
long term care for, 242–244, 243t
operations for, 238–239
organ distribution and, 231–232
preservation of ideal transplant
status for, 83–84
prognosis with, 245–246
psychosocial considerations with,
245
timing of referral for, 232–233

M

Magnesium deficiency, 106
Magnetic resonance imaging (MRI),
289
in hepatobiliary disease, 122
Marijuana smoking, 66
Maxillary antrostomy, for sinusitis,
74–75
Maximum voluntary ventilation
(MVV), exercise and, 181
Measles immunization, 57
Mechanical ventilation, in terminal
care, 272–273
Meconium ileus, 25–26, 135–137,
136f
liver disease associated with, 27
surgical therapy for, 215–218, 217f
Meconium ileus equivalent, 128–129,
130f, 131
surgical therapy for, 218
Meconium peritonitis, fetal, 25
Meconium plug syndrome, 26, 138f,
138–139
Medium chain triglycerides (MCTs),
in formula feedings, 110
Membrane stabilizers, for
inflammation, 71